（案例版）

药理学学习指导

主　编　乐　江　杨哲琼　敖　英
副主编　陈　效

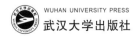

武汉大学出版社

图书在版编目(CIP)数据

药理学学习指导：案例版 / 乐江,杨哲琼,敖英主编；陈效副主编. --武汉：武汉大学出版社,2025.3. -- ISBN 978-7-307-24874-8

Ⅰ.R96

中国国家版本馆 CIP 数据核字第 2025FM2152 号

责任编辑：何青霞　　责任校对：鄢春梅　　版式设计：马　佳

出版发行：武汉大学出版社　　（430072　武昌　珞珈山）
（电子邮箱：cbs22@whu.edu.cn　网址：www.wdp.com.cn）
印刷：湖北诚齐印刷股份有限公司
开本：787×1092　1/16　　印张：17.75　　字数：419 千字　　插页：1
版次：2025 年 3 月第 1 版　　2025 年 3 月第 1 次印刷
ISBN 978-7-307-24874-8　　定价：53.00 元

版权所有，不得翻印；凡购我社的图书，如有质量问题，请与当地图书销售部门联系调换。

编委会

主　编　乐　江　杨哲琼　敖　英

副主编　陈　效

编　委　(按姓氏笔画排序)

叶少剑　乐　江　杨哲琼　邹玉莲　陈　效

敖　英　奚瑾磊　谢先飞　鄢友娥

前　言

药理学是研究药物与机体(包含病原体)相互作用规律及其机制的科学,是连接基础医学、药学、临床医学之间的桥梁学科。对于医学生而言,深入研习药理学,有助于熟练掌握药物的药理效应、代谢过程、临床应用以及不良反应等相关知识,为精准制定临床治疗方案奠定坚实的基础。

为了将基础医学的理论基石与临床医学的实践应用紧密相连,《药理学学习指导(案例版)》应运而生。传统的学习过程中,学生往往陷入理论与实践相互割裂的困境,难以将抽象的药理知识有效运用于实际临床病例。本书以执业医师考纲为核心,紧密围绕药理学核心知识点展开,精心筛选与设计各章节的案例。案例学习能够将晦涩的药理学理论具体化,通过让学生身临其境地感受药物在疾病治疗中的应用场景,深刻理解药物的作用机制、疗效及不良反应等核心要点。这不仅有助于激发学生的学习兴趣与主动性,更能有效培养他们的临床思维能力、分析问题与解决问题的能力,帮助他们在未来的临床实践中迅速做出科学合理的用药决策。每个案例均配有详细的分析与解答,引导学生逐步深入思考,从案例中提炼药理知识要点,帮助学生举一反三和知识内化。同时,本指南注重与教材的有机结合,确保案例学习与课堂教学相互补充、相得益彰,帮助学生全面系统地掌握药理学知识体系。

本书的编写工作得到了多所医学院校一线药理学教育工作者的鼎力支持,历经数月的精心雕琢与悉心打磨,终于顺利完稿。本书共分为四十四章,包括第一章至第四章药理学总论(鄢友娥编写)、第五章至第十一章传出神经系统药物(杨哲琼编写)、第十二章至第十九章中枢神经系统药物(乐江编写,其中邹玉莲参与编写第十八章至第十九章)、第二十章至第二十七章心血管系统药物（敖英编写第二十章至第二十三章，叶少剑编写第二十五章和第二十七章，谢先飞编写第二十四章和第二十六章）、第二十八章至第三十章内脏系统药物（奚瑾磊编写）、第三十一章至第三十三章内分泌系统药物（敖英编写）和第三十四章至第四十四章抗菌、抗肿瘤、抗寄生虫、免疫功能调节药（陈效编写）。期盼本书能为药理学教学与学习贡献绵薄之力，助力莘莘学子成长成才。

在编写本书的漫长征程中，我们广泛参阅了众多国内外药理学领域的经典教材与前沿研究文献，其中包括 *Goodman and Gilman's The Pharmacological Basis of Therapeutics*（McGraw Hill）、*Katzung's Basic and Clinical Pharmacology*（McGaw Hill）、*Brenner and Stevens' Pharmacology*（Elsevier）以及国内极具影响力的药理学教材等。在此，我们向这些著作的原作者们致以最诚挚的敬意与感谢。

尽管在编写过程中，我们全体编写人员始终秉持精益求精的态度，力求尽善尽美，但鉴于案例学习本身所具有的丰富多样性与高度复杂性，书中难免会存在一些瑕疵与不足之处。我们怀着诚挚而谦逊的心，敬请药理学前辈、同行专家以及同学们批评指正。

乐　江

2024 年 12 月 7 日于武汉

目 录

第一章　药理学总论——绪言 …………………………… 001
第二章　药物代谢动力学 ………………………………… 003
第三章　药物效应动力学 ………………………………… 011
第四章　影响药物效应的因素 …………………………… 015
第五章　传出神经系统药理概论 ………………………… 017
第六章　胆碱受体激动药 ………………………………… 020
第七章　抗胆碱酯酶药和胆碱酯酶复活药 ……………… 025
第八章　胆碱受体阻断药（Ⅰ）——M胆碱受体阻断药 …… 033
第九章　胆碱受体阻断药（Ⅱ）——N胆碱受体阻断药 …… 039
第十章　肾上腺素受体激动药 …………………………… 044
第十一章　肾上腺素受体阻断药 ………………………… 050
第十二章　全身麻醉药 …………………………………… 056
第十三章　局部麻醉药 …………………………………… 062
第十四章　镇静催眠药 …………………………………… 067
第十五章　抗癫痫药和抗惊厥药 ………………………… 073
第十六章　治疗中枢神经系统退行性疾病药 …………… 079
第十七章　抗精神失常药 ………………………………… 084
第十八章　镇痛药 ………………………………………… 093
第十九章　解热镇痛抗炎药 ……………………………… 099
第二十章　离子通道概论及钙通道阻滞药 ……………… 106
第二十一章　抗心律失常药 ……………………………… 111
第二十二章　作用于肾素-血管紧张素系统的药物 ……… 118
第二十三章　利尿药 ……………………………………… 123
第二十四章　抗高血压药 ………………………………… 132
第二十五章　治疗心力衰竭的药物 ……………………… 138

第二十六章	调血脂药与抗动脉粥样硬化药	145
第二十七章	抗心绞痛药	150
第二十八章	作用于血液及造血系统的药物	156
第二十九章	作用于呼吸系统的药物	166
第三十章	作用于消化系统的药物	173
第三十一章	肾上腺皮质激素类药物	182
第三十二章	甲状腺激素及抗甲状腺药	188
第三十三章	胰岛素及其他降血糖药	193
第三十四章	抗菌药物概论	200
第三十五章	β-内酰胺类抗生素	208
第三十六章	大环内酯类抗菌药和林可霉素	216
第三十七章	氨基苷类抗菌药	222
第三十八章	四环素与氯霉素类	229
第三十九章	人工合成抗菌药	235
第四十章	抗真菌药和抗病毒药	243
第四十一章	抗结核药及抗麻风病药	250
第四十二章	抗寄生虫药	257
第四十三章	抗恶性肿瘤药物	264
第四十四章	影响免疫功能的药物	271

参考文献 …… 276

第一章 药理学总论——绪言

知识要点

一、药理学的性质与任务

1. 药物与毒物

(1)药物(drug):可以改变或查明机体的生理功能及病理状态,用于预防、诊断和治疗疾病的物质。

(2)毒物(poison):是指在较小剂量即对机体产生毒害作用,损害人体健康的化学物质。

(3)药物和毒物之间并无严格界限,药物剂量过大也可产生毒性反应。

2. 药理学

药理学是研究药物与机体(含病原体)相互作用及其作用规律的学科。

(1)研究内容:①药物效应动力学(药效学,pharmacodynamics):研究药物对机体的作用及作用机制,包括药物的药理作用、作用机制、临床应用、不良反应等。②药物代谢动力学(药动学,pharmacokinetics):研究药物在机体的影响下所发生的变化及其规律,即药物的体内过程(包括吸收、分布、代谢、排泄)和血药浓度随时间变化的规律。

(2)学科任务:阐明药物的作用及作用机制,为临床合理用药、发挥药物最佳疗效以及降低不良反应提供理论依据;研究开发新药,发现药物新用途;为其他生命科学研究提供重要的科学依据和研究方法。

二、新药开发与研究过程

1. 新药

新药(new drugs)指化学结构、药品组分和药理作用不同于现有药品的药物。

2. 研究过程

(1)临床前研究。主要由药物化学和药理学相关内容组成,前者包括药物制备工艺路线、理化性质及质量控制标准等,后者包括以符合《实验动物管理条例》的实验动物为研究对象的药效学、药动学及毒理学研究。

(2)临床研究。包括四个阶段:①Ⅰ期临床试验:在20~30例正常成年志愿者身上进行的药理学及人体安全性试验,这是新药人体试验的起始阶段。②Ⅱ期临床试验:随机双盲对照临床试验,主要是对新药的有效性及安全性作出初步评价,并推荐临床给药剂量,观察病例不少于 100 例。③Ⅲ期临床试验：扩大的多中心临床试验，目的是对新药的有效性、安全性进行社会性考察，观察例数一般不应少于 300 例。④Ⅳ期临床试验：药物上市后在社会人群大范围内继续进行的新药安全性和有效性评价，是在广泛长期使用的条件下考察疗效和不良反应，也叫售后调研，该期对最终确定新药的临床价值有重要意义。

第二章 药物代谢动力学

知识要点

一、药物的体内过程

1. 吸收

吸收(absorption)：指药物从用药部位进入血液循环的过程。

口服给药：最常用的给药途径。

注射给药：静脉注射、肌肉注射、皮下注射等。

呼吸道吸入给药：气雾剂。

局部用药：如脂溶性药物经皮给药。

舌下给药：可在很大程度上避免首过消除。

首过消除(first-pass elimination)：指药物经过肠粘膜及肝脏时被部分灭活，使进入体循环的药量减少的现象。为了避免首过效应，通常采用舌下给药和直肠给药。

2. 分布

分布(distribution)：指药物吸收后从血液循环到达机体各部位和组织的过程。

影响药物在体内分布的因素：

(1) 组织器官血流量：药物先分布到血流量大的组织，再分布到血流量少的组织。

(2) 血浆蛋白结合率：高血浆蛋白结合率的药物合用易发生药物相互作用。

(3) 组织细胞结合：药物组织分布出现选择性。

(4) 体液 pH 与药物解离度：可用于药物解毒。

(5) 体内屏障：血脑屏障、胎盘屏障、血眼屏障。

3. 代谢

代谢(metabolism)：指药物在体内发生化学结构的改变，是药物在体内消除的重要途径，又称生物转化(biotransformation)。药物经代谢过程后，并不一定意味着药物作用被中止。药物可能被转化为具有药理学活性的代谢物甚至是药物被活化，也可能是被转化为毒性代谢物或者无活性代谢物。

步骤：

Ⅰ相反应：氧化、还原和水解反应，使极性增加。

Ⅱ相反应：结合反应，葡萄糖醛酸、硫酸、谷胱甘肽、甘氨酸等与药物或其代谢物的极性基团结合，极性进一步增加。

肝药酶：促进体内药物生物转化的酶，主要是肝脏微粒体细胞色素 P-450 酶系统（又称肝药酶）。酶活性受多因素影响，致使药物作用的个体差异大。药物也可能对肝药酶产生诱导作用和抑制作用。

4. 排泄

排泄（excretion）：指药物原形或其代谢产物通过排泄器官或分泌器官排出体外的转运过程。生物转化与排泄统称为消除。

（1）肾脏排泄：是大多数药物的主要排泄途径。弱酸性药物在碱性尿液中解离多，重吸收少，排泄快，而在酸性尿液中解离少，重吸收多，排泄慢；弱碱性药物则相反。改变尿液 pH 值可以改变药物的排泄速度，用于药物中毒的解毒或增强疗效。

（2）消化道排泄：部分药物经胆汁排入肠腔可再经小肠上皮细胞重吸收经肝脏进入血液循环，这种肝脏、胆汁、小肠间的循环称肠肝循环（enterohepatic circulation）。

（3）其他排泄途径：汗液、唾液、泪液、乳汁等。

二、药物代谢动力学重要参数

1. 房室模型

房室模型（compartment model）是目前最常用的药动学模型。房室模型是将整个机体视为一个系统，并将该系统按动力学特性划分为若干个房室（compartments），把机体看成由若干个房室组成的一个完整的系统。根据药物在体内的动力学特性，房室模型可分为一室模型、二室模型和多室模型。

一室模型（one-compartment model）：体内药物瞬时在各部位达到动态平衡，各组织药物转运速度相同或相似。

二室模型（two-compartment model）：某些部位的药物浓度可以和血液中的浓度迅速达到平衡，而在另一些部位需要一段时间才能完成。

多室模型：若在上述二室模型的基础上还有一部分组织、器官或细胞内药物的分布更慢，则可以从周边室中划分出第三房室，由此形成三室模型。按此方法，可以将在体内分布速率有多种水平的药物按多室模型（multiple compartment model）进行处理。

2. 药物消除动力学

一级动力学消除（first-order elimination kinetics）：即线性动力学过程，体内药物按恒定比例消除。

零级动力学消除（zero-order elimination kinetics）：即非线性动力学过程，体内药物按恒定的速率消除。

混合消除动力学：在高浓度或高剂量使用药物时，因消除能力饱和，先按零级动力学消除，浓度降低后再按一级动力学消除。

3. 多次用药的稳态血浆浓度（steady-state plasma concentration，Css）

多次给药后药物达 Css 的时间取决于药物的消除半衰期。改变给药剂量或频率只能改变体内药物总量或峰浓度与谷浓度之差，不能改变到达 Css 的时间。

4. 重要参数

消除半衰期(half time，$t_{1/2}$)：血浆药物浓度降低一半所需要的时间。根据 $t_{1/2}$ 可确定给药间隔时间；根据 $t_{1/2}$ 可以预测连续给药后达到 Css 的时间以及停药后药物从体内消除所需要的时间。

清除率(clearance，CL)或总体(血浆)清除率：机体消除器官在单位时间内清除药物的血浆容积。在一级动力学消除中，CL 是一个恒定值；而在零级动力学消除中，CL 是可变的。

表观分布容积(apparent volume of distribution，V_d)：血浆和组织内药物分布达到平衡后，体内药物按此时的血浆药物浓度在体内分布时所需的体液容积。$V_d = A(\text{mg})/C(\text{mg})/L$，可估计药物的分布范围，以及计算产生期望药物浓度所需要的给药剂量。

生物利用度(bioavailability)：指药物经血管外途径给药后，吸收进入全身血液循环的相对量和速度，用 F 表示，计算公式为 $F = A/D \times 100\%$，其中 A 表示进入体循环的药量，D 表示服药剂量。绝对生物利用度：$F = $ 血管外给药 AUC/静脉给药 $AUC \times 100\%$。相对生物利用度：$F = $ 受试制剂 AUC/标准制剂 $AUC \times 100\%$ 是确定含量相同的不同制剂是否具有生物等效性的依据。

案例学习

学习要点：
(1)代谢环节产生药物相互作用影响药物效应。
(2)吸收、排泄环节产生药物相互作用影响药物效应。

关键词：吸收；分布；代谢；排泄；药物相互作用

案例一

一位 50 岁女性，患有高脂血症，服用辛伐他汀进行治疗。她平时喜欢喝橘子汁，服药 3 周后开始改喝葡萄柚汁，出现肌痛，检查发现肌酸磷酸激酶增加。医生建议：不喝葡萄柚汁。

两年后，该患者患过敏性皮炎，并服用特非那定进行治疗，1 天 2 次，治疗 2 年以上。因消化性溃疡，她又加服西咪替丁后去田间劳动，中途感觉不舒服，回家休息，但午饭后死亡。药物与葡萄柚汁一起服用时药-时曲线下面积(AUC)变化情况见图 2-1。

问答题

1. 病人在改服葡萄柚汁后为什么会出现肌痛？为何医生建议不喝葡萄柚汁？
2. 从药物相互作用的角度讨论患者的死亡原因。

案例二

患者，女，59 岁，患 2 型糖尿病并发高血压、心房纤颤，每天接受胰岛素治疗控制血糖，接受地高辛治疗控制心功能。因单独胰岛素治疗对餐后高血糖、高尿糖难以控制，因此她增服阿卡波糖(50 mg/次，3 次/日)。4 个月后，患者突发严重心房纤颤，被紧急

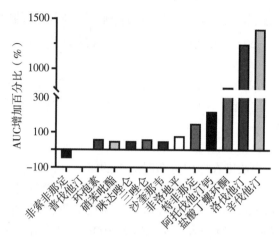

图 2-1 药物与葡萄柚汁一起服用时药-时曲线下面积(AUC)变化情况

送往医院就诊。经检查,患者血浆中地高辛浓度仅为 0.24 ng/mL,低于有效浓度(0.8~2.0 ng/mL)。因此,停用阿卡波糖,检查发现地高辛浓度升至 1.7 ng/mL。当再次服用阿卡波糖后,血浆中地高辛浓度又再次下降。

一年后,为了治疗支气管炎,服用克拉霉素。给药第三天,患者出现呕吐和精神不正常而住院。服用克拉霉素前的地高辛血药浓度为 0.95 ng/mL(正常范围),入院时升高到 3.8 ng/mL。停用克拉霉素后症状缓解。入院后第 4 天,地高辛血药浓度恢复正常。心电图也恢复正常。

◎ 问答题

1. 从药物相互作用的角度,讨论患者突发严重心房纤颤的原因。
2. 从药物相互作用的角度,讨论患者出现呕吐和精神不正常的原因。
3. 试分析案例中两次出现地高辛血药浓度变化的原因及机制。

📝 选择题

1. 一级动力学消除的特点为(　　)。
    A. 药物的半衰期不是恒定值　　B. 一种少数药物的消除方式
    C. 单位时间内实际消除的药量随时间递减　　D. 一种恒速消除动力学
    E. 其消除速度与初始血药浓度高低有关
2. 以下给药途径中,最易受到首过消除影响的是(　　)。
    A. 吸入给药　　B. 舌下给药　　C. 口服给药　　D. 直肠给药　　E. 皮下注射
3. 药物在体内开始作用的快慢取决于(　　)。
    A. 分布　　B. 吸收　　C. 转化　　D. 排泄　　E. 代谢
4. 按一级动力学消除的药物,其半衰期(　　)。
    A. 随给药剂量而变　　B. 随血药浓度而变　　C. 固定不变
    D. 随给药途径而变　　E. 随给药剂型而变
5. 为迅速达到稳态血浆浓度,可采取下列哪一个措施?(　　)

A. 每次用药量加倍　　　B. 缩短给药间隔时间　　　C. 每次用药量减半
D. 延长给药间隔时间　　E. 首次剂量加倍，而后按其原来的间隔时间给予原剂量

6. 药物的半衰期主要取决于(　　)。
   A. 吸收速度　　　　　　B. 消除速度　　　　　　C. 血浆蛋白结合率
   D. 剂量　　　　　　　　E. 药物的表观分布容积(V_d)

7. 在碱性尿液中弱酸性药物(　　)。
   A. 解离多，重吸收少，排泄快　　　　B. 解离少，重吸收多，排泄快
   C. 解离多，重吸收多，排泄快　　　　D. 解离少，重吸收多，排泄慢
   E. 以上都不对

8. 促进药物生物转化的主要酶系统是(　　)。
   A. 葡萄糖醛酸转移酶　　B. 单胺氧化酶　　　　　C. 细胞色素 P450 酶系统
   D. 辅酶Ⅱ　　　　　　　E. 水解酶

9. 某药物与肝药酶抑制剂合用后其效应(　　)。
   A. 减弱　　　B. 增强　　　C. 不变　　　D. 消失　　　E. 以上都不对

10. 临床最常用的给药途径是(　　)。
    A. 静脉注射　　B. 雾化吸入　　C. 口服给药　　D. 肌肉注射　　E. 动脉给药

Case study

Key points:
(1) The impact of drug interactions in metabolic processes on drug action.
(2) The impact of drug interactions in the absorption and excretion process on drug action.

Key words: absorption; distribution; metabolism; excretion; drug interactions

Case 1

A 50-year-old female with hyperlipidemia was treated with simvastatin. She changed her habit of drinking orange juice and began to drink grapefruit juice after 3 weeks. Then she developed muscle soreness. During the examination, an increased creatine phosphokinase is identified. The doctor advises: don't drink grapefruit juice.

After two years, this patient suffered from allergic dermatitis. She had been taking terfenadine twice a day for more than 2 years. She began to take cimetidine because of peptic ulcer. She went to work in the field after taking cimetidine. and felt uncomfortable, then she went home to rest, but died after lunch.

Figure 2-2 shows that examples of AUC changes over baseline when the drug was given with grapefruit juice.

◎ **Essay questions**
1. Why did the patient suffer from muscle soreness when switching to grapefruit juice? Why did the doctor recommend not drinking grapefruit juice?
2. Please discuss the cause of death of the patient from the perspective of drug interaction.

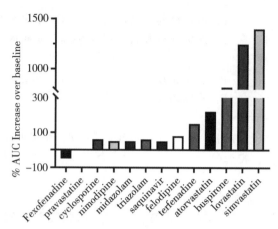

Figure 2-2 Examples of area under the curve (AUC) changes over baseline when the drug was given with grapefruit juice

Case 2

The 59-year-old female patient, who has been suffering from type 2 diabetes mellitus complicated with hypertension and atrial fibrillation, received insulin therapy to control blood glucose and digoxin to control heart function. It's ineffective to control postprandial hyperglycemia and high urine glucose by insulin treatment alone, so acarbose (50 mg, 3 times/day) was added in prescription. 4 months later, this patient was sent to hospital with sudden severe atrial fibrillation. After examination, the concentration of digoxin was only 0.24 ng/mL in plasma, lower than effective concentrations (0.8-2.0 ng/mL). After withdrawing acarbose, the concentration of digoxin rose to 1.7 ng/mL. The blood concentration of digoxin fell when taking acarbose again.

After one year, this patient took clarithromycin for the treatment of bronchitis. After treatment for 3 days, this patient appeared symptoms of vomiting and psychosis. Before taking clarithromycin, her concentration of digoxin in plasma was 0.95 ng/mL (normal range), and increased to 3.8 ng/mL when sent to hospital. Symptoms relieve after withdrawing clarithromycin. Four days later, her plasma concentration of digoxin returned to normal. The electrocardiogram returned to normal too.

◎ **Essay questions**

1. Please discuss the cause of severe atrial fibrillation from the perspective of drug interaction.
2. Please discuss the cause of vomiting and psychosis from the perspective of drug interaction.
3. Discuss the cause and mechanism of the changes of the concentration of digoxin in this case.

Multiple-choice questions

1. The characteristic of the first-order elimination kinetics is that (   ).
   A. the half-life of a drug is not constant

B. it's a way of eliminating a few drugs

C. the amount of drug actually eliminated per unit time decreases with time

D. it is a constant rate elimination kinetics

E. the speed of its elimination is related to the initial blood concentration

2. Among the following routes of administration, which one is most susceptible to first-pass elimination? (　　)

　　A. Inhalation administration　　　　B. Sublingual administration

　　C. Oral administration　　　　　　　D. Rectal administration

　　E. Subcutaneous injection

3. How quickly the drug starts working in the body depends on? (　　)

　　A. Distribution　　B. Absorption　　C. Transformation

　　D. Excretion　　　E. Metabolism

4. The half-life of a drug which is eliminated by first-order elimination kinetics (　　).

　　A. varies with dose administered　　B. varies with blood concentration

　　C. permanent　　　　　　　　　　　D. varies depending on the route of administration

　　E. varies with the dosage form administered

5. Which of the following measures can be taken to quickly achieve steady-state blood concentration? (　　)

　　A. Double the dose each time　　　　B. Shorten the dosing interval

　　C. Halve the dosage each time　　　　D. Extend the dosing interval

　　E. Double the first dose, and give the original dose at its original intervals

6. The half-life of a drug depends mainly on (　　).

　　A. absorption rate　　　　　　　　　B. elimination rate

　　C. plasma protein binding rate　　　　D. dose

　　E. apparent volume of distribution (V_d) of the drug

7. Weakly acidic drugs in alkaline urine have (　　).

　　A. more dissociation, less reabsorption, faster excretion

　　B. less dissociation, more reabsorption, faster excretion

　　C. more dissociation, more reabsorption, faster excretion

　　D. less dissociation, more reabsorption, slower excretion

　　E. none of the above

8. The major enzyme system that promote drug biotransformation is (　　).

　　A. glucuronyl transferase　　　　　　B. monoamine oxidase enzyme

　　C. cytochrome P450 enzyme system　　D. coenzyme Ⅱ

　　E. hydrolase

9. The effect of a drug combined with a hepatic microsomal enzyme inhibitor (　　).

　　A. weakens　　　　B. enhances　　　　C. stays the same

　　D. disappears　　　E. none of the above

10. The most commonly used route of administration in clinical practice is (   ).
    A. intravenous injection
    B. aerosol inhalation
    C. oral administration
    D. intramuscular injection
    E. arterial administration

第二章案例学习和选择题答案

第三章 药物效应动力学

知识要点

一、不良反应

不良反应(adverse reaction)：凡不符合用药目的，并给患者带来不适或痛苦的反应。包括：

(1)副作用(side reaction)：在治疗剂量下出现的与治疗目的无关的作用，是药物固有的作用，并且是可以预知的。

(2)毒性反应(toxic reaction)：在剂量过大或用药时间过长，药物在体内蓄积过多时发生的危害性反应，一般比较严重。

(3)后遗效应(residual effect)：停药后血药浓度下降至阈浓度以下时所残存的药理效应。

(4)停药反应(withdrawal reaction)：突然停药后原有疾病(或症状)的加剧，又称反跳反应(rebound reaction)。

(5)变态反应(allergic reaction)：又称过敏反应(hypersensitive reaction)，是药物引起的免疫反应，反应的严重程度差异大，反应性质与药物原有药理效应无关，发生反应与否与所用药物剂量无关，拮抗药解救无效。停药后反应逐渐消失，再用时可再发。

(6)特异质反应(idiosyncratic reaction)：为非免疫反应，多为先天遗传异常。症状与药物固有作用基本一致，药理性拮抗药救治可能有效。

二、药物剂量与效应的关系

剂量-效应关系(dose-effect relationship)：药物效应与剂量在一定范围内成比例，简称量效关系；量-效曲线(dose-effect curve)：以药物剂量(或浓度)为横坐标、以效应强度为纵坐标作图，则得量-效曲线。

1. 量反应

量反应(graded response)：药理效应可用连续性数量值表示的反应，可用具体数量或最大反应的百分率表示。

(1)最小有效剂量(最小有效浓度)：引起药理效应的最小剂量或最小药物浓度，亦称阈剂量或阈浓度。

(2)最大效应(maximal effect，Emax)：药物所能达到的最大效应，当剂量增加到一定程度时，再增加药物剂量或浓度而其效应不再继续增强，也称效能(efficacy)。

(3)效价强度：达到相同药理效应时所需要的相对药物剂量，所需要的剂量越大，则效价强度越小。

2. 质反应

质反应(qualitative response)：是指药物的效应表现为反应性质的变化，即全或无、阳性或阴性。

(1)半数有效量(ED_{50})：能引起50%的实验动物出现阳性反应的药物剂量。

(2)半数致死量(LD_{50})：引起50%的实验动物死亡所用的药物剂量。

(3)治疗指数(TI)：药物的 LD_{50}/ED_{50} 的比值，用于表示药物的安全性，但不完全可靠。

三、药物和受体

1. 受体的概念和特性

受体是一类介导细胞信号转导的功能蛋白质，能与相应的配体分子特异结合，传递信息，引起生物效应。其特性包括灵敏性、特异性、饱和性、可逆性及多样性。

2. 受体与药物间的相互作用

(1)占领学说：受体只有与药物结合才能被激活并产生效应，药理效应的强度与药物占领受体数目成正比，当受体全部被占领时出现最大效应。药物与受体结合不仅需要亲和力(affinity)，还需要有内在活性(intrinsic activity)。

(2)亲和力：药物与机体的结合能力。

(3)内在活性：药物与受体结合后所产生效应的能力。

3. 作用于受体的药物分类

(1)激动药(agonist)：是指对受体既有亲和力又有内在活性的药物，分为完全激动药和部分激动药。完全激动药(full agonist)有较强亲和力和较强内在活性($\alpha=1$)；部分激动药(partial agonist)有较强亲和力和较弱内在活性($0<\alpha<1$)，与激动药合用还可拮抗激动药的部分效应。

(2)拮抗药(antagonist)：有较强的亲和力，但无内在活性的药物。分为竞争性拮抗药(competitive antagonist)和非竞争性拮抗药(noncompetitive antagonist)。竞争性拮抗药与受体结合是可逆的，使激动药 E_{max} 不变，但量-效曲线平行右移；非竞争性拮抗药与受体结合牢固，使激动药 E_{max} 下降，量-效曲线非平行右移。拮抗参数 pA_2：当激动药与拮抗药合用时，若2倍浓度激动药所产生效应恰好等于未加入拮抗药时激动药的效应，则所加入拮抗药的摩尔浓度的负对数值为 pA_2。

选择题

1. 药物产生副作用的药理学基础是(　　)。
   A. 用药剂量过大　　　B. 血药浓度过高　　　C. 药物作用的选择性低
   D. 药物在体内蓄积　　E. 机体对药物敏感性高

2. 药物安全范围指的是(　　)。

A. ED_{50} 与 LD_{50} 的比值　　B. LD_{50} 与 ED_{50} 的比值　　C. LD_5 与 ED_{95} 的比值
D. ED_{95} 与 LD_5 的比值　　E. ED_{95} 和 LD_5 之间的距离

3. 以下关于药物副作用的说法正确的是（　　）。
   A. 与药物结构无关　　B. 属于药物固有药理作用　　C. 不可逆
   D. 超剂量使用药物才会出现　　E. 长时间使用药物才会出现

4. 药物的治疗指数是指（　　）。
   A. ED_{50}/TD_{50} 的比值　　B. TD_{10}/ED_{90} 的比值　　C. LD_{50}/ED_{50} 的比值
   D. ED_{95}/LD_5 的比值　　E. ED_{50}/LD_{50} 的比值

5. 药物与受体结合后，可激动受体，也可阻断受体，取决于（　　）。
   A. 药物是否具有亲和力　　B. 药物的酸碱度　　C. 药物是否具有内在活性
   D. 药物的脂溶性　　E. 药物的解离度

6. 药物的何种不良反应与用药剂量的大小无关？（　　）
   A. 副作用　　B. 毒性作用　　C. 继发反应　　D. 变态反应　　E. 后遗效应

7. 药物与受体结合能力主要取决于（　　）。
   A. 药物作用强度　　B. 药物的极性大小　　C. 药物与受体是否具有亲和力
   D. 药物分子量大小　　E. 药物的脂溶性

8. 下列哪个不是竞争性拮抗剂具有的特点？（　　）
   A. 使激动药量-效曲线平行右移　　B. 使激动药的最大效应降低
   C. 竞争性拮抗作用是可逆的　　D. 拮抗参数 pA_2 越大，拮抗作用越强
   E. 最大效能不变

9. 肌注阿托品治疗胆绞痛，引起视力模糊的作用被称为（　　）。
   A. 毒性反应　　B. 副反应　　C. 应激反应　　D. 变态反应　　E. 停药反应

10. 半数有效量是指（　　）。
    A. 引起50%动物产生毒性反应的剂量　　B. 治疗剂量一半所引起的效应
    C. 能引起最大效应所需剂量的一半　　D. 能引起最大效应的50%所用的剂量
    E. 产生50%有效血药浓度的剂量

Multiple-choice questions

1. The pharmacological basis of drug side effects is(　　).
   A. excessive dosage
   B. high blood concentration
   C. low selectivity of drug action
   D. drug accumulation in the body
   E. high sensitivity of the body to the drug

2. What is the safety range of a drug? (　　)
   A. The ratio of ED_{50} to LD_{50}
   B. The ratio of LD_{50} to ED_{50}
   C. The ratio of LD_5 to ED_{95}
   D. The ratio of ED_{95} to LD_5
   E. The range between ED_{95} and LD_5

3. Which of the following statements about side reactions of drug is correct? (　　)
   A. They are unrelated to the structure of the drug

B. They are inherent pharmacological effects of the drug

C. They are irreversible

D. They only occur when drugs are used in excessive doses

E. They only occur when drugs are used for a long time

4. The therapeutic index of a drug is( ).

 A. the ratio of ED_{50}/TD_{50}
 B. the ratio of TD_{10}/ED_{90}
 C. the ratio of LD_{50}/ED_{50}
 D. the ratio of ED_{95}/LD_5
 E. the ratio of ED_{50}/LD_{50}

5. After binding to the receptor, a drug may either activate or block the receptor, depending on ( ).

 A. the affinity of the drug
 B. the pH of the drug
 C. the intrinsic activity of the drug
 D. the lipid solubility of the drug
 E. the dissociation degree of drugs

6. What kind of adverse reactions of drugs are not related to the dosage? ( )

 A. Side effects
 B. Toxic effects
 C. Secondary reactions
 D. Allergic reactions
 E. Residual effect

7. The ability of drugs binding to receptors depends mainly on( ).

 A. the strength of drug action
 B. the polarity of drugs
 C. whether the drug and receptor have affinity
 D. the size of drug molecular weight
 E. the lipid solubility of the drug

8. Which of the following is not the characteristic of competitive antagonism? ( )

 A. To move the dose-effect curve of agonist parallel to the right
 B. To reduce the maximum effect of agonist
 C. Competitive antagonism is reversible
 D. The greater the antagonism parameter pA_2, the stronger the antagonism
 E. Maximum efficiency remains unchanged

9. The effect of intramuscular injection of atropine in the treatment of biliary colic, which causes blurred vision, is called( ).

 A. toxic reactions
 B. side effects
 C. stress reactions
 D. allergic reactions
 E. withdrawal reaction

10. The median effective dose is( ).

 A. the dose that causes 50% of the animals to have a toxic reaction
 B. the effect caused by half the therapeutic dose
 C. half the dose needed to cause the maximum effect
 D. the dose that causes 50% of the maximum effect
 E. the dose that causes 50% of the effective blood concentration

第三章选择题答案

第四章 影响药物效应的因素

知识要点

一、药物因素

1. 药物剂型和给药途径

药物可制成溶液剂、糖浆剂、片剂、胶囊、颗粒剂、注射剂、气雾剂、栓剂等用于各种不同给药途径的剂型。给药途径影响药物吸收、产生效应的速度和时间。药物产生效应的速度通常是：静脉注射>吸入>肌肉注射>皮下注射>直肠>口服>贴皮。

2. 药物相互作用（drug interaction）

药物相互作用主要表现在两方面。一是不改变药物在体液中的浓度但影响药理作用，表现为药物效应动力学的改变，其结果有使原有效应增强的协同作用（synergism）和使原有效应减弱的拮抗作用（antagonism）两种。二是通过影响药物的吸收、分布、代谢和排泄，改变药物在作用部位的浓度从而影响药物的作用，表现为药物代谢动力学的改变。

二、机体因素

1. 年龄

年龄对药物作用的影响主要表现在：①新生儿和老年人体内药物代谢与肾排泄功能较低，药物可能会蓄积；②药物效应靶点的敏感性发生改变；③老年人的特殊生理因素（如心血管反射减弱）和病理因素（如体温过低）对药物的反应性会发生变化；④机体成分的构成比例变化（如老年人脂肪在机体中所占比例增大），导致药物分布容积发生相应的改变；⑤老年人常需服用更多的药物，发生药物相互作用的概率相应增加。

2. 性别

女性体重一般轻于男性，在使用治疗指数低的药物时，为维持相同效应，女性可能需要的剂量更小。女性脂肪的比例比男性高，而水的比例比男性低，这会影响药物的分布和药理作用。

3. 遗传因素

遗传是药物代谢和效应的决定因素。

（1）遗传多态性：又称基因多态性，由同一正常人群中的同一基因位点上具有多种等位基因引起，并由此导致多种表型。表型是在环境影响下基因型所产生的机体的物理表现和可见性状，是个体间药物代谢和反应差异的表现。

(2) 种族差异：种族因素包含遗传和环境两方面。不同种族具有不同的遗传背景（如不同的基因型及相同基因型的不同分布频率）。不同的地理环境、文化背景、食物来源和饮食习惯都会对药物代谢酶的活性和作用靶点的敏感性产生影响，导致一些药物的代谢和反应存在种族差异（racial/ethnic difference）。

(3) 个体差异：人群中即使各方面条件都相同，但仍有少数人对药物的反应性不同，这种差异被称为个体差异。

(4) 特异质反应：是一种性质异常的药物反应，通常是有害的，甚至是致命的。反应是否发生常与剂量无关，即使很小剂量也会发生。

4. 疾病状况

疾病本身能导致药物代谢动力学和药物效应动力学的改变。肝、肾功能损伤易引起药物体内蓄积，产生过强或过久的药物作用，甚至发生毒性反应。回肠或胰腺疾病、慢性心功能不全或肾病综合征均可导致药物吸收减少。

5. 心理因素-安慰剂效应

安慰剂（placebo）一般指由本身没有特殊药理活性的中性物质如乳糖、淀粉等制成的外形似药的制剂。从广义上讲，安慰剂还包括那些本身没有特殊作用的医疗措施如假手术等。安慰剂产生的效应称为安慰剂效应（placebo effect）。

6. 长期用药引起的机体反应性变化

(1) 耐受性（tolerance）和耐药性（drug resistance）：耐受性为机体在连续多次用药后对药物的反应性降低，增加剂量可恢复反应，停药后耐受性可消失。耐药性是指病原体或肿瘤细胞对反复应用的化学治疗药物的敏感性降低，也称抗药性。

(2) 依赖性（dependence）：依赖性指长期应用某种药物后，机体对这种药物产生生理性或精神性的依赖和需求。生理依赖性（physiological dependence）也称躯体依赖性（physical dependence），即停药后患者产生身体戒断症状（abstinent syndrome）。精神依赖性（psychological dependence）是指停药后患者表现出主观不适，无客观症状和体征。

(3) 停药症状（withdrawal symptom）或停药综合征（withdrawal syndrome）：患者在长期反复用药后突然停药可使原有疾病症状加重。

第五章 传出神经系统药理概论

知识要点

一、传出神经的分类

外周神经系统按照传统的解剖学分类及所支配器官和组织见图 5-1。

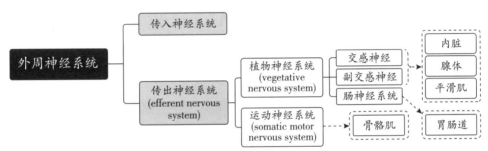

图 5-1 传出神经系统分类(解剖学分类)

按传出神经末梢释放递质分类及分布见图 5-2。

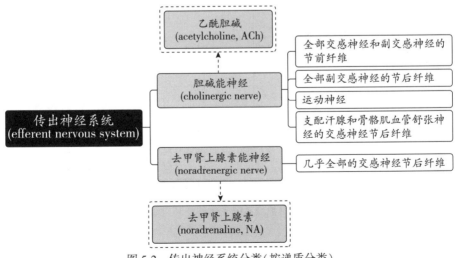

图 5-2 传出神经系统分类(按递质分类)

二、传出神经系统受体的分型

传出神经系统的受体可分成胆碱受体和肾上腺素受体(图5-3)。

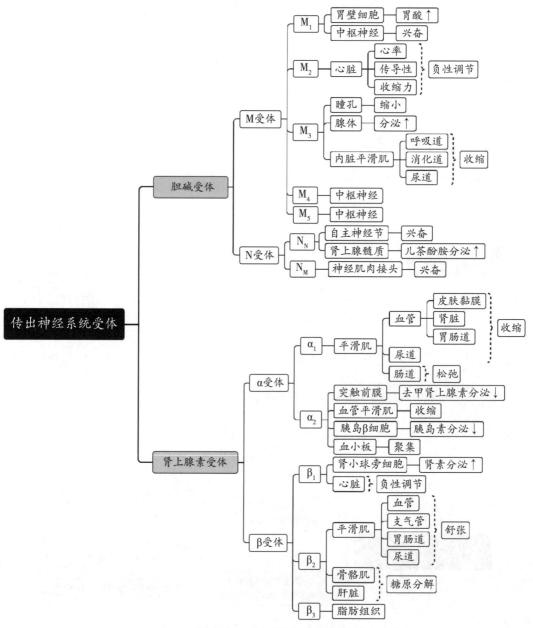

图5-3　传出神经系统受体种类和组织分布

三、传出神经递质的合成、储存、释放及作用的消失

乙酰胆碱和去甲肾上腺素的药动学过程见表 5-1。

表 5-1　　　　　　　　　　乙酰胆碱和去甲肾上腺素的药动学过程

	乙酰胆碱	去甲肾上腺素
合成	胆碱+乙酰辅酶 A→乙酰胆碱	酪氨酸→多巴→多巴胺→去甲肾上腺素
贮存	与 ATP 及囊泡蛋白共存于囊泡内	
释放	胞裂外排(需 Ca^{2+} 参与)、量子化释放	
代谢	被胆碱酯酶(AChE)水解	神经元摄取——贮存型摄取 非神经元摄取——代谢型摄取 (儿茶酚氧位甲基转移酶 COMT、单胺氧化酶 MAO)

四、传出神经系统的生理功能

1. 胆碱能神经兴奋时的效应

(1) M 受体兴奋时的效应包括心脏抑制、血管扩张、腺体分泌、胃肠和支气管平滑肌收缩、瞳孔缩小等;

(2) N 受体兴奋时的效应包括骨骼肌收缩、神经节兴奋、肾上腺髓质分泌增加。

2. 去甲肾上腺素能神经兴奋时的效应

(1) α 受体兴奋时的效应包括皮肤黏膜及内脏血管收缩、瞳孔扩大、汗腺分泌;

(2) β 受体兴奋时的效应包括心脏兴奋、骨骼肌血管和冠状动脉扩张、支气管平滑肌松弛。

传出神经系统药物导图见图 5-4。

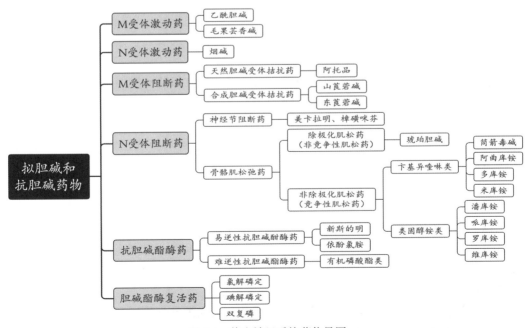

图 5-4　传出神经系统药物导图

第六章 胆碱受体激动药

知识要点

一、M 胆碱受体激动药

1. 药品分类

(1) 胆碱酯类(choline esters)：乙酰胆碱(acetylcholine，ACh)、醋甲胆碱(methacholine)、卡巴胆碱(carbachol)和氯贝胆碱(bethanechol)。

(2) 生物碱类(alkaloids)：毛果芸香碱(pilocarpine)、槟榔碱(arecoline)、毒蕈碱(muscarine)和震颤素(oxotremorine)。

2. 作用机制

与 M 胆碱受体结合并产生与神经递质乙酰胆碱相似的作用。

3. 药理作用

大多数胆碱酯类对 M、N 胆碱受体均有兴奋作用，但以 M 胆碱受体为主；生物碱类则主要兴奋 M 胆碱受体。

以乙酰胆碱为例，其药理作用包括：

(1) 心血管系统：①舒张血管；②减弱心肌收缩力；③减慢心率；④减慢房室结和浦肯野纤维传导；⑤缩短心房不应期。

(2) 胃肠道：兴奋胃肠道平滑肌，使其收缩幅度、张力和蠕动增加，能促进胃、肠分泌，引起恶心、嗳气、呕吐、腹痛及排便等症状。

(3) 泌尿道：使泌尿道平滑肌蠕动增加，膀胱逼尿肌收缩，使膀胱最大自主排空压力(maimal voluntary voiding pressure)增加，降低膀胱容积，同时膀胱三角区和外括约肌舒张，导致膀胱排空。

(4) 其他：

①腺体：使泪腺、气管和支气管腺体、唾液腺、消化道腺体和汗腺分泌增加。

②眼：局部滴眼可使瞳孔括约肌收缩，瞳孔缩小，睫状肌收缩，调节近视。

③神经节和骨骼肌：作用于自主神经节 N_N 胆碱受体和骨骼肌神经肌肉接头的 N_M 胆碱受体，引起交感和副交感神经节兴奋及骨骼肌收缩。此外，因肾上腺髓质受交感神经节前纤维支配，故 N_N 胆碱受体激动能引起肾上腺素释放。

④支气管：兴奋颈动脉体和主动脉体化学受体，可收缩支气管。

⑤中枢：不易通过血脑屏障，故外周给药很少产生中枢作用。

4. 临床应用

代表药物毛果芸香碱，能选择性地激动 M 胆碱受体，对眼和腺体的作用较明显。滴眼后能引起缩瞳、降低眼内压和调节痉挛等作用，主要用于青光眼和虹膜炎的治疗。

5. 不良反应

过量可出现 M 胆碱受体过度兴奋症状，可用阿托品对症处理。滴眼时应压迫内眦，避免药液流入鼻腔增加吸收而产生不良反应。

二、N 胆碱受体激动药

1. 药品分类

烟碱(nicotine，尼古丁)、洛贝林(lobeline，山梗菜碱)、合成化合物二甲铵(tetramethylammonium，TMA)和二甲基苯哌嗪(1,1-dimethyl-4-phenylpiperazinium，DMPP)。

2. 作用机制

与 N 胆碱受体结合并产生与神经递质乙酰胆碱相似的作用。

3. 药理作用

双相性作用于自主神经节 N_N 和神经肌肉接头的 N_M 胆碱受体(先兴奋后抑制)。

4. 临床应用

无临床实用价值，有毒理学意义。

案例学习

学习要点：
(1) 青光眼的治疗措施。
(2) 毛果芸香碱的药理作用及其机制。

关键词： 青光眼；毛果芸香碱；眼内压

案例

大学生费某，男，24 岁。通宵联网游戏 3 天，今晨双眼胀痛、头痛、恶心、视物模糊前来就诊。测得左眼眼压 38 mmHg，右眼眼压 41 mmHg。双眼混合充血，角膜水肿呈雾状浑浊，前房显著变浅，前房角闭塞，周边前房<1/3 CT。瞳孔竖椭圆形散大，对光反射消失，眼球指压坚硬如石。临床诊断为双眼原发性急性闭角型青光眼。治疗：①20%甘露醇注射液 250 mL，30 min 内快速静脉滴注，6 h 后重复给药一次。②1%毛果芸香碱滴眼剂，双眼每次各 1 滴，每 5~10 min 一次，瞳孔缩小后每 6 h 一次。③乙酰唑胺 0.25 g，每日 3 次，首剂加倍。

问答题

1. 毛果芸香碱治疗青光眼的作用机制？
2. 毛果芸香碱对视力的影响及其机制？

选择题

1. 下列有关乙酰胆碱的说法正确的是(　　)。

A. 致血管扩张的作用主要与激动 M_2 胆碱受体有关
B. 可致泌尿道平滑肌松弛
C. 可致心收缩力减弱
D. 可通过血脑屏障
E. 致骨骼肌收缩作用与激动 N_N 胆碱受体有关

2. 以下毛果芸香碱对眼睛的作用的描述正确的是(　　)。
A. 瞳孔缩小，升高眼内压，调节痉挛
B. 瞳孔缩小，降低眼内压，调节痉挛
C. 瞳孔扩大，升高眼内压，调节麻痹
D. 瞳孔扩大，降低眼内压，调节麻痹
E. 瞳孔缩小，降低眼内压，调节麻痹

3. 对于乙酰胆碱，下列叙述错误的是(　　)。
A. 激动 M 型和 N 型胆碱受体
B. 无临床实用价值
C. 作用广泛
D. 选择性较高
E. 化学性质不稳定

4. 毛果芸香碱滴眼后，对视力的影响是(　　)。
A. 视近物清楚，视远物模糊
B. 视近物模糊，视远物清楚
C. 视近物、远物均清楚
D. 视近物、远物均模糊
E. 以上都不对

5. 毛果芸香碱缩瞳机制是(　　)。
A. 阻断虹膜 α 受体，瞳孔开大肌松弛
B. 阻断虹膜 M 胆碱受体，瞳孔括约肌松弛
C. 激动虹膜 α 受体，瞳孔开大肌收缩
D. 激动虹膜 M 胆碱受体，瞳孔括约肌收缩
E. 抑制胆碱酯酶，使乙酰胆碱增多

6. 毛果芸香碱对眼调节作用的正确叙述是(　　)。
A. 睫状肌松弛，悬韧带放松，晶状体变凸
B. 睫状肌收缩，悬韧带拉紧，晶状体变扁平
C. 睫状肌收缩，悬韧带放松，晶状体变凸
D. 睫状肌松弛，悬韧带拉紧，晶状体变扁平
E. 睫状肌收缩，悬韧带放松，晶状体变扁平

7. 乙酰胆碱与毛果芸香碱比较，下列说法正确的是(　　)。
A. 在体内都极易被乙酰胆碱酯酶水解
B. 都可激动 N 受体
C. 都可减少出汗
D. 都可促进胃肠蠕动
E. 都可引起心动过速

8. 影响眼睛视力调节的肌肉为(　　)。
A. 瞳孔开大肌　B. 瞳孔括约肌　C. 睫状肌　D. 上直肌　E. 上斜肌

9. 不属于 N 胆碱受体激动药的是(　　)。
A. 烟碱　　B. 琥珀胆碱　　C. 洛贝林　　D. 四甲铵　　E. 二甲基苯哌嗪

10. 乙酰胆碱的舒张血管作用与下列哪种物质有关？(　　)
A. 前列腺素　B. 缓激肽　C. 多巴胺　D. 组胺　E. 一氧化氮

Case study

Key points:
(1) Therapeutic measures for glaucoma.
(2) Pharmacological effects of pilocarpine and its mechanisms.

Key words: glaucoma; pilocarpine; intraocular pressure

Case

Fei, a 24-year-old male college student. He came to the clinic this morning with distension, headache, nausea, and blurred vision in both eyes after playing online games overnight for 3 days. The intraocular pressure of the left eye was 38 mmHg, and that of the right eye was 41 mmHg. Both eyes were mixed and congested, corneal edema was foggy and cloudy, the anterior chamber was significantly shallow, the anterior chamber angle was occluded, and the peripheral anterior chamber was<1/3 CT. The pupils were vertically elliptical and dilated, and light reflexes disappeared, and the eyeballs were hard as a stone when finger-pressure was applied. Clinical diagnosis: primary acute angle-closure glaucoma in both eyes. Treatment: ① 20% mannitol injection 250 mL, rapid intravenous drip within 30 min, repeat administration once after 6 h. ② 1% hairy fruit rutabaga eye drops, 1 drop in each eye each time, every 5-10 min, every 6 h after pupil dilation. ③ acetazolamide 0.25 g, 3 times a day, the first dose is doubled.

Essay questions

1. What is the mechanism of action of pilocarpine in the treatment of glaucoma?
2. What is the effect of pilocarpine on vision and its mechanism?

Multiple-choice question

1. Which of the following statements about acetylcholine is true? (   )
   A. Its vasodilatory effect is primarily due to its antagonism of the M_2 cholinergic receptor
   B. It relaxes the smooth muscle of the urinary tract
   C. It lowers cardiac contractility
   D. It can cross the blood-brain barrier
   E. Its contractile effects on skeletal muscle are due to its agonism of N_N cholinergic receptors
2. Which of the following statements about pilocarpine's effects on the eye is correct? (   )
   A. Miosis, increasing intraocular pressure, and accommodation spasm
   B. Miosis, decreasing intraocular pressure, and accommodation spasm
   C. Mydriasis, increasing intraocular pressure, and accommodation paralysis
   D. Mydriasis, decreasing intraocular pressure, and accommodation paralysis
   E. Miosis, decreasing intraocular pressure, and accommodation paralysis
3. In the case of acetylcholine, the following statement is incorrect(   ).

A. agonizes M and N cholinergic receptors   B. not clinically useful

C. wide range of actions   D. higher selectivity

E. chemically unstable

4. The effect on visual acuity after eye drops of Hirschsprung's disease is (   ).

    A. clear vision for near objects and blurred vision for distant objects

    B. blurred vision for near objects and clear vision for distant objects

    C. sight of near objects and distant objects are clear

    D. both near and far objects are blurred

    E. none of the above

5. The mechanism of pupil constriction of Hirschsprung's base is (   ).

    A. blocking iris α-receptor and relaxing the pupil opening muscle

    B. blocking iris M cholinergic receptor and relaxing pupil sphincter

    C. agonizing iris α-receptor, contraction of the pupil opening muscle

    D. agonize iris M choline receptor, pupil sphincter contraction

    E. inhibits cholinesterase and increases acetylcholine.

6. The correct description of the effect of Hirsutine on eye regulation is (   ).

    A. ciliary muscle relaxation, suspensory ligament relaxation, lens convexity

    B. the ciliary muscle contracts, the suspensory ligament tightens, and the lens flattens

    C. the ciliary muscle contracts, the suspensory ligament relaxes, and the lens becomes convex

    D. ciliary muscle relaxes, suspensory ligament tightens, lens flattens

    E. the ciliary muscle contracts, the suspensory ligament relaxes, and the lens flattens

7. Acetylcholine and rutaecarpine, the following statements (   ) are correct.

    A. in the body are very easy to be hydrolyzed by acetylcholinesterase

    B. both can agonize N receptors

    C. both can reduce sweating

    D. both can promote gastrointestinal motility

    E. both can cause tachycardia

8. The muscle that affects the visual adjustment of the eye is (   ).

    A. pupil opening muscle   B. pupillary sphincter   C. ciliary muscle

    D. superior rectus muscle   E. superior oblique muscle

9. N-choline receptor agonists are not classified as (   ).

    A. niacin   B. succinylcholine   C. lobelin

    D. tetramethylammonium   E. dimethylphenylpiperazine

10. Which of the following substances is involved in the vasodilatory effect of acetylcholine? (   )

    A. Prostaglandins   B. Bradykinin   C. Dopamine

    D. Histamine   E. Nitric oxide

第六章案例学习和选择题答案

第七章 抗胆碱酯酶药和胆碱酯酶复活药

知识要点

一、药品分类

1. 易逆性抗胆碱酯酶药

新斯的明（neostigmine）、吡斯的明（pyridostigmine）、依酚氯胺（edrophonium chloride）、安贝氯铵（ambenonium chloride）、毒扁豆碱（physostigmine）、地美溴铵（demecarium bromide）等。

2. 难逆性抗胆碱酯酶药（有机磷酸酯类）

农业和环境卫生杀虫剂：敌百虫（dipterex）、乐果（rogor）、马拉硫磷（malathion）、敌敌畏（DDVP）、内吸磷（systox E，1059）和对硫磷（parathion，605）等；战争毒气：沙林（sarin）、梭曼（soman）和塔崩（tabun）等；缩瞳药：乙硫磷（echothiophate iodide）和异氟磷（isoflurophate）等。

3. 胆碱酯酶复活药

氯解磷定（pralidoxime chloride，PAM-CL）、碘解磷定（pralidoxime iodide，PAM）、双复磷等。

二、药理作用及机制

抗胆碱酯酶药可与AChE结合形成复合物，使得AChE失去活性。因复合物水解较慢，故抗胆碱酯酶药可致胆碱能神经末梢释放的ACh堆积，产生拟胆碱作用，使得M和N型胆碱受体兴奋。抗胆碱酯酶药可分为易逆性抗胆碱酯酶药和难逆性抗胆碱酯酶药。

易逆性抗胆碱酯酶药如新斯的明，药理作用有：①眼：收缩瞳孔括约肌及睫状肌，降低眼内压。②胃肠道：增加胃酸分泌，促进肠道活动，促进肠内容物的排出。③对骨骼肌的兴奋作用强：主要是通过抑制神经肌肉接头处的AChE，有一定直接兴奋作用。④其他：低剂量即可增强神经冲动所致的腺体分泌作用，还可影响心血管系统。

难逆性抗胆碱酯酶药如有机磷酸酯类，可与AChE牢固结合，结合位点为AChE的酯解部位——丝氨酸的羟基上。有机磷酸酯类的磷原子具有亲电子性，可与羟基上具有亲核性的氧原子共价键结合，形成难以水解的磷酰化AChE，使AChE失去水解ACh的能力，造成体内ACh大量积聚而引起一系列对胆碱能神经突触、胆碱能神经肌肉接头和中枢神经系统的毒性症状。其症状主要包括：①胆碱能神经突触（M样症状）：首先出现眼和呼吸道症状，表现为瞳孔明显缩小、眼球疼痛、睫状肌痉挛、眼眉疼痛，腺体分泌增加，胸腔紧缩，呼吸困难，呕吐、腹痛、腹泻等；②胆碱能神经肌肉接头（N样症状）：不自主肌束抽搐、震颤；③中枢神经系统症状：中枢性呼吸麻痹，血管运动中枢抑制，血压下降。

磷酰化胆碱酯酶性质稳定，故作用持久。中毒后若不及时抢救，AChE则易"老化"，即磷酰化AChE的磷酰化基团上的一个烷氧基断裂，生成更为稳定的单烷氧基磷酰化AChE。

胆碱酯酶复活药可恢复AChE的活性，与磷酰化胆碱酯酶结合成复合物，复合物再裂解形成磷酰化氯解磷定，使胆碱酯酶游离而复活。亦可直接与体内游离的有机磷酸酯类结合，成为无毒的磷酰化氯解磷定从尿中排出，从而阻止游离的毒物继续抑制AChE活性。

三、临床应用

低剂量易逆性抗胆碱酯酶药可用于重症肌无力、腹气胀、尿潴留、青光眼及竞争性神经肌肉阻滞药中毒的解救及阿尔茨海默病。难逆性抗胆碱酯酶药如有机磷酸酯类则主要用作农业杀虫剂。胆碱酯酶复活药用于救治有机磷农药中毒，可明显减轻N样症状，对骨骼肌痉挛的抑制作用最为明显；对中枢神经系统的中毒症状也有一定改善作用；但对M样症状影响较小，故应与阿托品合用，以控制症状。

四、不良反应

以新斯的明为代表的易逆性抗胆碱酯酶药的不良反应主要与胆碱能神经过度兴奋有关，其表现可参考难逆性抗胆碱酯酶药有机磷酸酯类农药中毒的症状。

治疗剂量的氯解磷定毒性较小，肌内注射局部有轻微疼痛。静脉注射过快（>500 mg/min）可出现头痛、眩晕、乏力、视物模糊、恶心及心动过速。剂量过大（>8 g/24h）时，其本身也可以抑制AChE，使神经肌肉传导阻滞，严重者呈癫痫样发作、抽搐、呼吸抑制。

案例学习

学习要点：
(1) 肌无力的治疗措施。
(2) 新斯的明、毒扁豆碱的药理作用及其机制。
(3) 有机磷酸酯类中毒的治疗措施。
(4) 阿托品和解磷定救治有机磷酸酯类中毒的作用机制。

关键词：肌无力；新斯的明；毒扁豆碱；有机磷酸酯类中毒；解磷定。

案例一

1399年，明朝燕王朱棣发动了夺取侄子建文皇帝朱允炆皇位的战争。1400年，朱棣带兵远征离开了北平，朱允炆突然派兵包围了北平城。冬天刮着西北风，燕王妃徐仪华和长子朱高炽组织城里的将士和百姓坚守。朱高炽跑上跑下，每天都全身大汗。朱高炽开始还挺精神，可是没过几天，就变得精神萎靡、全身无力，但是他还是强打着精神和大家一起守城。后来朱棣带兵回救北平，打败了围城部队，才解了围。朱高炽自这次战役后，变得越来越肥胖、嗜睡、无力。经太医刘纯诊断，朱高炽是由于过度受风，患上了痿症。刘纯使用补中益气汤给朱高炽治疗，症状不但未见缓解，反而日渐严重。在朱棣当了皇帝之后，想要放弃长子朱高炽，而立老二朱高煦为太子。尽管在皇后徐仪华的坚持以及众大臣的游说下，朱棣还是"立嫡以长"，立了朱高炽为皇太子，但朱棣还是十分厌恶朱高炽肥胖、无力的样子。自1409年，朱棣常住北平，让朱高炽在南京处理国家政务，仍时常对其加以责骂，使得朱高炽的病情日益加重。太医刘纯为尽快治愈太子，于一年冬天在南京利用服刑的犯人制作了痿症模型，并试用了不同的治疗方法，找到了有效治疗痿症的中药组方"苏厥散"。1411年，刘纯上奏明朝永乐皇帝朱棣，报告了这个研究成果。这时的太子朱高炽已卧床不起，于是刘纯马上使用新方法对太子进行治疗。经过三个多月的治疗，朱高炽的痿症被彻底治愈。

现代医学明确了痿症的病因，即劳累受凉导致了周围神经炎，进而诱发肌无力的症状。在西方，1672年英国医生托马斯·威利斯发现了肌无力这种疾病。至1934年，英国医生玛丽·布罗德福特·沃克开始尝试对肌无力的病人进行治疗。她发现肌无力病人的症状类似筒箭毒碱中毒表现，因此，沃克医生给那些行动不便的病人服用了一种解毒剂——毒扁豆碱。结果令人震惊——几分钟之内，病人就能站起来并走过房间。尽管她的发现意义重大，但遭到了科学界的嘲笑，因为这种治疗方法改善重症肌无力症状的速度太快、效果太好，令人难以置信。直到许多年后，科学界才开始承认她的研究成果。

至20世纪60年代，医学界才明确了肌无力的发病机理：肌无力是神经肌肉接头处胆碱能受体的自身免疫性抗体抑制了突触的传递能力导致的。但是血液中为什么出现这种抗体，至今原因不明。现代医学使用切除胸腺、肌注新斯的明等办法能够缓解无力的症状，但是仍容易复发。

◎ 问答题
1. 为什么筒箭毒碱中毒和重症肌无力会产生相似的症状？
2. 毒扁豆碱如何改善重症肌无力的症状？
3. 为什么对每一位出现肌无力的病人使用毒扁豆碱是危险的？
4. 毒扁豆碱还有哪些其他治疗用途？

案例二

患者王某，女，33岁。与家人发生口角，服敌百虫300 mL左右，20分钟后出现腹痛、恶心、呕吐、多汗，2小时后陷入昏迷，送入急诊。检查发现，患者神志不清、胡言乱语，双眼上翻、瞳孔为针尖样大小。面部肌肉抽搐，口角流涎，呼吸可闻及浓重的大蒜味。大小便失禁。双肺可闻及散在湿啰音。呼吸24次/分，SpO_2 95%，心率66次/分，血压96/54 mmHg。血清胆碱酯酶：326 U/L。临床诊断为：重度急性有机磷酸酯类中毒。治疗：①抽出胃液和毒物，并用微温的2%碳酸氢钠溶液或1%盐水反复洗胃，直至洗出液中不含农药味，随后给予硫酸镁导泻。②阿托品10 mg静脉注射，每5分钟重复给药1次。达"阿托品化"后1 mg每1~2小时给药1次，中毒情况好转后逐步减量。③氯解磷定

2 g 静脉注射，随后以 0.5 g 每 2 小时使用 1 次，中毒情况好转后逐步减量。

◎ 问答题

1. 有机磷酸酯类中毒治疗措施的作用原理？
2. 解救有机磷中毒时阿托品与解磷定反复应用的原因及注意事项有哪些？

选择题

1. 某病人患重症肌无力多年，现急诊入院，主诉突发手部无力、复视以及吞咽困难。突发症状可能与自行变动药物治疗方案有关。为了鉴别病人所出现的症状是药物使用量不足引起的重症肌无力危象或药物过量导致的胆碱能危象，应选择(　　)。
   A. 阿托品　　B. 吡斯的明　　C. 依酚氯铵　　D. 毒扁豆碱　　E. 解磷定

2. 患者在田间喷洒敌敌畏，由于防护不当出现以下中毒症状，立即使用阿托品解救，不能得到缓解的症状是(　　)。
   A. 腹痛　　B. 针尖样瞳孔　　C. 肌震颤　　D. 出汗　　E. 流涎

3. 筒箭毒碱过量中毒，应选用(　　)解救。
   A. 卡巴胆碱　　B. 新斯的明　　C. 多库铵　　D. 碘解磷定　　E. 阿托品

4. 琥珀胆碱的肌肉松弛作用机制是(　　)。
   A. 促进乙酰胆碱灭活
   B. 抑制运动神经末梢释放乙酰胆碱
   C. 中枢性骨骼肌松弛作用
   D. 终板膜持续过度去极化
   E. 抑制乙酰胆碱酯酶活性

5. 下面有关新斯的明的叙述，错误的是(　　)。
   A. 口服吸收少，且不规则
   B. 不易透过血脑屏障
   C. 可直接激动 N、M 受体
   D. 属难逆性抗胆碱酯酶药
   E. 生物利用度很低

6. 碘解磷定对下面哪种农药解毒效果最差？(　　)
   A. 马拉硫磷　　B. 敌百虫　　C. 乐果　　D. 对硫磷　　E. 内吸磷

7. 新斯的明的药理作用不包括(　　)。
   A. 使骨骼肌收缩力增强　　B. 兴奋胃肠道平滑肌　　C. 使支气管平滑肌收缩
   D. 导致心动过速　　E. 使腺体分泌增加

8. 有机磷酸酯类中毒症状中，不属于 M 样症状的是(　　)。
   A. 瞳孔缩小　　B. 流涎、流泪　　C. 腹痛、腹泻
   D. 肌肉震颤　　E. 小便失禁

9. 新斯的明的禁忌证是(　　)。
   A. 青光眼　　B. 阵发性室上性心动过速　　C. 重症肌无力
   D. 机械性肠梗阻　　E. 尿潴留

10. 某病人被诊断为重症肌无力，可考虑用吡斯的明或新斯的明进行治疗，但两者均可能引起(　　)。
    A. 支气管舒张　　B. 调节麻痹　　C. 腹泻
    D. 腹气胀　　E. 胃酸分泌减少

Case study

Key points:

(1) Therapeutic measures for myasthenia gravis.

(2) Pharmacological effects of neostigmine, toxaphene and their mechanisms.

(3) Therapeutic measures for organophosphate poisoning.

(4) The mechanism of action of atropine and antiphosphidine in the treatment of organophosphate poisoning.

Key words: myasthenia gravis; neostigmine; toxaphene; organophosphate poisoning; antiphosphate

Case 1

In 1399, Zhu Di, King of Yan in the Ming Dynasty in China, launched a war to seize the throne of his nephew, Emperor Zhu Yunwen. In 1400, Zhu Di left Beiping with an expedition when Zhu Yunwen unexpectedly dispatched troops to surround the city. When the wind blew from the northwest in the winter, Zhu Di's consort, Xu Yihua and her eldest son, Zhu Gaochi, rallied the soldiers and residents of the city to hold out. Every day, Zhu Gaochi ran up and down, sweating profusely. Zhu Gaochi was initially fairly energetic, but after a few days, he grew feeble, yet he still fought alongside everyone else to defend the city. Later, Zhu Di returned forces to Beiping and defeated the besieging army to lift the siege. Since this battle, Zhu Gaochi has become increasingly obese, lethargic and impotent, and diagnosed with Flaccidity Syndrome by Liu Chun, the Imperial Doctor, as a result of burnout and wind exposure. Liu Chun used Buzhong Yiqi Decoction to treat Zhu Gaochi, but the symptoms worsened rather than improved. When Zhu Di became Emperor, he sought to depose his eldest son, Zhu Gaochi, and install his second son, Zhu Gaoxu, as Crown Prince. Because of the empress Xu Yihua's pleas and ministers' lobbying, Zhu Di followed the tradition by naming Zhu Gaochi, as the crown prince, but Zhu Di is still unhappy with Zhu Gaochi's obesity and frail appearance. Since 1409, Zhu Di has frequently lived in Beiping and entrusted governmental duties to Zhu Gaochi in Nanjing, yet he still often scolded him, worsening Zhu Gaochi's condition. To cure the prince as soon as possible, Liu Chun, the Imperial Doctor, created a model of Flaccidity Syndrome using prisoners in Nanjing in during the winter of one year and tried various treatments until he discovered an effective treatment for Flaccidity Syndrome in the Chinese herbal formula "Su Jue San". In 1411, Liu Chun reported the findings of this research to Emperor Zhu Di, the Emperor Yongle of the Ming Dynasty. At that time, the crown prince Zhu Gaochi was already bedridden, so Liu Chun used the new method to treat him right away. Zhu Gaochi was cured after more than three months of treatment.

According to modern medicine, Muscle weakness symptoms of Flaccidity Syndrome are produced by peripheral neuritis induced by exhaustion and cold exposure. In the West, the disease of myasthenia gravis was discovered in 1672 by the English physician Thomas Willis. By 1934, the English physician Mary Broadfoot Walker began to treat patients with muscle weakness symptoms. Dr. Walker discovered that the symptoms of patients with myasthenia gravis were similar to the those of tubocurare poisoning, so she gave an antidote, physostigmine, to her immobile patients. The results were startling—within minutes, her patients were able to rise and walk across the room. Despite the significance of her accomplishment, it is largely ridiculed by the scientific community because the treatment improves the symptoms of myasthenia gravis too rapidly and effectively to be believable. It is not until many years later that the scientific community comes to accept her findings.

The pathogenesis of myasthenia gravis was not clear to the medical community until the 1960s: myasthenia gravis is caused by autoimmune antibodies directed against cholinergic receptors at the neuromuscular junction, which inhibit the ability of synapses to transmit. The reason for the presence of such antibodies in the blood, however, is still unknown. Modern medicine treats the symptoms of muscle weakness with methods such as thymus gland removal and intramuscular neostigmine, but it is still prone to recurrence.

◎ **Essay questions**

1. Why do tubocurare poisoning and myasthenia gravis produce similar symptoms?
2. How does physostigmine improve the symptoms of myasthenia gravis?
3. Why is it dangerous to administer physostigmine to every patient presenting with muscle weakness?
4. What are the other therapeutic uses of physostigmine?

Case 2

Patient Wang, female, 33 years old. After a verbal argument with her family, she took about 300 mL of trichlorfon, and 20 minutes later, she developed abdominal pain, nausea, vomiting, and excessive sweating, and fell into a coma 2 hours later, and was admitted to the emergency room. Examination revealed that the patient was delirious and rambling, with upturned eyes and pinpoint pupils. Facial muscles were twitching, salivation was observed at the corners of the mouth, and a strong odor of garlic could be detected on breathing. Incontinence. Scattered wet rhonchi could be heard in both lungs. Respiration 24 times/min, SpO_2 95%, heart rate 66 times/min, blood pressure 96/54 mmHg. serum cholinesterase: 326 U/L. Clinical diagnosis: severe acute organophosphate poisoning. Treatment: ①Gastric fluid and poison were withdrawn and the stomach was washed repeatedly with slightly warm 2% sodium bicarbonate solution or 1% saline water until the washed out fluid did not smell of pesticide, followed by magnesium sulfate for diarrhea. ②Atropine 10 mg was given intravenously, and the administration of the drug was repeated once every 5 minutes. 1mg every 1-2 hours after "atropinization", gradually tapering off after improvement. ③Chlorpheniramine 2 g IV, followed by 0.5 g every 2 hours, gradually tapering off after improvement.

◎ **Essay questions**
1. What is the rationale behind the therapeutic measures for organophosphate poisoning?
2. What ate the reasons and precautions for the repeated application of atropine and dephosphidine in the rescue of organophosphate poisoning?

✎ Multiple-choice questions

1. A patient who has had myasthenia gravis for many years is admitted to the hospital as an emergency due to sudden onset of hand weakness, diplopia, and dysphagia. A change in medication regimen could be the cause of the sudden onset of symptoms. Which drug should be used to determine whether the patient's symptoms are due to a myasthenia gravis crisis or a cholinergic crisis caused by an overdose? (   )
   A. Atropine   B. Pyridostigmine   C. Edrophonium chloride
   D. Physostigmine   E. Pyraloxime

2. A man spraying dichlorvos in a field develops the following poisoning symptoms due to insufficient protection. Which of the following symptoms can't be relieved by tropine, the antidote(   ).
   A. abdominal pain   B. pinpoint pupils   C. muscle tremor
   D. sweating   E. salivation

3. Which antidote is used for tubocurarine overdose poisonings? (   )
   A. Carbachol   B. Neostigmine   C. Doxacurium
   D. Pralidoxime iodide E. Atropine

4. What is the mechanism by which succinylcholine causes muscle relaxation? (   )
   A. Enhancement of acetylcholine inactivation
   B. Inhibition of acetylcholine release from motor nerve endings
   C. Centrally acting muscle relaxation
   D. Sustained hyperdepolarization of the endplate membrane
   E. Inhibition of acetylcholinesterase

5. Which of the following description of neostigmine is incorrect? (   )
   A. It is poorly and irregularly absorbed orally
   B. It is not easy to cross the blood-brain barrier
   C. It can directly agonize N_M receptors
   D. It is a refractory anticholinesterase drug
   E. Low bioavailability

6. Which of the following pesticides does iodophosphamide have the worst detoxification effect? (   )
   A. Malathion   B. Trichlorfon   C. Parathion
   D. Parathion   E. Phosphorus endosulfan

7. The pharmacological effects of neostigmine do not include (　　).
   A. increasing the contractility of skeletal muscle
   B. exciting the smooth muscle of gastrointestinal tract
   C. constriction of bronchial smooth muscle
   D. causing tachycardia
   E. increase the secretion of glands
8. Among the symptoms of organophosphate poisoning, the one that does not belong to M-like symptoms is (　　).
   A. pupil narrowing　　　B. salivation and tearing　　C. abdominal pain, diarrhea
   D. muscle tremor　　　　E. urinary incontinence
9. The contraindication of neostigmine is (　　).
   A. glaucoma　　　　　　　　　　　　B. paroxysmal supraventricular tachycardia
   C. myasthenia gravis　　　　　　　　D. mechanical intestinal obstruction
   E. urinary retention
10. A patient diagnosed with myasthenia gravis may be considered for treatment with pyridostigmine or neostigmine, but both may cause (　　).
    A. bronchodilation　　　　　　　　B. regulatory paralysis
    C. diarrhea　　　　　　　　　　　　D. abdominal gas and distension
    E. decreased gastric acid secretion

第七章案例学习和选择题答案

第八章 胆碱受体阻断药（Ⅰ）
——M胆碱受体阻断药

📖 知识要点

一、药品分类

(1) 阿托品及其类似生物碱：阿托品(atropine)、东莨菪碱(scopolamine)和山莨菪碱(anisodamine)。

(2) 阿托品的合成代用品：①合成扩瞳药，后马托品(homatropine)、托吡卡胺(tropicamide)、环喷托酯(cyclopentolate)和尤卡托品(eucatropine)；②合成解痉药，异丙托溴铵(ipratropium bromide)、溴丙胺太林(propantheline bromide)、溴甲东莨菪碱(scopolamine methylbromide)、溴甲后马托品(homatropine methylbromide)、溴化甲哌佐酯(mepenzolate bromide)、双环维林(dicyclomine)、黄酮哌酯(flavoxate)和奥昔布宁(oxybutynin)等；③选择性M胆碱受体阻断药，哌仑西平(pirenzepine)、索利那新(solifenacin)等。

二、作用机制

M胆碱受体阻断药(muscarinic cholinoceptor blocker)能阻碍乙酰胆碱(ACh)或胆碱受体激动药与平滑肌、心肌、腺体、外周神经节和中枢神经系统的M胆碱受体结合，而拮抗其拟胆碱作用，表现出胆碱能神经被阻断或抑制的效应，通常对N胆碱受体兴奋作用影响较小。但是，阿托品及其类似药物的季铵类衍生物等具有较强的拮抗N胆碱受体的活性，可干扰外周神经节或神经肌肉的传递。在中枢神经系统如脊髓、皮质和皮质下中枢，也存在胆碱能神经递质传递以及M和N胆碱受体的激动效应，大剂量或毒性剂量的阿托品及其相关药物通常对中枢神经系统具有先兴奋后抑制的作用，季铵类药物由于较难透过血脑屏障，对中枢神经系统的影响很小。

三、药理作用

阿托品对M胆碱受体有较高选择性，但对各种M受体亚型的选择性较低；大剂量时也有阻断神经节N受体的作用。阿托品的作用非常广泛，随剂量增加可依次出现腺体分泌减少、瞳孔扩大和调节麻痹、胃肠道和膀胱平滑肌抑制、心率加快等现象，大剂量可出现中枢作用。

山莨菪碱药理作用与阿托品相似，但其中枢兴奋作用很弱。东莨菪碱具有较强的抑制中枢和抑制腺体分泌作用，有防晕、止吐和抗帕金森病作用。

四、临床应用

阿托品用于各种内脏绞痛、虹膜睫状体炎、缓慢型心律失常、感染性休克、解救有机磷酸酯类中毒等。由于副作用太多，已被一些合成的药物取代，如合成扩瞳药（后马托品）、合成解痉药（溴丙胺太林）、选择性 M 受体阻断药（哌仑西平）等。

山莨菪碱主要用于感染性休克和内脏平滑肌绞痛。东莨菪碱主要用于麻醉前给药、防治晕动病等。

五、不良反应

不良反应与其选择性低所致广泛的 M 受体阻断作用有关，禁用于青光眼及前列腺肥大者。

案例学习

学习要点：
(1) 阿托品的不良反应。
(2) 阿托品化和阿托品中毒的区别。
关键词： 阿托品；阿托品化；阿托品中毒

案例

患者张某，男，34 岁，拟行双侧腋下汗腺切除术。术前各项常规检查指标均正常，心率 68 次/分。上午 10 时患者注射阿托品等麻醉前用药后进入手术室等待，监测发现其心率为 150 次/分，患者自述心悸、口干，面色潮红，无明显精神症状。详细询问患者既往病史，答复以前未曾出现过类似情况，初步考虑可能是术前过于紧张所致。遂静脉推注丙泊酚 50 mg，继以 400 mg/h 维持。患者逐渐入睡，其心率略有下降，但仍维持在 130 次/分左右。鉴于患者心率持续偏快，且原因不明，故将手术推迟，待其苏醒后送回病房，床边监测其心率仍在 140 次/分左右。怀疑术前误用大剂量阿托品，随嘱主管医师核查术前用药情况。经查，因电子处方选择错误（错行），术前医嘱有误，将 0.5 mg 的阿托品误开成了 10 mg 的阿托品，护士亦未考虑到剂量过大而直接执行医嘱。当天回病房后患者述双眼视物模糊、口干、心慌、烦躁，查双侧瞳孔散大。未予特殊处理，至傍晚病情逐渐好转，第二天完全恢复正常。

问答题

1. 患者注射大剂量阿托品后为什么会出现心悸、口干、颜面潮红、视物模糊等症状？
2. 阿托品中毒和阿托品化的区别？

选择题

1. 对阿托品的作用最敏感的效应器是（　　）。
   A. 心脏　　B. 腺体　　C. 胃肠道、膀胱平滑肌　　D. 骨骼肌　　E. 瞳孔
2. 阿托品对眼睛的作用表现为（　　）。
   A. 瞳孔缩小，眼内压升高，调节痉挛，视近物清楚
   B. 瞳孔扩大，眼内压升高，调节痉挛，视远物清楚
   C. 瞳孔扩大，眼内压降低，调节麻痹，视近物清楚
   D. 瞳孔缩小，眼内压降低，调节麻痹，视近物清楚
   E. 瞳孔扩大，眼内压升高，调节麻痹，视远物清楚
3. 阿托品对眼的调节作用表现为（　　）。
   A. 睫状肌松弛，悬韧带放松，晶状体变凸
   B. 睫状肌收缩，悬韧带拉紧，晶状体变扁平
   C. 睫状肌收缩，悬韧带放松，晶状体变凸
   D. 睫状肌收缩，悬韧带拉紧，晶状体变扁平
   E. 睫状肌松弛，悬韧带拉紧，晶状体变扁平
4. 东莨菪碱不用于治疗（　　）。
   A. 晕动病　　B. 震颤麻痹　　C. 呕吐　　D. 青光眼　　E. 麻醉前给药
5. 阿托品解除平滑肌痉挛，效果最好的是（　　）。
   A. 支气管平滑肌痉挛　　B. 胃肠道平滑肌痉挛　　C. 胆道平滑肌痉挛
   D. 输尿管平滑肌痉挛　　E. 子宫平滑肌兴奋
6. 阿托品用作全身麻醉前给药的主要目的是（　　）。
   A. 增强麻醉　　B. 镇静　　C. 防心动过缓
   D. 减少呼吸道腺体分泌　　E. 辅助骨骼肌松弛
7. 对山莨菪碱叙述错误的是（　　）。
   A. 其人工合成品为 654-2　　B. 平滑肌解痉作用与阿托品相似
   C. 解除血管痉挛，改善微循环　　D. 具有较强的中枢抗胆碱作用
   E. 青光眼禁用
8. 阿托品的不良反应不包括（　　）。
   A. 口干、乏汗　　B. 排尿困难　　C. 心率加快　　D. 瞳孔扩大　　E. 视远物模糊
9. 阿托品最适于治疗以下哪种休克（　　）。
   A. 感染性休克　　B. 过敏性休克　　C. 心源性休克　　D. 失血性休克　　E. 疼痛性休克
10. 阿托品抗感染中毒性休克的主要原因是（　　）。
    A. 解除血管痉挛，改善微循环，增加重要脏器的血流量
    B. 解除迷走神经对心脏的抑制　　C. 解除胃肠绞痛
    D. 兴奋中枢神经　　E. 升高血压

Case study

Key points:
(1) Adverse effects of atropine.
(2) Difference between atropinization and atropine poisoning.

Key words: atropine; atropinization; atropine poisoning

Case

Patient Zhang, male, 34 years old, was to undergo bilateral axillary sweat gland excision. Preoperative routine examination indicators were normal, heart rate 68 times / min. At 10 am., the patient was injected with atropine and other preanesthetic drugs, and entered the operating room to wait for the operation, where he was monitored and found to have a heart rate of 150 beats/min, with palpitations, a dry mouth, and a flushed complexion, and no obvious psychiatric symptoms. The patient was asked about his past medical history and replied that he had not experienced similar symptoms before, so he was initially considered to be too nervous before the operation. Propofol was injected intravenously at 50mg and maintained at 400mg/h. The patient gradually fell asleep. The patient gradually fell asleep, and his heart rate decreased slightly, but remained around 130 beats/min. Given that the patient's heart rate continued to be fast and the cause was unknown, the operation was postponed and the patient was sent back to the ward after awakening, and his heart rate was still around 140 beats/min on bedside monitoring. The patient was suspected of misuse of high-dose atropine, and the physician in charge was instructed to check the preoperative medication. It was found that, due to a mistake in the selection of the electronic prescription (wrong line), the preoperative medical advice was wrongly prescribed from 0.5 mg of atropine to 10 mg of atropine, and the nurse directly carried out the medical advice without considering the high dose. After returning to the ward, the patient reported blurred vision in both eyes, dry mouth, panic, irritability, and bilateral pupil dilation. No special treatment was given, and the patient's condition gradually improved in the evening and returned to normal the next day.

◎ Essay questions

1. Why did the patient experience palpitations, dry mouth, facial flushing and blurred vision after high-dose atropine injection?
2. What is the difference between atropine poisoning and atropinization?

Multiple-choice question

1. The effector most sensitive to the action of atropine is (   ).
   A. heart　　　　　B. glands　　　C. gastrointestinal tract, bladder smooth muscle
   D. skeletal muscle　　E. pupil

2. The effect of atropine on the eyes is manifested as (　　).
   A. pupil narrowing, increased intraocular pressure, spasm, clear vision of near objects
   B. pupil dilation, increased intraocular pressure, spasm, clear vision
   C. pupil dilation, decreased intraocular pressure, regulation paralysis, clear vision of near objects
   D. dilated pupil, decreased intraocular pressure, regulation paralysis, clear vision of near objects
   E. pupil dilation, increased intraocular pressure, regulation paralysis, clear vision of distant objects

3. The regulatory effect of atropine on the eye is manifested as (　　).
   A. ciliary muscle relaxation, suspensory ligament relaxation, lens convexity
   B. the ciliary muscle contracts, the suspensory ligament tightens, and the lens flattens
   C. the ciliary muscle contracts, the suspensory ligament relaxes, and the lens becomes convex
   D. ciliary muscle contracts, suspensory ligament tightens, lens flattens
   E. the ciliary muscle relaxes, the suspensory ligament tightens, and the lens flattens

4. Scopolamine is not used to treat (　　).
   A. motion sickness　　B. tremor paralysis　　C. vomiting
   D. glaucoma　　E. administration before anesthesia

5. Atropine relieves smooth muscle spasm and is most effective in (　　).
   A. bronchial smooth muscle spasm　　B. gastrointestinal smooth muscle spasm
   C. biliary tract smooth muscle spasm　　D. ureteral smooth muscle spasm
   E. uterine smooth muscle excitation

6. The main purpose of atropine is to be administered before general anesthesia (　　).
   A. enhancement of anesthesia　　B. sedation
   C. anti-bradycardia　　D. to reduce the secretion of respiratory glands
   E. to assist skeletal muscle relaxation

7. What is wrong with the description of scopolamine? (　　)
   A. The synthetic product is 654-2
   B. Smooth muscle antispasmodic effect is similar to that of atropine
   C. Relieve vasospasm and improve microcirculation
   D. Strong central anticholinergic effect
   E. Glaucoma prohibited

8. Adverse effects of atropine do not include (　　).
   A. dry mouth, lack of sweat　　B. difficulty in urination　　C. increased heart rate
   D. pupil dilation　　E. blurred vision

9. Atropine is most suitable for the treatment of which of the following types of shock? (　　)
   A. Infectious shock　　B. Anaphylactic shock　　C. Cardiogenic shock
   D. Hemorrhagic shock　　E. Painful shock

10. The main reason for atropine anti-infective toxic shock is (   ).
    A. relieve vasospasm, improve microcirculation and increase blood flow to important organs
    B. release the inhibition of vagus nerve to the heart
    C. relieving gastrointestinal colic
    D. excite the central nervous system
    E. elevate blood pressure

第八章案例学习和选择题答案

第九章　胆碱受体阻断药（Ⅱ）
——N胆碱受体阻断药

> 知识要点

一、药品分类

（1）神经节阻断药（N_N受体阻断药）：如美卡拉明（mecamylamine）、樟磺咪芬（trimethaphan camsylate）。

（2）骨骼肌松弛药（N_M受体阻断药，神经肌肉阻滞药）：除极化肌松药和非除极化肌松药。

①除极化型肌松药（非竞争性肌松药）：如琥珀胆碱（suxamethonium, succinylcholine, 司可林）。

②非除极化型肌松药（竞争性肌松药）：如筒箭毒碱、阿曲库铵（atracurium）、多库铵（doxacurium）和米库铵（mivacurium）。

二、药理作用及机制

神经节阻断药能选择性地与神经节细胞的N_N胆碱受体结合，竞争性地阻断ACh与受体结合，使ACh不能引起神经节细胞去极化，从而阻断了神经冲动在神经节中的传递。

去极化型肌松药与神经肌肉接头后膜的胆碱受体结合，产生与ACh相似但较持久的去极化作用，使神经肌肉接头后膜的N_M胆碱受体不能对ACh起反应，此时神经肌肉的阻滞方式已由去极化转变为非去极化，前者为Ⅰ相阻断，后者为Ⅱ相阻断，从而使骨骼肌松弛。

非去极化型肌松药能与ACh竞争神经肌肉接头的N_M胆碱受体，能竞争性阻断ACh的去极化作用，使骨骼肌松弛。

三、临床应用

神经节阻断药用于：麻醉时控制血压，以减少手术区出血；有效地防止主动脉瘤手术中因手术剥离而撕拉组织所造成的交感神经反射，使病人血压不致明显升高。

除极化型肌松药（临床常用药物仅有琥珀胆碱）对喉肌松弛作用较强，静脉注射给药适用于气管内插管、气管镜、食管镜检查等短时操作，静脉滴注可用于较长时间手术。

非除极化型肌松药临床上可作为麻醉辅助药，用于胸腹手术和气管插管等。

四、不良反应

樟磺咪芬可以诱发组胺释放，使其心血管反应（即降压作用）更为明显。

琥珀胆碱的不良反应包括窒息（过量致呼吸肌麻痹）、眼压升高、肌束颤动、血钾升高、心血管反应（可兴奋迷走神经及副交感神经节，产生心动过缓、心脏骤停以及室性节律障碍；亦可兴奋交感神经节使血压升高）、恶性高热、增加腺体分泌、促进组胺释放等作用。

筒箭毒碱作用时间较长，用药后不易逆转，如剂量过大，可致膈肌麻痹、呼吸停止。

案例学习

学习要点：
(1) 琥珀胆碱中毒的治疗措施。
(2) 除极化型肌松药和非除极化型肌松药的区别。

关键词： 肌无力；琥珀胆碱；新斯的明

案例

朱某，男，24岁，昨晚于夜市食用红烧狗肉两份，凌晨因腹胀、腹痛、恶心、呕吐入院急诊。查体诉肩胛、胸腹部肌肉疼痛，肌张力降低，血检报告血钾升高。检验其打包带回的食物，发现琥珀胆碱成分。治疗：0.9%氯化钠溶液5000 mL洗胃，拔管前注入20%甘露醇溶液60 mL。洗胃结束后，静脉滴注5%葡萄糖溶液500 mL×2瓶，每瓶加能量合剂1支、20 mg呋塞米1支，并监测血钾和患者肌张力状态。

问答题

1. 琥珀胆碱中毒为什么会引起血钾升高？
2. 琥珀胆碱中毒引起的肌无力能否用新斯的明治疗？为什么？

选择题

1. 应用琥珀胆碱后，肌松作用最明显的部位是（　　）。
   A. 颈部及四肢肌肉　B. 舌肌　　C. 颜面肌　　D. 腹部肌肉　　E. 背部肌肉
2. 属于除极化型肌松药的是（　　）。
   A. 筒箭毒碱　　B. 琥珀胆碱　　C. 多库铵　　D. 东莨菪碱　　E. 阿曲库铵
3. 解救琥珀胆碱过量中毒的药物是（　　）。
   A. 新斯的明　　B. 乙酰胆碱　　C. 泮库铵　　D. 碘解磷定　　E. 以上都不是
4. 筒箭毒碱过量中毒，解救的药物是（　　）。
   A. 阿托品　　B. 新斯的明　　C. 烟碱　　D. 碘解磷定　　E. 以上都不是
5. 对于琥珀胆碱叙述不正确的是（　　）。
   A. 琥珀胆碱属于除极化型肌松药　　B. 对全身骨骼肌产生相同程度的松弛作用
   C. 琥珀胆碱作用时间短暂　　D. 琥珀胆碱由假性胆碱酯酶水解灭活

E. 过量可导致呼吸麻痹
6. 关于筒箭毒碱叙述错误的是（　　）。
   A. 属于非除极化型肌松药
   B. 具有神经节阻滞作用
   C. 经常作为麻醉辅助用药使用
   D. 不良反应较多
   E. 阿曲库铵是其同类药物
7. 琥珀胆碱的肌肉松弛作用机制是（　　）。
   A. 促进乙酰胆碱灭活
   B. 抑制运动神经末梢释放乙酰胆碱
   C. 中枢性骨骼肌松弛作用
   D. 终板膜持续过度除极化
   E. 抑制乙酰胆碱酯酶活性
8. 以下哪项不是琥珀胆碱的不良反应（　　）。
   A. 肌肉酸痛　B. 眼内压降低　C. 恶性高热　D. 血钾升高　E. 呼吸肌麻痹
9. 琥珀胆碱的临床应用不包括（　　）。
   A. 气管内插管　B. 气管镜检查　C. 食管镜检查　D. 辅助麻醉　E. 严重哮喘
10. 关于恶性高热，以下说法错误的是（　　）。
    A. 属于遗传病
    B. 死亡率高
    C. 是筒箭毒碱独有的不良反应
    D. 可使用丹曲林治疗
    E. 需迅速给予降温、吸氧、纠正酸中毒等处理

Case study

Key points：
(1) Treatment of succinylcholine poisoning.
(2) Differences between depolarizing and non-depolarizing muscarinic agents.

Key words：Myasthenia gravis；Succinylcholine；Neostigmine

Case

Zhu, male, 24 years old, consumed two servings of braised dog meat at the night market last night and was admitted to the emergency room in the early morning with abdominal distension, abdominal pain, nausea and vomiting. Physical examination complained of scapular, thoracic and abdominal muscle pain, decreased muscle tone, and blood tests reported elevated potassium. Examination of the food he packed and brought back revealed succinylcholine content. Treatment: gastric lavage with 5000 mL of 0.9% sodium chloride solution, injection of 60 mL of 20% mannitol solution before extubation. at the end of gastric lavage, intravenous infusion of 5% dextrose solution 500 mL×2 vials, each vial with 1 vial of Energy Compound, and 1 vial of 20 mg furosemide. Blood potassium and patient's dystonic status were also monitored.

◎ **Essay questions**
1. Why does succinylcholine poisoning cause an increase in blood potassium?
2. Can muscle weakness caused by succinylcholine poisoning be treated with neostigmine? Why?

Multiple-choice questions

1. After the application of succinylcholine, the most pronounced myorelaxation is in (　　).
   A. neck and limb muscles　　B. lingual muscles　　C. facial muscles
   D. abdominal muscles　　E. back muscles
2. Depolarizing muscarinic drugs (　　).
   A. d-tubocurarine　　B. succinylcholine　　C. docuronium
   D. scopolamine　　E. atracurium
3. The antidote to succinylcholine overdose is (　　).
   A. neostigmine　　B. acetylcholine　　C. pancuronium
   D. dephosphoryl iodine　　E. none of the above
4. The antidote to an overdose of d-tubocurarine is (　　).
   A. atropine　　B. neostigmine　　C. niacin
   D. dephosphoryl iodine　　E. none of the above
5. Succinylcholine is incorrectly described as (　　).
   A. succinylcholine is a depolarizing muscle relaxant
   B. it produces the same degree of relaxation in skeletal muscle throughout the body
   C. succinylcholine has a short duration of action
   D. succinylcholine is inactivated by hydrolysis of pseudocholinesterase
   E. overdose can cause respiratory paralysis
6. What is wrong with the narration of the d-tubocurarine? (　　)
   A. It belongs to non-polarizing muscle relaxants
   B. It has ganglionic blocking effect
   C. It is often used as auxiliary drug for anesthesia
   D. There are many adverse reactions
   E. Atracurium is a similar drug
7. The mechanism of muscle relaxation of succinylcholine is (　　).
   A. promoting the inactivation of acetylcholine
   B. inhibit the release of acetylcholine from motor nerve endings.
   C. centralized skeletal muscle relaxation
   D. continuous overdepolarization of the endplate membrane
   E. inhibition of acetylcholinesterase activity
8. Which of the following is not an adverse effect of succinylcholine? (　　)
   A. Muscle pain　　B. Decreased intraocular pressure
   C. Malignant hyperthermia　　D. Elevation of potassium
   E. Paralysis of respiratory muscles
9. The clinical application of succinylcholine does not include (　　).
   A. endotracheal intubation　　B. tracheoscopy　　C. esophagoscopy

D. auxiliary anesthesia   E. severe asthma
10. About malignant hyperthermia, the wrong statement is (　　).
    A. genetic diseases
    B. ghe mortality rate is high
    C. it is a unique adverse reaction of the alkaloids of the cylinder arrow
    D. dantrolene can be used for treatment
    E. it needs to be treated with rapid cooling, oxygenation and correction of acidosis.

第九章案例学习和选择题答案

第十章　肾上腺素受体激动药

知识要点

一、肾上腺素受体激动药分类和代表药（图 10-1）

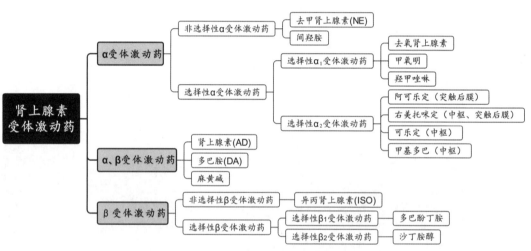

图 10-1　肾上腺素受体激动药分类和代表药

二、α_1、α_2 受体激动药

去甲肾上腺素（noradrenaline，NA；norepinephrine，NE）可由去甲肾上腺素能神经末梢释放，也可由肾上腺髓质少量分泌。

1. 药理作用

（1）血管：非选择性激动 α_1 和 α_2 受体。激动血管的 α_1 受体，使血管收缩，特别是使小动脉和小静脉收缩。皮肤黏膜血管收缩最明显，其次是对肾脏血管；对脑、肝、肠系膜甚至骨骼肌的血管也都有收缩作用。

（2）心脏：激动心脏的 β_1 受体，作用较肾上腺素弱，使心肌收缩力加强，心率加快，传导加速，心输出量增加。在整体情况下由于血压下降，反射性兴奋迷走神经，可使心率减慢。

(3)血压：小剂量滴注时由于心脏兴奋，收缩压升高；较大剂量时使外周阻力明显增高。

(4)其他：对机体代谢的影响较弱，只有在大剂量时才出现血糖升高。

2. 临床应用

(1)休克：神经源性休克早期、药物中毒引起的低血压。

(2)上消化道出血：食管、胃底静脉扩张或消化性溃疡引起的出血。

(3)药物中毒性低血压：中枢抑制药(镇静催眠药、吩噻嗪类抗精神病药)中毒引起的低血压。

3. 不良反应

(1)局部组织缺血性坏死：静脉滴注时间过长、浓度过高或药液漏出血管，可引起局部缺血性坏死。

(2)急性肾功能衰竭：滴注时间过长或剂量过大，可使肾脏血管剧烈收缩，肾血流量减少，出现少尿、无尿及急性肾功能衰竭。

三、α、β受体激动药

肾上腺素(adrenaline，AD；epinephrine)是肾上腺髓质的主要激素，能激动α和β两类受体，产生较强的α和β作用，其对β受体作用略大于对α受体作用，对α受体作用没有NA强，对β受体作用没有异丙肾上腺素强。去甲肾上腺素转化为肾上腺素的过程见图10-2。

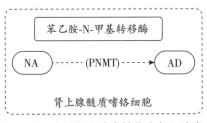

图 10-2 去甲肾上腺素转化为肾上腺素

1. 药理作用

(1)心脏：作用于心肌、传导系统和窦房结的$β_1$受体，加强心肌收缩性，加快传导，加快心率，提高心肌的兴奋性。

(2)血管：在小动脉及毛细血管前括约肌上$α_1$受体密度高，作用较强，而静脉和大动脉的受体密度低，作用较弱。

(3)血压：皮下注射治疗量(0.5~1 mg)或低浓度静脉滴注(10~30 μg/min)时，收缩压升高，促进肾素的分泌。

(4)支气管：激动支气管平滑肌$β_2$受体，发挥强大舒张作用，并能抑制肥大细胞释放过敏性物质(如组胺等)，还可使支气管黏膜血管收缩，降低毛细血管的通透性，有利于消除支气管黏膜水肿。

(5)代谢：能提高机体代谢率，在治疗剂量下可使耗氧量升高 20%～30%。降低外周组织对葡萄糖摄取的作用（$β_2$ 受体）；激活甘油三酯酶，加速分解脂肪，使血液中游离脂肪酸升高（$β_3$ 受体）。

2. 临床应用

（1）心脏骤停：溺水、麻醉和手术过程中的意外以及药物中毒、传染病和心脏传导阻滞等所致的心脏骤停。

（2）过敏性休克：药物（如青霉素、链霉素、普鲁卡因等）或异体蛋白（如免疫血清、人体白蛋白、细胞色素等）引起的过敏性休克。

（3）支气管哮喘：支气管哮喘的急性发作。肾上腺素激动 $β_2$ 受体，激活腺苷酸环化酶，使 cAMP 增加，扩张支气管。

（4）与局麻药配伍及局部止血：肾上腺素加入局麻药注射液中，可延缓局麻药的吸收，减少吸收中毒的可能性，同时又可延长麻醉时间。

3. 不良反应

用量过大或皮下注射误入血管内或静脉注射太快，可引起血压骤升，甚至发生脑溢血，也可发生心律失常。

四、$β_1$、$β_2$ 受体激动药

异丙肾上腺素是人工合成品，对 β 受体有很强的激动作用，对 $β_1$、$β_2$ 受体没有选择性。

1. 药理作用

（1）对心脏的作用：具有典型的 $β_1$ 受体激动作用，表现为正性肌力和正性频率作用，缩短收缩期和舒张期。

（2）对血管和血压的影响：激动 $β_2$ 受体，使骨骼肌血管舒张，对肾血管和肠系膜血管舒张作用较弱，对冠状血管也有舒张作用。

（3）对支气管平滑肌的作用：激动 $β_2$ 受体，舒张支气管平滑肌的作用比肾上腺素的略强，也具有抑制组胺等过敏性物质释放的作用。

（4）其他：能增加组织的耗氧量，不易通过血脑屏障，中枢兴奋作用弱。

2. 临床应用

（1）支气管哮喘：舌下或喷雾给药，用于控制支气管哮喘急性发作，疗效快而强。

（2）心脏骤停：适用于心室自身节律缓慢、高度房室传导阻滞或窦房结功能衰竭而并发的心脏骤停。

（3）房室传导阻滞：治疗Ⅱ度房室传导阻滞，采用舌下含药或静脉滴注给药。

3. 不良反应

不良反应有心悸、头晕。如剂量过大，可致心肌耗氧量增加，易引起心律失常。

案例学习

学习要点：

（1）了解拟交感物质对外周器官组织的作用。

(2)掌握主要肾上腺素受体激动剂的治疗作用和不良反应。

关键词：肾上腺素；去甲肾上腺素；异丙肾上腺素

案例

王某，男，55 岁，饮酒 30 余年。昨晚与 3 位朋友聚餐，饮用啤酒 3 箱。今晨突发胃痛、呕血，量约 100 mL，为暗红色血液，混有食物残渣，遂来院急诊。测生命体征基本平稳，初步判断为急性酒精性胃溃疡，根据患者情况先紧急给予冰盐水加去甲肾上腺素口服。收住院后，注射用生长抑素加强止血，降低门脉压力，同时注射艾司奥美拉唑钠抑制胃酸分泌、保护胃黏膜治疗，并给予葡萄糖注射液、维生素 C 注射液、氯化钾注射液，加强补液及对症处理。

◎ 问答题

1. 口服去甲肾上腺素为什么可以止血？
2. 去甲肾上腺素的主要不良反应是什么？

选择题

1. 青霉素引起过敏性休克时，首选哪种药物进行抢救？（　　）
   A. 多巴胺　　B. 去甲肾上腺素　　C. 肾上腺素　　D. 葡萄糖酸钙　　E. 氯化钠
2. 以下哪种药物可用于治疗上消化道出血？（　　）
   A. 麻黄碱　　B. 多巴胺　　C. 去甲肾上腺素　　D. 甲氧胺　　E. 异丙肾上腺素
3. 给予酚妥拉明，再给予肾上腺素后血压可出现什么样的变化？（　　）
   A. 升高　　B. 降低　　C. 不变　　D. 先降后升　　E. 先升后降
4. 一位 25 岁患感染性休克的病人，被给予低剂量多巴胺静脉滴注给药，可能会出现以下哪种情况？（　　）
   A. 降低心输出量　　B. 降低收缩压　　C. 增加肾血流量
   D. 产生明显的外周血管收缩　　E. 明显升高舒张压
5. 与去甲肾上腺素相比，间羟胺和甲氧胺经由下列哪种酶代谢？（　　）
   A. 儿茶酚氧位甲基转移酶　　B. 单胺氧化酶　　C. 单加氧酶
   D. 以上都是　　E. 以上都不是
6. 下列哪种描述最准确？（　　）
   A. α-肾上腺素受体激动剂可用来减少黏膜充血
   B. α-肾上腺素受体激动剂用于治疗支气管痉挛
   C. β-肾上腺素受体激动剂用于减少手术出血
   D. $β_2$-肾上腺素能受体激动剂是用来延长局部麻醉作用
   E. β-肾上腺素受体激动剂用于缓解心肌缺血
7. 肾上腺素哪种作用可被哌唑嗪阻断？（　　）
   A. 支气管扩张　　B. 增加心搏量　　C. 心率增加　　D. 扩瞳　　E. 增加骨骼肌血流
8. 下列哪种情况不适宜使用 β-肾上腺素受体拮抗剂？（　　）
   A. 支气管哮喘　　B. 心律失常　　C. 高血压　　D. 缺血性心脏病

E. 甲状腺功能亢进
9. 对于突触前膜受体的描述正确的是(　　)。
   A. 激动突触前膜 α_2 受体，去甲肾上腺素释放增加
   B. 激动突触前膜 α_2 受体，去甲肾上腺素释放减少
   C. 激动突触前膜 β_2 受体，去甲肾上腺素释放减少
   D. 阻断突触前膜 β_2 受体，去甲肾上腺素释放增加
   E. 存在于突触前膜的 β 受体主要是 β_1 和 β_2
10. 滴注去甲肾上腺素外漏，最佳的处理方式是(　　)。
    A. 局部注射局部麻醉药　　B. 肌肉注射酚妥拉明　　C. 局部注射酚妥拉明
    D. 局部注射 β 受体阻断药　　E. 局部用氟轻松软膏

Case study

Key points：
(1) Outline the effects of sympathomimetic agents on peripheral organ systems.
(2) Describe the therapeutic and adverse effects of the major sympathomimetic drugs.

Key words：epinephrine；norepinephrine；isoprenaline

Case

Wang, male, 55 years old, has a history of alcohol consumption for more than 30 years. Last night he had a dinner with 3 friends and consumed 3 cases of beer. This morning, he came to the emergency room with stomach pain and vomited blood, about 100 mL of dark red blood mixed with food residue. Vital signs were basically stable, and the preliminary judgment was acute alcoholic gastric ulcer, according to the patient's condition, ice saline with norepinephrine was given orally. After admission to the hospital, injection of growth inhibitor to strengthen hemostasis and reduce portal pressure, while injection of esomeprazole sodium to inhibit gastric acid secretion and protect the gastric mucosa treatment, and glucose injection, vitamin C injection, potassium chloride injection to strengthen rehydration and symptomatic treatment.

◎ **Essay questions**
1. Why can oral norepinephrine stop gastrointestinal bleeding?
2. What are the main adverse effects of norepinephrine?

Multiple-choice questions

1. Which drug should be used to treat penicillin-induced anaphylactic shock? (　　)
   A. Dopamine　　　　　B. Norepinephrine　　　　C. Epinephrine
   E. Calcium gluconate　　D. Sodium chloride
2. Which of the following drugs can be used to treat upper gastrointestinal bleeding? (　　)
   A. Ephedrine　B. Dopamine　C. Norepinephrine　D. Methoxamine　E. Isoprenaline

3. What will happen to the blood pressure after taking phentolamine and then epinephrine? ( )
   A. Increase   B. Decrease   C. No change
   D. Decrease and then increase   E. Increase and then decrease
4. A 25-year-old man is noted to be in septic shock. A low-dose dopamine infusion is administered and will likely result in which of the following? ( )
   A. Decrease cardiac output   B. Decrease systolic blood pressure
   C. Increase renal blood flow   D. Produce significant peripheral vasoconstriction
   E. Significantly increase diastolic blood pressure
5. In contrast to norepinephrine, metaraminol and methoxamine are metabolized by which of the following? ( )
   A. COMT (Catechol-O-methyl transferase)   B. MAO (monoamine oxidase)
   C. MO (monooxygenase)   D. All   E. None
6. Which of the following is the most accurate statement? ( )
   A. α-Adrenoceptor sympathomimetic agonists are used to reduce mucous membrane congestion
   B. α-Adrenoceptor agonists are used to treat bronchospasm
   C. β-Adrenoceptor agonists are used to reduce surgical bleeding
   D. $β_2$-Adrenoceptor agonist agents are used to prolong local anesthesia
   E. β-Adrenergic receptor agonists are used for the relief of myocardial ischemia
7. Which of the following actions of epinephrine are blocked by prazosin? ( )
   A. Bronchial dilation   B. Increased cardiac stroke volume   C. Increased heart rate
   D. Mydriasis   E. Increased blood flow to skeletal muscle
8. Which of the following is the least likely clinical use for β-adrenoceptor antagonists? ( )
   A. Benign prostatic hypertrophy   B. Cardiac arrhythmias   C. Hypertension
   D. Ischemic heart disease   E. Hyperthyroidism
9. The correct description of presynaptic membrane receptors is ( ).
   A. the activation of presynaptic membrane $α_2$ receptors increases norepinephrine release
   B. the activation of presynaptic membrane $α_2$ receptors decreases norepinephrine release
   C. the activation of presynaptic membrane $β_2$ receptors decreases norepinephrine release
   D. the activation of presynaptic membrane $β_2$ receptors increases norepinephrine release
   E. the β-receptors present in the presynaptic membrane are mainly $β_1$ and $β_2$
10. Leakage of a norepinephrine drip is best managed by ( ).
    A. local injection of local anesthetic
    B. intramuscular injection of phentolamine
    C. local injection of phentolamine
    D. local injection of β-blocker
    E. topical skin relaxant ointment

第十章案例学习和选择题答案

第十一章　肾上腺素受体阻断药

知识要点

一、肾上腺素受体阻断药分类和代表药（图11-1）

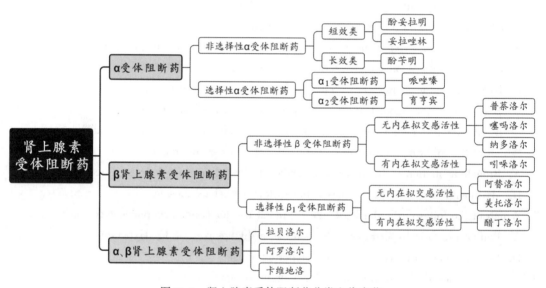

图11-1　肾上腺素受体阻断药分类和代表药

二、α_1、α_2 肾上腺素受体阻断药

α_1、α_2 肾上腺素受体阻断药有酚妥拉明和妥拉唑林。

1. 药理作用

(1) 血管：舒张血管，其机制主要是对血管平滑肌 α_1 受体的阻断作用和直接舒张血管作用。

(2) 心脏：兴奋心脏。

(3) 其他：有拟胆碱作用，可兴奋胃肠道平滑肌；有组胺样作用。

2. 临床应用

(1) 外周血管痉挛性疾病；

(2) 去甲肾上腺素静脉滴注外漏；
(3) 肾上腺嗜铬细胞瘤的鉴别诊断及该病诱发的高血压危象和手术前的准备；
(4) 休克；
(5) 急性心肌梗死和充血性心力衰竭；
(6) 药物引起的高血压；
(7) 其他：妥拉唑林还可用于治疗新生儿的持续性肺动脉高压症。

3. 不良反应

直立性低血压，胃肠平滑肌兴奋所致的腹痛、腹泻、呕吐和诱发溃疡病等。

三、β肾上腺素受体阻断药

1. 药理作用

(1) β受体阻断作用如下：
①心血管系统：阻断心脏$β_1$受体，减慢心率，使心收缩力减弱、心排出量减少、心肌耗氧量下降、血压稍降低，延缓心房和房室结的传导；
②支气管平滑肌：阻断$β_2$受体，使平滑肌收缩，气道阻力增加；
③代谢：抑制交感神经兴奋所引起的脂肪分解；
④肾素：阻断肾小球旁器细胞的$β_1$受体而抑制肾素释放。
(2) 内在拟交感活性。
(3) 膜稳定作用。
(4) 其他：普萘洛尔有抗血小板聚集作用；噻吗洛尔有降低眼内压作用。

2. 临床应用

(1) 心律失常；
(2) 心绞痛和心肌梗死；
(3) 高血压；
(4) 充血性心力衰竭；
(5) 辅助治疗甲状腺功能亢进及甲状腺危象，噻吗洛尔常局部用药治疗青光眼。

3. 不良反应

(1) 心血管反应：可引起重度心功能不全、完全性房室传导阻滞、心脏骤停、外周血管收缩甚至痉挛以及肺水肿等。
(2) 诱发或加剧支气管哮喘：非选择性β受体阻断药对支气管平滑肌的$β_2$受体的阻断作用，使支气管平滑肌收缩，呼吸道阻力增加，诱发或加剧支气管哮喘。
(3) 反跳现象：长期应用突然停药可引起原来的病情加重。
(4) 其他：偶见眼-皮肤黏膜综合征，个别患者有幻觉、失眠和抑郁症状。

4. 禁忌证

禁用于严重左室心功能不全、窦性心动过缓、重度房室传导阻滞和支气管哮喘的病人。

四、α、β受体竞争性阻断药

α、β受体竞争性阻断药有拉贝洛尔，其药理作用为对β受体的阻断作用强于对α受体的阻断作用，用于中、重度高血压和心绞痛。

案例学习

学习要点：
掌握 α 肾上腺素受体和 β 肾上腺素受体拮抗剂的治疗作用和不良反应。
关键词： 儿茶酚胺；单胺氧化酶；酚妥拉明；肾上腺素受体

案例

李先生 10 年前被确诊抑郁症，经常感到绝望和缺乏生活动力。他试过多种疗法，但症状均无明显改善。最近，医生给他开了一种抗抑郁的新药——异丙烟肼。这种药物的作用机制是通过抑制脑内的单胺氧化酶（MAO）———种负责儿茶酚胺类降解的酶。作为一种新药，其潜在副作用还需更多临床用药观察。所以医生叮嘱他，服药期间如有任何不适，即刻联系医生处理。

因为饱受抑郁症折磨，李先生满怀希望地开始服用这种新型药物。用药几周后，李先生感觉自己精神焕发，摆脱了 10 年来病痛的阴影。高兴之余，李先生广邀亲朋，设宴庆祝。答谢来宾之际，李先生喝下了满满一杯葡萄酒。宴会结束后，李先生感觉到剧烈的头痛、恶心。记起医生的嘱咐，他马上请一位朋友迅速将他送到医院。在急诊室，医生发现他的血压升高到 230/160 mmHg。医生推断他可能是高血压危象发作，便立刻使用了酚妥拉明（一种 α 肾上腺素受体拮抗剂），使他的血压很快降为正常。医生随后对李先生进行了进一步检查，证实了他的症状是由 MAO 抑制剂和葡萄酒之间的相互作用所致。

◎ **问答题**

1. 儿茶酚胺经什么酶代谢？不同的儿茶酚胺代谢酶亚型以何种儿茶酚胺作为其特异性底物？
2. 如何解释 MAO 抑制剂和葡萄酒之间相互作用的机制？
3. 酚妥拉明是如何发挥降压作用的？

选择题

1. 医生给一位患高血压的 34 岁男子开了拉贝洛尔。该药对心血管系统的作用是其对以下哪种受体拮抗作用的结果？（   ）
   A. α 肾上腺素受体   B. β 肾上腺素受体   C. α 肾上腺素受体和 β 肾上腺素受体
   D. 毒蕈碱胆碱 M 受体   E. 烟碱 N 受体
2. 以下哪种药物可用于治疗甲亢？（   ）
   A. 酚妥拉明   B. 普萘洛尔   C. 噻吗洛尔   D. 拉贝洛尔   E. 妥拉唑林
3. 酚妥拉明的不良反应不包括（   ）。
   A. 心动过缓   B. 低血压   C. 诱发溃疡病   D. 心绞痛   E. 腹痛、腹泻
4. 有关普萘洛尔叙述错误的是（   ）。
   A. 口服吸收好   B. 不易通过血脑屏障   C. 可分泌于乳汁中

D. 用药需从小剂量开始   E. 易透过胎盘
5. 下列哪一种药物主要用于治疗青光眼？（   ）
   A. 阿替洛尔   B. 吲哚洛尔   C. 拉贝洛尔   D. 普萘洛尔   E. 噻吗洛尔
6. 外周血管痉挛性疾病可选用（   ）。
   A. 山莨菪碱   B. 异丙肾上腺素   C. 间羟胺   D. 普萘洛尔   E. 酚妥拉明
7. 普萘洛尔没有下述哪一种作用？（   ）
   A. 抑制肾素分泌   B. 增加糖原分解   C. 抑制脂肪分解
   D. 降低心脏耗氧量   E. 增加呼吸道阻力
8. 下列关于噻吗洛尔的描述中，不正确的是（   ）。
   A. 减少房水生成   B. 属于β受体阻断药   C. 可治疗青光眼
   D. 无调节痉挛作用   E. 有缩瞳作用
9. 选择性 β_1 受体阻断药是（   ）。
   A. 普萘洛尔   B. 噻吗洛尔   C. 美托洛尔   D. 吲哚洛尔   E. 纳多洛尔
10. β受体阻断药不可用于治疗（   ）。
    A. 快速型心律失常   B. 高血压   C. 心绞痛   D. 支气管哮喘   E. 甲亢

Case study

Key points：
Describe the therapeutic uses and adverse effects of α-adrenoceptor antagonists and β-adrenoceptor antagonists.

Key words：catecholamines；monoamine oxidase；phentolamine；adrenoceptor

Case

Mr. Lihas been diagnosed with depression for 10 years, and he always feel hopelessness and lack of motivation. He has tried several different medications to relieve his symptoms, but nothing seems to help. Recently, his doctor has prescribed iproniazid, a new medication which has beneficial effects in depression by inhibiting an enzyme in the brain called monoamine oxidase (MAO). MAO is one of the enzymes responsible for catecholamine degradation. Since iproniazid is a new drug just coming to the market, its potential adverse effects are not well defined. So, his doctor advises him to report any unusual effects of the medication.

In order to get rid of thetorment of depression, Mr. Li began to take the new drug with hope. Within a few weeks, he begins to feel motivated and energetic for the first time in 10 years. To celebrate being freed from the shadow of 10 years of pain, Mr. Li holds a reception and invites all his friends and relatives. As he stands up to give thanks to his attendees, Mr. Li takes a full glass of his favorite wine. At the end of the party, Mr. Li has a severe headache and nausea. Recalling his doctor's warning, Mr. Li asks a friend drive him to the nearest hospital. In the emergency department, Mr. Li's blood pressure is found to be as high as 230/160 mmHg. Recognizing that

Mr. Li is experiencing a hypertensive emergency, the doctor quickly administers phentolamine (an α-adrenoceptor antagonist). Mr. Li's blood pressure quickly goes down to normal. The doctor then carries out a further examination of Mr. Li, confirming that his symptoms were caused by the interaction of wine with MAO inhibitors.

◎ **Essay questions**

1. Which enzymes metabolize catecholamines? What are the specificities of isoforms of these enzymes for the various catecholamines?
2. What is the mechanistic explanation for the interaction of MAO inhibitors with red wine?
3. How did phentolamine lower Mr. Li's blood pressure?

Multiple-choice questions

1. A 34-year-old man is prescribed labetalol for hypertension. The effect on the cardiovascular system is a result of its action as an antagonist at which of the following? (　　)
   A. α-Adrenoceptors
   B. β-Adrenoceptors
   C. Both α-adrenoceptors and β-adrenoceptors
   D. Muscarinic cholinoreceptors
   E. Nicotinic Receptors
2. Which of the following drugs can be used to treat hyperthyroidism? (　　)
   A. Phentolamine   B. Propranolol   C. Timolol
   D. Labetalol   E. Tolazoline
3. Adverse effects of phentolamine do not include (　　).
   A. bradycardia   B. hypotension   C. induced ulcer disease
   D. angina pectoris   E. abdominal pain, diarrhea
4. What is wrong with the description of propranolol? (　　)
   A. Good oral absorption
   B. It is not easy to pass the blood-brain barrier
   C. It can be secreted in breast milk
   D. The drug should be started from a small dose
   E. Easy to cross the placenta
5. Which of the following drugs is mainly used in the treatment of glaucoma? (　　)
   A. Atenolol   B. Indolol   C. Labetalol
   D. Propranolol   E. Timolol
6. Peripheral vasospastic disease can use (　　).
   A. scopolamine   B. isoprenaline   C. mesalamine
   D. propranolol   E. phentolamine
7. Which of the following does propranolol not do? (　　)
   A. Inhibit renin secretion
   B. Increase glycogenolysis
   C. Inhibit lipolysis
   D. Decrease cardiac oxygen consumption
   E. Increase respiratory resistance
8. The following description of timolol is incorrect (　　).
   A. decreases atrial water production
   B. it is a β-blocker

C. it can treat glaucoma D. no regulation of spasticity

E. it has the effect of pupil constriction

9. Selective β_1-blocking drugs are （　　）.

  A. propranolol B. timolol C. metoprolol

  D. indolol E. nadolol

10. Beta-blocking drugs should not be used to treat （　　）.

  A. tachyarrhythmias B. hypertension C. angina pectoris

  D. bronchial asthma E. hyperthyroidism

第十一章案例学习和选择题答案

第十二章　全身麻醉药

知识要点

一、药品分类

1. 吸入麻醉药
(1) 挥发性液体：如乙醚(ether)、氟烷(halothane)、异氟烷(isoflurane)。
(2) 挥发性气体：如氧化亚氮(nitrous oxide，笑气)。

2. 静脉麻醉药
(1) 丙泊酚(propofol，异丙酚)。
(2) NMDA 受体抑制剂：如氯胺酮(ketamine)。
(3) 巴比妥类：如硫喷妥钠(thiopental sodium)。
(4) 苯二氮䓬类：如咪达唑仑(midazolam)。

二、药理作用及机制

全身麻醉药属于中枢抑制性药物，通过抑制兴奋性突触和增强抑制性突触的传递功能而发挥作用。全身麻醉药能可逆性抑制中枢神经系统功能，引起暂时性感觉和反射消失，产生镇痛、肌松、催眠、遗忘、意识消失、抑制异常应激反应等诸多方面作用。

全身麻醉药的药理学机制不完全相同，主要作用于配体门控离子通道。绝大多数全身麻醉药可以与 $GABA_A$ 受体结合，增加 $GABA_A$ 受体对神经递质 GABA 的敏感性，使得 Cl^- 通道开放，神经细胞膜超极化，发挥中枢神经系统抑制作用。全身麻醉药的镇痛作用可能与多种神经递质受体相关，包括 $GABA_A$ 受体、NMDA 受体、甘氨酸受体、阿片受体和烟碱受体等。

丙泊酚增加 $GABA_A$ 受体对神经递质 GABA 的敏感性，抑制中枢兴奋性神经递质谷氨酸的 NMDA 受体，从而抑制兴奋性突触和增强抑制性突触的传递功能，发挥麻醉作用。

氯胺酮为 NMDA 受体的特异性阻断药，可阻断痛觉刺激向丘脑、新皮质传导，发挥镇痛作用。氯胺酮引起意识模糊以及短暂性记忆缺失，但意识并未完全消失，常有梦幻，肌张力增加，血压上升，此状态又称为分离麻醉(dissociative anesthesia)。

硫喷妥钠、咪达唑仑药理作用机制见第十四章镇静催眠药。

三、临床应用

吸入麻醉药经呼吸道肺泡吸收，通过调节吸入气体中的全身麻醉药浓度(分压)控制麻醉深度。吸入麻醉药在肺泡气体中的浓度越高，患者肺通气量和肺血流量越大，药物吸收速率就越快，起效越迅速。

静脉麻醉药通过静脉注射或滴注给药，与吸入麻醉药相比，无诱导期，迅速进入麻醉状态，无呼吸道刺激性，但不易于掌握麻醉深度。

目前，全身麻醉药单独应用都不够理想。为达到满意的外科手术条件以及镇痛效果，多采用复合麻醉，即同时或先后应用两种以上麻醉药物或其他辅助药物。

（1）麻醉前给药：术前常用镇静催眠药，如苯巴比妥或地西泮，消除患者紧张情绪。

（2）基础麻醉：常用于小儿麻醉。进入手术室前给予较大剂量催眠药，达到深睡状态，减少麻醉药使用剂量。

（3）诱导麻醉：应用诱导期短的硫喷妥钠或氧化亚氮，迅速进入第三期外科麻醉期，然后改用其他药物维持麻醉。

（4）合用肌松药：在麻醉时，合用肌松药满足手术时肌肉松弛的要求。

（5）低温麻醉：用于脑手术和心血管手术。合用氯丙嗪配合物理降温，使体温下降至 28～30℃，降低心、脑等生命器官的耗氧量。

（6）控制性降压：常用于止血难度大的脑科手术。抬高手术部位，合用短效血管扩张药硝普钠或钙拮抗药，降低血压，减少出血。

（7）神经安定镇痛术（神经安定麻醉）：用于外科小手术。常用氟哌利多与芬太尼合剂，静脉注射，使患者意识模糊，痛觉消失，自主动作停止。在此基础上，可加用氧化亚氮及肌松药，以达到满意麻醉效果。

四、不良反应

麻醉深度分为四期：第一期（镇痛期）、第二期（兴奋期）、第三期（外科麻醉期，可细分为四级）、第四期（延髓麻醉期）。病人通常在第三期一至三级进行手术。临近第四级时，病人出现明显呼吸抑制，血压下降，即麻醉深度达到延髓生命中枢，必须立即停药，进行人工呼吸，心脏按压，争分夺秒全力进行复苏。

案例学习

学习要点：
（1）麻醉的严重并发症。
（2）恶性高热的治疗措施。
关键词： 麻醉；恶性高热；琥珀胆碱

案例

一名23岁男性患者需要进行嵌顿性腹股沟疝手术，麻醉方法采用全身麻醉。患者进入手术室后，首先建立外周静脉通路，给予硫喷妥钠行静脉麻醉，再合用骨骼肌松弛药物琥珀胆碱。患者迅速出现血压上升，心动过速，全身骨骼肌强直性收缩和恶性高热。生化检查结果显示，患者出现了高钾血症和酸中毒。

◎ 问答题

1. 患者在麻醉过程中出现异常并发症的最可能原因是什么？
2. 患者应立即使用哪一种药物治疗？

✎ 选择题

1. 关于全身麻醉药的药理学作用，下列描述正确的是(　　)。
   A. 只消除疼痛，不影响意识　　　　B. 意识丧失，骨骼肌松弛
   C. 不可逆性抑制中枢神经系统功能　D. 阻断钠离子通道
   E. 不产生遗忘

2. 关于吸入麻醉药的药理学作用，下列描述正确的是(　　)。
   A. 吸入麻醉药的起效速度仅取决于药物在肺泡气体中的浓度
   B. 血/气分布系数小的吸入麻醉药，麻醉诱导时间短
   C. 脑/血分布系数小的吸入麻醉药，麻醉持续时间长
   D. 吸入麻醉药不会引起延髓抑制效应
   E. 吸入麻醉药不会经肝脏代谢

3. 关于静脉麻醉药丙泊酚的药理学作用，下列描述正确的是(　　)。
   A. 抑制迷走神经反射　　　　　　　B. 对心血管系统有明显的兴奋作用
   C. 不易透过血脑屏障，起效速度慢　D. 抑制咽喉反射，有利于气管插管
   E. 抑制 $GABA_A$ 受体

4. 关于静脉麻醉药氯胺酮的药理学作用，下列描述正确的是(　　)。
   A. 抑制脑干和边缘系统　　　　　　B. 对心血管系统有明显的兴奋作用
   C. 不易产生短暂性记忆缺失　　　　D. 引起意识完全消失
   E. 兴奋 NMDA 受体

5. 关于全身麻醉药的不良反应，下列描述错误的是(　　)。
   A. 乙醚因刺激粘液分泌，易引起吸入性肺炎
   B. 反复使用氟烷可导致肝损伤
   C. 过大浓度使用地氟烷可诱发喉头痉挛
   D. 氧化亚氮代谢产物可导致肾损伤
   E. 硫喷妥钠可诱发支气管和喉头痉挛

6. 关于吸入麻醉药氧化亚氮的药理学特征，下列描述错误的是(　　)。
   A. 绝大多数经肺以原形排出体外
   B. 脂溶性低，起效慢
   C. 麻醉效能低，需与其他麻醉药配伍使用
   D. 对肝肾功能无影响
   E. 镇痛作用强，患者感觉舒适愉悦

7. 起效最快的吸入麻醉剂是(　　)。
   A. 氟烷　　B. 乙醚　　C. 七氟烷　　D. 恩氟烷　　E. 地氟烷

8. 外科小手术可采用神经安定麻醉，常配伍使用(　　)。

A. 氟哌利多与芬太尼　　B. 硫喷妥钠与芬太尼　　C. 氧化亚氮与咪达唑仑
D. 恩氟烷与咪达唑仑　　E. 氟哌利多与硫喷妥钠

9. 一名 20 岁男性患者，多汗、心动过速、呼吸急促，收缩压 200 mmHg，舒张压 115 mmHg，肝肾功能正常，肺部影像正常，MRI 发现上腹部有一肿块，儿茶酚胺筛查阳性，诊断为嗜铬细胞瘤。患者手术麻醉过程中禁用(　　)。
   A. 氟烷　　B. 地氟烷　　C. 七氟烷　　D. 咪达唑仑　　E. 硫喷妥钠

10. 一名 38 岁二胎妈妈，孕 38 周入院，B 超检查发现胎盘位置异常，为中央性前置胎盘，伴有胎盘植入。患者拟采用全身麻醉行剖宫产术，手术麻醉过程中禁用(　　)。
    A. 氟烷　　B. 地氟烷　　C. 七氟烷　　D. 咪达唑仑　　E. 硫喷妥钠

Case study

Key points：
(1) Serious complications of anesthesia.
(2) Therapeutic measures for malignant hyperthermia.

Key words：anesthesia；malignant hyperthermia；succinylcholine

Case

A 23-year-old male patient required surgery for an incarcerated inguinal hernia with general anesthesia. After the patient was admitted to the operating room, peripheral venous access was first established. Thiopental sodium was administered intravenously for anesthesia and then the patient was treated with skeletal muscle relaxant succinylcholine. The patient rapidly developed hypertension, tachycardia and malignant hyperthermia. Biochemical results showed that the patient had hyperkalemia and acidosis.

◎ **Essay questions**
1. What is the most likely cause for this unusual complication of anesthesia in the patient?
2. Which medication should the patient be treated with immediately?

Multiple-choice questions

1. Which following statement about the pharmacological effect of general anesthetics is accurate? (　　)
   A. They only eliminate pain and do not affect consciousness
   B. They cause loss of consciousness and skeletal muscle relaxation
   C. They irreversibly depress central nervous system function
   D. They block sodium channels
   E. They do not cause amnesia

2. Which following statement about the pharmacological effect of inhaled anesthetics is accurate? (　　)

A. The time for onset of inhaled anesthetics depends only on the alveolar anesthetic concentration

B. Inhaled anesthetic with low blood/gas partition coefficient has a rapid onset of anesthesia

C. Inhaled anesthetic with low brain/blood partition coefficient has a long duration of anesthesia

D. Inhaled anesthetics do not induce medullary depression

E. Inhaled anesthetics are not metabolized by the liver

3. Which following statement about the pharmacological effect of intravenous anesthetic propofol is accurate? (   )

   A. It inhibits vagal reflexes

   B. It has a marked excitatory effect on the cardiovascular system

   C. It does not easily cross the blood-brain barrier and has a slow onset of action

   D. It inhibits the gag reflex, facilitating tracheal intubation

   E. It inhibits $GABA_A$ receptor

4. Which following statement about the pharmacological effect of intravenous anesthetic ketamine is accurate? (   )

   A. It inhibits the brainstem and limbic system

   B. It has a marked excitatory effect on the cardiovascular system

   C. It does not easily produce transient memory loss

   D. It causes a complete loss of consciousness

   E. It excites NMDA receptors

5. Which following statement about the adverse effects of general anesthetics is incorrect? (   )

   A. Ether is prone to cause aspiration pneumonia due to stimulation of mucus secretion

   B. Repeated use of halothane can lead to liver injury

   C. Excessive concentration of desflurane can induce laryngospasm

   D. The metabolite from nitrous oxide can cause kidney injury

   E. Thiopental sodium can induce bronchospasm and laryngospasm

6. Which following statement about the pharmacologic profile of inhaled anesthetic nitrous oxide is incorrect? (   )

   A. Most of it is eliminated via the lung as a prototype

   B. It has low lipid solubility and slow onset of action

   C. It has low anesthetic efficacy and needs to be combined with other anesthetics

   D. It has no effect on liver and kidney function

   E. It has a strong analgesic effect, and patients feel comfortable and pleasant

7. Which inhaled anesthetic has the most rapid onset of anesthesia? (   )

   A. Halothane   B. Ether   C. Sevoflurane
   D. Enflurane   E. Desflurane

8. Which combination is appropriate for neuroleptanesthesia in minor surgery? (   )
   A. Droperidol and fentanyl
   B. Thiopental sodium and fentanyl
   C. Nitrous oxide and midazolam
   D. Enflurane and midazolam
   E. Droperidol and thiopental sodium

9. A 20-year-old male patient with excessive sweating, tachycardia, shortness of breath, systolic blood pressure of 200 mmHg, and diastolic blood pressure of 115 mmHg. Hepatic and renal function are normal, and lung imaging is normal. MRI imaging shows an epigastric mass. The catecholamine screening is positive, and he is diagnosed with pheochromocytoma. Which of the following drugs should be contraindicated during anesthesia for surgery? (   )
   A. Halothane
   B. Desflurane
   C. Sevoflurane
   D. Midazolam
   E. Thiopental sodium

10. A 38-year-old woman in labor with her second child is admitted to the hospital at 38 weeks of gestation. The ultrasound examination reveals the central placenta previa with placental implantation. The patient is to undergo a cesarean section under general anesthesia. Which of the following drugs should be contraindicated during anesthesia for surgery? (   )
    A. Halothane
    B. Desflurane
    C. Sevoflurane
    D. Midazolam
    E. Thiopental sodium

第十二章案例学习和选择题答案

第十三章 局部麻醉药

知识要点

一、药品分类

(1) 酯类：如普鲁卡因(procaine)、丁卡因(tetracaine)。
(2) 酰胺类：如利多卡因(lidocaine)。

二、药理作用及机制

局部麻醉药可使神经冲动阈电位升高、传导速度减慢、动作电位幅度降低，甚至丧失兴奋性及传导性。局部麻醉药阻断神经冲动的强度与神经组织的解剖特点有关。在低浓度时可对无髓鞘的交感、副交感神经节后纤维显效，高浓度才能对有髓鞘的感觉和运动神经纤维产生作用。首先消失的是持续性钝痛（如压痛），其次是短暂性锐痛。神经冲动传导的恢复则按相反的顺序进行。

局部麻醉药的作用机制相同，以非解离型形式进入神经细胞内，与 Na^+ 通道特异性结合位点结合，产生阻滞作用。

三、临床应用

1. 表面麻醉

局部麻醉药涂于黏膜表面，麻醉黏膜下神经末梢。用于眼、鼻、口腔、咽喉、气管、食管和泌尿生殖道黏膜的浅表手术。

2. 浸润麻醉

局部麻醉药溶液注入皮下或手术视野附近的组织，使局部神经末梢麻醉。根据需要可在溶液中加少量肾上腺素，减缓局部麻醉药的吸收，延长作用时间。

3. 神经阻滞麻醉

局部麻醉药注射到外周神经干附近，使该神经所分布的区域麻醉，常用于口腔和四肢手术。为延长麻醉时间，也可将布比卡因和利多卡因合用。

4. 蛛网膜下腔麻醉

蛛网膜下腔麻醉又称脊髓麻醉或腰麻。麻醉药注入腰椎蛛网膜下腔，首先被阻断的是交感神经纤维，其次是感觉纤维，最后是运动纤维。常用于下腹部和下肢手术。

5. 硬膜外麻醉

麻醉药注入硬膜外腔，沿着神经鞘扩散，穿过椎间孔阻断神经根。硬膜外腔不与颅腔相通，故药物不扩散至脑组织，无腰麻时头痛或脑脊膜刺激现象。硬膜外麻醉也可引起外周血管扩张、血压下降及心脏抑制，可应用麻黄碱防治。

6. 区域镇痛

围术期镇痛的有效方法，通常与阿片类药物联合应用，可减少阿片类药物的用量。

7. 常用药物

(1)普鲁卡因又名奴佛卡因(novocaine)，普鲁卡因黏膜穿透力弱，一般不用于表面麻醉，可用于浸润麻醉、神经阻滞麻醉、硬膜外麻醉。可引起过敏反应，故用药前应做皮肤过敏试验，但皮试阴性者仍可发生过敏反应。能对抗磺胺类药物的抗菌作用，故应避免与磺胺类药物同时应用。

(2)利多卡因又名赛罗卡因(xylocaine)，利多卡因可用于浸润麻醉、神经阻滞麻醉、硬膜外麻醉，有全能麻醉药之称。因其在蛛网膜下腔分布不均，蛛网膜下腔麻醉慎用。本药也可用于心律失常的治疗。

(3)丁卡因又称地卡因(dicaine)，丁卡因黏膜穿透力强，常用于表面麻醉，如咽喉喷雾麻醉。

四、不良反应

1. 毒性反应

局部麻醉药引起的全身毒性反应，主要表现为中枢神经系统和心血管系统的毒性。

(1)中枢神经系统：局部麻醉药对中枢神经系统的作用是先兴奋后抑制。这是由于中枢抑制性神经元对局部麻醉药比兴奋性神经元更为敏感，首先被阻断，出现脱抑制症状。初期表现为眩晕、多言、震颤，甚至发生阵挛性惊厥；之后转为抑制症状，进入昏迷和呼吸衰竭状态。中毒早期，注射地西泮可加强中枢抑制，防止惊厥发作；中毒晚期，维持呼吸。

(2)心血管系统：局部麻醉药对心肌细胞膜具有膜稳定作用，可降低心肌兴奋性，传导减慢，不应期延长；引起血压下降甚至休克等心血管反应。局部麻醉药对心血管的作用常滞后于中枢神经系统的作用，偶有少数人应用小剂量局部麻醉药突发心室纤颤导致死亡。应采用分次小剂量注射的麻醉方法，小儿、孕妇、肾功能不全患者应适当减量。

2. 变态反应

普鲁卡因麻醉前应做皮试，用药时可先给予小剂量，若患者无特殊主诉和异常再给予适当剂量。一旦发生变态反应立即停药，并适当应用肾上腺皮质激素、肾上腺素、抗组胺药等对症处理。

3. 其他不良反应

局部麻醉药用于椎管内阻滞时，可能诱发神经损害，原有神经系统疾病、脊髓外伤或炎症等可能会加重。

案例学习

学习要点：

(1)局部麻醉药的不良反应。

(2)处理不良反应的紧急措施。

关键词：局部麻醉药；不良反应

案例

一名29岁妇女分娩，医生计划硬膜外麻醉以缓解疼痛。在行硬膜外穿刺时，不小心穿破硬膜，只能将麻醉方式变更为连续腰麻。手术过程中，患者出现了血压明显下降和心律失常。

◎ 问答题

1. 患者在麻醉过程中出现异常情况的最可能原因是什么？
2. 患者应立即采用哪些治疗措施？

选择题

1. 局部麻醉药的作用机制是（   ）。
   A. 阻断电压依赖性钙离子通道　　B. 阻断配体门控型钙离子通道
   C. 阻断配体门控型钠离子通道　　D. 阻断电压依赖性镁离子通道
   E. 阻断电压依赖性钠离子通道
2. 关于利多卡因的特征，下列哪一项描述正确？（   ）
   A. 安全范围窄　　B. 具有抗心律失常作用　　C. 具有扩张血管作用
   D. 不会引起心脏毒性　　E. 用于蛛网膜下腔麻醉
3. 已知利多卡因的pK_a是7.9，普鲁卡因的pK_a是8.9，感染组织的pH值为6.3。下列哪一项描述正确？（   ）
   A. 普鲁卡因比利多卡因更易解离　　B. 利多卡因比普鲁卡因更易解离
   C. 普鲁卡因主要为非解离型形式　　D. 普鲁卡因组织穿透力更强
   E. 普鲁卡因麻醉效果更好
4. 关于局部麻醉药的不良反应，下列哪一项描述错误？（   ）
   A. 对中枢神经系统的作用是先兴奋后抑制
   B. 减弱心肌收缩力，不应期延长
   C. 加重神经系统炎症反应
   D. 外周血管阻力增加
   E. 诱发阵挛性惊厥
5. 下列哪一种局部麻醉药易引起过敏反应？（   ）
   A. 普鲁卡因　　B. 利多卡因　　C. 丁卡因　　D. 布比卡因　　E. 左布比卡因
6. 下列哪一种局部麻醉药起效速度最快？（   ）
   A. 普鲁卡因　　B. 利多卡因　　C. 丁卡因　　D. 布比卡因　　E. 罗哌卡因
7. 影响局部麻醉药作用的因素不包括（   ）。
   A. 神经干或神经纤维的粗细　　B. 麻醉方式　　C. 局部麻醉药的剂量
   D. 局部麻醉药的解离常数　　E. 首关消除
8. 关于局部麻醉药的描述，下列哪一种是错误的？（   ）

A. 局麻作用是可逆的 B. 硬膜外麻醉用药量较腰麻大
C. 加入肾上腺素，可延长作用时间 D. 皮试阴性者仍可发生过敏反应
E. 对温觉没有影响

9. 一名儿童需要采用表面麻醉实施鼻咽部浅表手术，适宜选择下列哪种药物？（ ）
   A. 普鲁卡因   B. 利多卡因   C. 丁卡因   D. 布比卡因   E. 罗哌卡因
10. 一名20岁男性患者需要拔除智齿，为延长利多卡因麻醉时间，可合用下列哪种药物？
    （ ）
    A. 肾上腺素   B. 阿托品   C. 去甲肾上腺素   D. 异丙肾上腺素   E. 多巴胺

Case study

Key points：
(1) Adverse drug reactions of local anesthesia.
(2) Management of adverse drug reactions.

Key words： local anesthesia; adverse drug reaction

Case

A 29-year-old woman was in labor and the doctor planned an epidural anesthesia to relieve the pain. During the epidural puncture, the dura was accidentally punctured and the anesthesia had to be changed to continuous spinal anesthesia. During the procedure, the patient experienced a significant drop in blood pressure and cardiac arrhythmia.

◎ **Essay questions**
1. What is the most likely cause of the patient's abnormalities during anesthesia?
2. What therapeutic measures should be applied immediately to the patient?

Multiple-choice questions

1. The mechanism of action of local anesthetics is (   ).
   A. blocking voltage-dependent calcium channels
   B. blocking ligand-gated calcium channels
   C. blocking ligand-gated sodium channels
   D. blocking voltage-dependent magnesium channels
   E. blocking voltage-dependent sodium channels
2. Which of the following descriptions of the characteristics of lidocaine is correct？（ ）
   A. Has a narrow safety profile   B. Has an antiarrhythmic effect
   C. Has a vasodilatory effect   D. Does not cause cardiotoxicity
   E. Used in subarachnoid anesthesia
3. It is known that the pK_a of lidocaine is 7.9, the pK_a of procaine is 8.9, and the pH of the infected tissue is 6.3. Which of the following descriptions is correct？（ ）

A. Procaine ionizes more readily than lidocaine

B. Lidocaine ionizes more readily than procaine

C. Procaine is primarily a unionized form

D. Procaine has greater tissue penetration

E. Procaine is more effective in anesthesia

4. Which of the following descriptions of the adverse effects of local anesthetics is incorrect? (　　)

A. Local anesthetics act on the central nervous system with excitation followed by depression

B. Local anesthetics reduce myocardial contractility and prolong the period of inactivity

C. Local anesthetics exacerbate the inflammatory response of the nervous system

D. Local anesthetics increase peripheral vascular pressure

E. Local anesthetics induce clonic seizure

5. Which of the following local anesthetics is prone to allergic reactions? (　　)

　　A. Procaine　　B. Lidocaine　　C. Tetracaine　　D. Bupivacaine　　E. Levobupivacaine

6. Which of the following local anesthetics has the fastest onset of action? (　　)

　　A. Procaine　　B. Lidocaine　　C. Tetracaine　　D. Bupivacaine　　E. Ropivacaine

7. Factors that affect the action of local anesthetics do not include (　　).

A. thickness of the nerve trunk or nerve fibers　　B. mode of anesthesia

C. the dose of local anesthetics　　D. pK_a of the local anesthetic

E. first pass elimination

8. Which of the following descriptions of local anesthetics is incorrect? (　　)

A. Actions are reversible

B. Epidural anesthesia requires a higher dose of drugs than spinal anesthesia

C. The addition of epinephrine can prolong the duration of action of local anesthetics

D. Negative skin test can still cause an allergic reaction

E. No effect on temperature sensation

9. Which of the following drugs would be appropriate for a child requiring surface anesthesia for a superficial nasopharyngeal surgery? (　　)

　　A. Procaine　　B. Lidocaine　　C. Tetracaine　　D. Bupivacaine　　E. Ropivacaine

10. Which of the following drugs would prolong lidocaine anesthesia in a 20-year-old male patient who needs to have his wisdom teeth removed? (　　)

　　A. Epinephrine　B. Atropine　　C. Norepinephrine　D. Isoprenaline　E. Dopamine

第十三章案例学习和选择题答案

第十四章　镇静催眠药

知识要点

一、苯二氮䓬类药物

1. 药品分类

(1) 长效类：如地西泮（diazepam）。

(2) 中效类：如劳拉西泮（lorazepam）。

(3) 短效类：如三唑仑（triazolam）。

2. 作用机制

苯二氮䓬类与$GABA_A$受体结合，诱导受体发生构象变化，增加$GABA_A$受体对神经递质 GABA 的敏感性，Cl^-通道的开放频率增加，神经细胞膜超极化，发挥中枢神经系统抑制作用。

3. 药理作用

(1) 抗焦虑作用：选择性作用于边缘系统中$GABA_A$受体，小剂量即可明显改善多种原因引起的焦虑。

(2) 镇静催眠作用：苯二氮䓬类能明显缩短入睡时间，显著延长睡眠持续时间，减少觉醒次数。

(3) 抗惊厥、抗癫痫作用：不能消除异常放电，可抑制放电向周围扩散。

(4) 中枢性肌肉松弛作用：可缓解大脑损伤所致的肌肉僵直。

(5) 其他：大剂量可致记忆缺失、血压下降、心率减慢。

4. 临床应用

(1) 焦虑症。

(2) 镇静催眠。

(3) 辅助治疗破伤风、子痫、小儿高热惊厥及药物中毒性惊厥。地西泮静脉注射是目前治疗癫痫持续状态的首选药物。

(4) 脑损伤所致肌僵直。

(5) 手术前用药以减少麻醉药使用剂量，以及心脏电击复律和各种内镜检查前用药。

5. 不良反应

最常见的不良反应是嗜睡、头晕、乏力和记忆力下降。长期应用可产生耐受性、依赖性和成瘾的问题，停用可出现反跳现象和戒断症状，表现为失眠、焦虑、兴奋、心动过速、呕吐、出汗及震颤，甚至惊厥。

静脉注射速度过快可引起呼吸和循环功能抑制，严重者可致呼吸及心搏停止。其他中枢抑制药和乙醇合用时，中枢抑制作用增强，加重嗜睡、昏睡、呼吸抑制、昏迷，严重者可致死。

苯二氮䓬类药物过量、中毒可用氟马西尼进行鉴别诊断和抢救。

氟马西尼特异地竞争性拮抗苯二氮䓬类衍生物与 $GABA_A$ 受体的结合位点，但对巴比妥类和其他中枢抑制药引起的中毒无效。

二、巴比妥类药物

1. 药品分类

（1）长效类：如苯巴比妥（phenobarbital）。

（2）中效类：如异戊巴比妥（amobarbital）。

（3）短效类：如司可巴比妥（secobarbital）。

（4）超短效类：如硫喷妥钠（thiopental sodium）。

2. 作用机制

巴比妥类影响多突触反应，属于中枢非特异性药物。巴比妥类模拟 GABA 的作用，增加 Cl^- 通道的开放时间，使细胞膜超极化，减弱或阻断谷氨酸受体介导的去极化反应，导致兴奋性被抑制。

3. 药理作用

（1）镇静催眠作用：少用。对睡眠结构影响明显，且安全性低。10 倍催眠量可引起呼吸中枢麻痹死亡。

（2）抗惊厥、抗癫痫作用：苯巴比妥有较强的抗惊厥及抗癫痫作用。

（3）麻醉：硫喷妥钠可用作静脉麻醉。

4. 临床应用

临床用于癫痫大发作和癫痫持续状态的治疗，也用于小儿高热、破伤风、子痫、脑膜炎、脑炎及中枢兴奋药引起的惊厥。

5. 不良反应

（1）最常见的不良反应是眩晕、困倦、精细运动不协调。长期连续服用成瘾，成瘾后停药可出现戒断症状，表现为激动、失眠、焦虑，甚至惊厥。

（2）抑制呼吸中枢，严重肺功能不全和颅脑损伤所致呼吸抑制者禁用。

（3）诱导肝药酶，易出现药物相互作用。

（4）巴比妥类过量中毒，氟马西尼无效。

案例学习

学习要点：

（1）特殊人群用药。

（2）镇静催眠药不良反应。

关键词：肝脏；药物代谢；镇静催眠药

案例

一位42岁的电脑程序员因久坐出现腰痛腿麻，无法入睡，严重影响工作或学习。MRI影像学检查发现腰椎间盘突出，拟进行手术。患者入院后，生化检查发现肝功能异常。

◎ 问答题

1. 患者可以使用哪种镇静催眠药物来缓解术前焦虑？
2. 患者术后感觉疼痛消失了，但不久又出现了。患者因为疼痛，睡眠质量差，希望使用镇静催眠药，医生需要告知他注意哪些风险？

选择题

1. 地西泮的作用机制是（　　）。
   A. 增强GABA与$GABA_A$受体的结合力，增加氯离子通道的开放时间
   B. 使$GABA_A$受体发生构象变化，增加氯离子通道的开放频率
   C. 可逆性抑制兴奋性神经递质的突触传递
   D. 不可逆性抑制兴奋性神经递质的突触传递
   E. 非特异性抑制多突触反应

2. 关于地西泮描述错误的是（　　）。
   A. 长期服用可产生依赖性和成瘾性   B. 影响睡眠结构
   C. 大剂量产生中枢性骨骼肌松弛   D. 久用突然停药可产生反跳性失眠
   E. 大剂量可用于抗癫痫

3. 不同巴比妥类药物起效时间存在差异的原因是（　　）。
   A. EC_{50}不同   B. 药物脂溶性不同   C. 肾脏排泄速度不同
   D. 血浆蛋白结合率不同   E. 肝脏代谢速度不同

4. 关于苯巴比妥描述错误的是（　　）。
   A. 可缓解焦虑   B. 影响睡眠结构   C. 连续应用产生耐受性
   D. 可使用氟马西尼逆转中枢抑制效应   E. 可用于癫痫大发作和癫痫持续状态

5. 与巴比妥类药物相比，关于苯二氮䓬类药物说法正确的是（　　）。
   A. 效能更大   B. 戒断症状更为严重   C. 严重影响肝脏代谢
   D. 更易出现中枢过度抑制 E. 安全范围更大

6. 下列说法准确的是（　　）。
   A. 苯巴比妥是首选的催眠药物   B. 苯巴比妥比硫喷妥钠脂溶性高
   C. 地西泮经肝脏代谢成无活性代谢物   D. 三唑仑为短效催眠药
   E. 氯硝西泮对癫痫持续状态无效

7. 关于药物不良反应，说法错误的是（　　）。
   A. 苯巴比妥由于耐受性要不断增加剂量
   B. 苯巴比妥对记忆的影响明显

C. 苯巴比妥治疗癫痫时无嗜睡现象

D. 苯巴比妥增强酒精对中枢神经系统的抑制作用

E. 苯巴比妥突然停药会有戒断症状

8. 苯巴比妥连续使用产生耐受性的主要原因是(   )。

  A. 肾脏排泄速度加快　　B. 诱导肝药酶　　　　C. 血浆蛋白减少

  D. 组织分布异常　　　　E. 转运体出现饱和现象

9. 一位19岁男性患者主诉很容易受到惊吓，担心无关紧要的事情，有时还会出现胃痉挛、失眠。病人没有药物滥用史，诊断为广泛性焦虑症。病人不适合使用下列哪种药治疗？(   )

  A. 苯巴比妥　　B. 度洛西汀　　C. 帕罗西汀　　D. 阿普唑仑　　E. 氯硝西泮

10. 一名38岁女性患者使用双氯芬酸钠镇痛，并服用地西泮治疗失眠，出现了中枢过度抑制。双氯芬酸与地西泮之间出现药物相互作用的原因最可能是(   )。

  A. 竞争性抑制肝药酶　　　　B. 竞争性抑制转运体　　　C. 竞争性结合血浆蛋白

  D. 竞争性结合 $GABA_A$ 受体　　E. 竞争性结合环氧化酶

Case study

Key points:

(1) Medication use in special populations.

(2) Adverse effects of sedative-hypnotics.

Key words: liver; drug metabolism; sedative-hypnotics

Case

A 42-year-old computer programmer complained of low back pain, numbness in a leg, and an inability to sleep due to a sedentary lifestyle, which seriously affected his work or study. An MRI imaging showed that he had a lumbar herniated disc. He was scheduled for surgery. After the patient was admitted to the hospital, biochemical tests found abnormal liver function.

◎ **Essay questions**

1. Which sedative-hypnotic medication can the patient use to relieve preoperative anxiety?

2. The patient felt that the pain disappeared after surgery, but it soon came back. He had poor sleep quality because of the pain and wanted to use a sedative-hypnotic drug. What risks does the doctor need to advise him to be aware of?

Multiple-choice questions

1. What is the mechanism of action of diazepam? (   )

  A. It enhances the binding of GABA to $GABA_A$ receptor and increases the opening of chloride channels

  B. It causes a conformational change in the $GABA_A$ receptor, increasing the frequency of chloride channel opening

C. It reversibly inhibits synaptic transmission of excitatory neurotransmitters

D. It irreversibly inhibits synaptic transmission of excitatory neurotransmitters

E. It non-specifically inhibits polysynaptic responses

2. Which following statement about diazepam is incorrect?（   ）

A. Long-term use of diazepam can produce dependence and addiction

B. Diazepam affects sleep structure

C. High doses of diazepam produce central relaxation of skeletal muscle

D. Sudden discontinuation of diazepam after long-term use can produce rebound insomnia

E. High dose of diazepam can be used for epilepsy treatment

3. What is the reason for the difference in the onset of action for barbiturates?（   ）

A. EC_{50} B. Lipid solubility

C. Rate of renal excretion   D. Plasma protein binding ratio

E. Hepatic metabolism

4. Which following statement about phenobarbital is incorrect?（   ）

A. It relieves anxiety

B. It affects sleep structure

C. It causes drug tolerance after long-term use

D. Its inhibitory effects on the central nervous system can be reversed by flumazenil

E. It can be used for generalized tonic-clonic seizures and status epilepticus

5. Which following statement about benzodiazepines is accurate when compared to barbiturates?（   ）

A. Benzodiazepines are more potent

B. Withdrawal symptoms of benzodiazepines are more severe

C. Benzodiazepines severely affect hepatic metabolism

D. Benzodiazepines are more prone to cause excessive CNS depression

E. Benzodiazepines have a greater range of safety

6. Which following statement is accurate?（   ）

A. Phenobarbital is the first choice of hypnotics

B. Phenobarbital has higher lipid solubility than sodium thiopental

C. Diazepam is metabolized by the liver into inactive metabolites

D. Triazolam is a short-acting hypnotic drug

E. Clonazepam is ineffective for status epilepticus

7. Which following statement about adverse drug reactions is incorrect?（   ）

A. Phenobarbital requires increasing doses due to tolerance

B. Phenobarbital affects memory

C. Phenobarbital does not cause drowsiness during epilepsy treatment

D. Phenobarbital enhances the depression of alcoholic beverages on the central nervous system

E. Abrupt discontinuation of phenobarbital causes withdrawal symptoms

8. What is the main reason for developing tolerance during continuous use of phenobarbital? (　　)

    A. Accelerated renal excretion

    B. Induction of hepatic drug-metabolizing enzymes

    C. Decreased plasma protein

    D. Abnormal tissue distribution

    E. Saturation of the transporter

9. A 19-year-old male patient complains of being easily startled, worrying about insignificant things, and sometimes experiencing stomach cramps and insomnia. The patient has no history of substance abuse and is diagnosed with generalized anxiety disorder. Which of the following medications is not appropriate for the treatment? (　　)

    A. Phenobarbital　　　　B. Duloxetine　　　　C. Paroxetine

    D. Alprazolam　　　　　E. Clonazepam

10. A 38-year-old female patient using diclofenac sodium for analgesia and diazepam for insomnia develops excessive CNS depression. What is the most likely cause for drug-drug interaction between diclofenac and diazepam? (　　)

    A. Competitive inhibition of hepatic drug-metabolizing enzymes

    B. Competitive inhibition of transporters

    C. Competitive binding to plasma proteins

    D. Competitive binding to $GABA_A$ receptors

    E. Competitive binding to cyclooxygenase

第十四章案例学习和选择题答案

第十五章 抗癫痫药和抗惊厥药

📖 知识要点

一、抗癫痫药

1. 药品

抗癫痫药主要有苯妥英钠(phenytoin sodium)，卡马西平(carbamazepine)，苯巴比妥(phenobarbital)，扑米酮(primidone)，乙琥胺(ethosuximide)，丙戊酸钠(sodium valproate)。癫痫主要发作类型、临床特征及治疗药物见表15-1。

表15-1　　癫痫主要发作类型、临床特征及治疗药物

发作类型	临床特征	治疗药物
单纯性局限性发作 (局灶性癫痫, partial seizures simple)	局部肢体运动或感觉异常	苯妥英钠、卡马西平、苯巴比妥
复合性局限性发作 (精神运动性发作, partial seizures, complex)	冲动性神经异常，不同程度意识障碍，无意识的运动，如唇抽动、摇头	卡马西平、苯妥英钠、扑米酮、丙戊酸钠
失神性发作(小发作, absence seizures)	多见于儿童，短暂的意识突然丧失	乙琥胺、丙戊酸钠
肌阵挛性发作 (myoclonic seizures)	部分肌群发生短暂的(约1秒)休克样抽动，意识丧失	丙戊酸钠
强直-阵挛性发作 (大发作, tonic-clonic seizures)	全身强直-阵挛性抽搐	苯妥英钠、卡马西平、丙戊酸钠
癫痫持续状态 (status epilepticus)	大发作持续状态，反复抽搐，昏迷	地西泮、苯妥英钠、苯巴比妥

2. 药理作用

苯妥英钠通过阻滞电压依赖性 Na^+ 通道、电压依赖性 Ca^{2+} 通道，抑制 Na^+、Ca^{2+} 内流以及抑制钙调素激酶系统，降低细胞膜的兴奋性，从而减少动作电位发生。苯妥英钠不能

抑制癫痫病灶异常放电，但可阻止异常放电向周围正常脑组织扩散，发挥抗癫痫作用。此外，苯妥英钠的膜稳定作用还可用于治疗神经痛和心律失常。

卡马西平阻滞电压依赖性 Na^+ 通道，抑制 T 型钙通道，从而抑制癫痫病灶及周围神经元放电；化学结构与丙米嗪类似，具有抗胆碱、抗抑郁，抑制神经肌肉接头传递作用；刺激抗利尿激素 ADH 分泌，发挥抗利尿作用。

3. 临床应用

苯妥英钠是局限性发作、强直-阵挛性发作（大发作）的首选药，对癫痫持续状态有效，对失神性发作（小发作）无效，还可治疗三叉神经痛、舌咽神经痛以及心律失常。

卡马西平是单纯性局限性发作、强直-阵挛性发作的首选药，复合性局限性发作和失神性发作有效；治疗三叉神经痛、舌咽神经痛，疗效优于苯妥英钠；用于治疗尿崩症、抑郁症、锂盐治疗无效的躁狂症。

苯巴比妥主要治疗强直-阵挛性发作及持续状态，也可用于局限性发作，对失神性发作无效。大剂量苯巴比妥有较强的中枢抑制作用，故不作为首选药。

扑米酮仅用于其他药物治疗无效的患者。与苯妥英钠、卡马西平合用具有协同作用，与苯巴比妥合用无明显协同效果。

乙琥胺是失神性发作的首选药，对其他类型癫痫无明显效果。可改善戊四氮诱发的阵挛性惊厥。

丙戊酸钠为广谱抗癫痫药，是癫痫大发作合并小发作的首选药。对癫痫大发作的效果不如苯妥英钠和苯巴比妥，但对上述药物治疗无效的患者仍有效；对癫痫小发作的效果强于乙琥胺，但因其肝毒性而不作为首选药；对精神运动性发作，疗效与卡马西平相似；对非典型的小发作，疗效不及氯硝西泮。

4. 不良反应

苯妥英钠口服可引起胃肠道刺激，静脉注射可致静脉炎；儿童和青少年多发牙龈增生，停药后可消退；用药剂量过大，可出现神经系统反应，如眼球震颤、眩晕、共济失调等，严重时可出现语言障碍、精神失常甚至昏迷；长期使用可引起血液系统反应，如因叶酸缺乏导致巨幼细胞贫血，可用甲酰四氢叶酸防治；骨骼系统反应，如低钙血症，儿童佝偻病，可用维生素 D 预防；过敏反应，如皮疹、血小板和粒细胞减少、再生障碍性贫血等；妊娠期用药致畸胎。

苯巴比妥不良反应见镇静催眠药章节。

扑米酮常见不良反应为嗜睡、眩晕、复视、共济失调等中枢神经系统症状；血液系统不良反应主要为白细胞、血小板减少、贫血等；少数患者可见荨麻疹、眼睑肿胀、呼吸困难、胸部紧绷等；肝功能、肾功能不全者禁用。

乙琥胺常见不良反应为胃肠道反应，其次是中枢神经系统不良反应，如焦虑、抑郁、意识丧失、幻听等，故精神病史患者慎用。少数患者出现嗜酸性粒细胞减少、粒细胞缺乏症、再生障碍性贫血。

丙戊酸钠的毒性为肝损伤，约 30%，偶见重症肝炎、急性胰腺炎和高氨血症。

二、抗惊厥药

1. 药品

抗惊厥药有硫酸镁(magnesium sulfate)。

2. 药理作用

1）注射给药

注射硫酸镁能抑制中枢及外周神经系统，使骨骼肌、心肌、血管平滑肌松弛。作用机制可能是由于 Mg^{2+} 和 Ca^{2+} 化学性质相似，可特异性地竞争 Ca^{2+} 结合位点，拮抗 Ca^{2+} 的作用。Mg^{2+} 松弛骨骼肌，抗惊厥；松弛血管平滑肌，血管扩张，血压下降。当 Mg^{2+} 过量中毒时，亦可用 Ca^{2+} 来解救。

2）口服给药

大量口服硫酸镁后，肠道难以吸收，使肠内容物渗透压增高，抑制肠内水分的吸收，增加肠容积而促进肠道推进性蠕动。此外，硫酸镁还有利胆作用。

3）外用热敷

硫酸镁外用，利用渗透压原理消炎去肿。

3. 临床应用

口服硫酸镁主要用于导泻、利胆，如外科术前或结肠镜检查前排空肠内容物、辅助排出一些肠道寄生虫或肠内毒物。

肌内注射或静脉滴注用于缓解子痫、破伤风等所致的惊厥以及治疗高血压危象。

案例学习

学习要点：

（1）癫痫发作类型。

（2）药源性癫痫。

关键词： 局限性发作；失神性发作；肌阵挛性发作；强直-阵挛性发作；癫痫持续状态

案例

一名 12 岁的男孩在父母的陪同下来到医院。5 年前，他不慎从台阶上摔下，一个月后出现抽搐症状，此后频繁发作。患儿接受药物治疗后，近日再次发作时，男孩突然大叫一声，意识丧失，跌倒在地，全身肌肉僵硬，上肢屈曲伸直，下肢强直伸直，双眼上翻，口唇发紫，持续十几秒后全身肌肉节律性抽动，约 2 分钟后，抽搐停止，逐渐恢复正常，醒后对发作过程无记忆。神经系统检查发现患儿存在水平眼球震颤、共济失调和构音障碍。

问答题

1. 该患儿的癫痫发作属于哪种类型？该发作类型首选何种药物治疗？

2. 分析该患儿出现神经系统检查异常的可能原因以及如何鉴别。

选择题

1. 以下药物可用于癫痫强直-阵挛性发作合并失神性发作的是（　　）。
   A. 苯妥英钠　　B. 卡马西平　　C. 乙琥胺　　D. 丙戊酸钠　　E. 硫酸镁
2. 以下药物可用于子痫的是（　　）。
   A. 苯妥英钠　　B. 卡马西平　　C. 乙琥胺　　D. 丙戊酸钠　　E. 硫酸镁
3. 以下药物对癫痫持续状态有效的是（　　）。
   A. 地西泮　　B. 卡马西平　　C. 乙琥胺　　D. 扑米酮　　E. 硫酸镁
4. 以下药物有明显中枢抑制作用的是（　　）。
   A. 苯妥英钠　　B. 卡马西平　　C. 乙琥胺　　D. 丙戊酸钠　　E. 苯巴比妥
5. 以下哪项不属于苯妥英钠的适应证？（　　）
   A. 癫痫持续状态　B. 低钙血症　　C. 三叉神经痛　　D. 舌咽神经痛　E. 心律失常
6. 以下哪项不属于卡马西平的药理作用？（　　）
   A. 抗癫痫　　B. 抗利尿　　C. 抗抑郁　　D. 增强细胞兴奋性
   E. 抑制神经肌肉接头传递作用
7. 卡马西平可用于治疗（　　）。
   A. 阿尔茨海默病　　　B. 帕金森病　　　C. 尿崩症
   D. 再生障碍性贫血　　E. 高血压
8. 关于扑米酮的描述，下列哪项不正确？（　　）
   A. 可用于治疗贫血　　B. 可引起白细胞减少　　C. 可引起嗜睡、共济失调
   D. 仅用于其他药物治疗无效的患者　　E. 与苯妥英钠合用有协同作用
9. 一名45岁男性患者，3年前患脑膜炎。患者最近经常出现幻觉，不停地摸头，眨眼，几分钟后恢复正常，被诊断为精神运动性发作。下列哪种药物可以用于治疗？（　　）
   A. 卡马西平　　B. 乙琥胺　　C. 丙米嗪　　D. 氯丙嗪　　E. 硫酸镁
10. 一名5岁小女孩，吃饭时突然筷子掉落，双目失神。父母呼喊她无反应，持续几秒钟后，恢复正常。女孩被诊断为失神性发作。下列哪种药物可以用于治疗？（　　）
    A. 苯妥英钠　　B. 卡马西平　　C. 硫酸镁　　D. 乙琥胺　　E. 扑米酮

Case study

Key points：
（1）Types of seizures.
（2）Drug-induced seizures.

Key words: partial seizures; absence seizures; myoclonic seizures; tonic-clonic seizures; status epilepticus

Case

A 12-year-old boy came to the hospital accompanied by his parents. Five years ago, he accidentally fell down the steps and developed convulsive symptoms a month later. He had frequent seizures since then. Recently, the boy had another seizure. He suddenly screamed, lost consciousness and fell to the ground. He had generalized muscle rigidity, flexion and extension of the upper limbs, tonic extension of the lower limbs, upturning of the eyes, and purpling of the mouth and lips, which lasted for ten seconds or so, followed by rhythmic convulsions throughout his body, and the seizure ceased and gradually returned to normal after about 2 minutes. He woke up with no memory of the course of the seizure. Neurologic examination revealed horizontal nystagmus, ataxia and dysarthria.

◎ **Essay questions**

1. Which seizure type does the boy have? What drug is preferred for this type of seizure?
2. Analyze the possible causes of the abnormal neurological examination for this child and how to identify them.

Multiple-choice questions

1. Which of the following drugs can be used for tonic-clonic seizures and absence seizures? ( )
   A. Phenytoin sodium   B. Carbamazepine   C. Ethosuximide
   D. Sodium valproate   E. Magnesium sulfate
2. Which of the following drugs can be used for eclampsia? ( )
   A. Phenytoin sodium   B. Carbamazepine   C. Ethosuximide
   D. Sodium valproate   E. Magnesium sulfate
3. Which of the following drugs can be used for status epilepticus? ( )
   A. Diazepam   B. Carbamazepine   C. Ethosuximide
   D. Primidone   E. Magnesium sulfate
4. Which of the following drugs has a significant inhibitory effect on the central nervous system? ( )
   A. Phenytoin sodium   B. Carbamazepine   C. Ethosuximide
   D. Sodium valproate   E. Phenobarbital
5. Which of the following is not an indication of phenytoin sodium? ( )
   A. Status epilepticus   B. Hypocalcemia   C. Trigeminal neuralgia
   D. Glossopharyngeal neuralgia   E. Arrhythmia
6. Which of the following is not a pharmacologic effect of carbamazepine? ( )
   A. Antiepileptic   B. Antidiuretic   C. Antidepressant
   D. Enhancement of cellular excitability
   E. Inhibition of neuromuscular junction transmission
7. Carbamazepine is used to treat ( ).
   A. Alzheimer's disease   B. Parkinson disease   C. diabetes insipidus
   D. aplastic anemia   E. hypertension

8. Which of the following descriptions of primidone is incorrect? （   ）
    A. It can be used to treat anemia
    B. It may cause leukopenia
    C. It may cause drowsiness and ataxia
    D. It is used only in patients who have failed with other drugs
    E. There is a synergistic effect in combination with phenytoin sodium
9. A 45-year-old male patient suffered from meningitis three years ago. Recently, he had been experiencing frequent hallucinations, constantly touching his head and blinking, then returning to normal after a few minutes. He was diagnosed with psychomotor epilepsy. Which of the following drugs can be used for treatment? （   ）
    A. Carbamazepine   B. Ethosuximide   C. Promethazine
    D. Chlorpromazine   E. Magnesium sulfate
10. A 5-year-old girl suddenly dropped her chopsticks while eating, and stared blankly. She became unresponsive to shouting from her parents, then returned to normal after a few seconds. She was diagnosed with absence seizures. Which of the following drugs can be used for treatment? （   ）
    A. Phenytoin sodium   B. Carbamazepine   C. Magnesium sulfate
    D. Ethosuximide   E. Primidone

第十五章案例学习和选择题答案

第十六章 治疗中枢神经系统退行性疾病药

知识要点

一、药品分类

(1) 多巴胺的前体药：如左旋多巴（levodopa，L-DOPA）。
(2) 氨基酸脱羧酶抑制药：如卡比多巴（carbidopa）。
(3) 抗胆碱药：如苯海索（trihexyphenidyl）。

二、作用机制

多巴胺因不易通过血脑屏障，不能用于治疗帕金森病（Parkinson disease，PD）。左旋多巴是多巴胺的前体，通过血脑屏障后，补充纹状体中多巴胺的不足而发挥治疗作用。

卡比多巴为芳香族 L-氨基酸脱羧酶抑制剂，不能通过血脑屏障，与 L-DOPA 合用时，抑制 L-DOPA 外周脱羧反应，促进其进入中枢神经系统。卡比多巴与 L-DOPA 合用可减少 L-DOPA 使用量，明显减少不良反应，减轻症状波动。

苯海索拮抗胆碱受体，减弱黑质-纹状体通路中乙酰胆碱的作用。

三、药理作用

L-DOPA 对肌肉僵直和运动困难的疗效好，对肌肉震颤的疗效差。左旋多巴起效慢，治疗作用与黑质-纹状体病损程度相关，轻症或较年轻患者疗效好，重症或年老体弱者疗效较差。

卡比多巴单独使用无效。

苯海索抗震颤效果好，也能改善肌肉强直。

四、临床应用

L-DOPA 可治疗各种类型 PD，不论年龄、性别差异和病程长短均适用，但对抗精神病药所引起的帕金森综合征（Parkinsonism）无效。

卡比多巴与 L-DOPA 组成的复方制剂称为心宁美。

苯海索对 PD 疗效有限，副作用较多，现已少用。临床上主要用于抗精神病药所致的帕金森综合征。

五、不良反应

1. L-DOPA 的早期反应

(1) 胃肠道反应：L-DOPA 刺激胃肠道和兴奋延髓催吐化学感受区 D_2 受体，引发恶心、呕吐，故 D_2 受体阻断药多潘立酮(domperidone)可对抗。

(2) 心血管反应：反馈性抑制交感神经末梢释放去甲肾上腺素，以及激动血管壁多巴胺受体，引发直立性低血压。

2. L-DOPA 的长期反应

(1) 运动过多症(hyperkinesia)：大量 L-DOPA 过度兴奋多巴胺受体，出现手足、躯体和舌的不自主运动，多巴胺受体拮抗药可减轻。

(2) 症状波动：与多巴胺储存能力下降有关。严重的称之为开-关反应(on-off response)，"开"时活动接近正常，而"关"时出现严重 PD 症状。

(3) 精神症状：可能与皮质和边缘系统多巴胺功能亢进有关，只能用非经典抗精神病药如氯氮平(clozapine)治疗。

苯海索的副作用与阿托品相同，但症状较轻，可能加重帕金森病患者伴有的痴呆症状，禁用于青光眼和前列腺肥大患者。

案例学习

学习要点：
(1) 左旋多巴用药原则。
(2) 帕金森病联合用药方案。

关键词： 帕金森病；左旋多巴；苯海索；MAO-B 抑制剂

案例

患者王某，68 岁，两年前出现左手手抖，不灵活，并不影响日常生活。近半年，患者的左脚出现无法控制的抖动。此外，他感到乏力，走路缓慢且一瘸一拐，行动能力明显下降。患者前往医院就诊，自述失去嗅觉已有多年，否认中毒等病史及家族史。体格检查发现，面部表情欠佳，左上肢肌张力稍增高；左手水平伸直时，可观察到轻微震颤；行走稍跛行，不自然；摆臂幅度减小。各项生化检测指标未发现明显异常。患者被诊断为帕金森病，使用左旋多巴进行治疗。由于疗效欠佳，患者自行增加到两倍剂量。增加剂量后，患者出现恶心、呕吐、站立时头晕乏力、手脚不自主异常运动、排尿困难等不适症状。患者前往医院复诊。

问答题

1. 患者为何出现异常情况？
2. 患者是否可以选择心宁美(卡比多巴/左旋多巴复方制剂)？患者可否加用苯海索(抗胆碱能药)或 MAO-B 抑制剂治疗？

选择题

1. 下列哪一种药物可增加左旋多巴疗效并减少不良反应？（　　）
   A. 氯丙嗪　　B. 维生素 B_6　　C. 阿托品　　D. 卡比多巴　　E. 苯海索
2. 下列哪一种关于卡比多巴的描述是正确的？（　　）
   A. 不可通过血脑屏障　　　　　　B. 增加中枢多巴胺释放
   C. 单用有较强的抗震颤作用　　　D. 抑制芳香族 L-氨基酸脱羧酶活性
   E. 激动多巴胺受体
3. 下列哪一种关于苯海索的描述是错误的？（　　）
   A. 抗胆碱作用弱于阿托品　　B. 可通过血脑屏障　　C. 促进多巴胺释放
   D. 抗震颤效果好　　　　　　E. 加重痴呆症状
4. 下列哪一种关于左旋多巴的描述是错误的？（　　）
   A. 属于前体药物　　　　B. 对老年患者效果好　　C. 对帕金森综合征无效
   D. 对轻症患者效果好　　E. 生物利用度低
5. 下列哪些药物可增强左旋多巴疗效？（　　）
   A. 苯海索　　B. 氯丙嗪　　C. 司来吉兰　　D. 卡比多巴　　E. 氯氮平
6. 下列哪一种药物不能和左旋多巴合用？（　　）
   A. 苄丝肼　　B. 维生素 B_6　　C. 司来吉兰　　D. 卡比多巴　　E. 托卡朋
7. 下列哪一种药物不能通过血脑屏障？（　　）
   A. 氯丙嗪　　B. 维生素 E　　C. 司来吉兰　　D. 苄丝肼　　E. 托卡朋
8. 关于左旋多巴的不良反应，下列哪一种描述是错误的？（　　）
   A. 刺激胃肠道　　　B. 舒张血管　　　C. 引起不自主异常运动
   D. 引起开关反应　　E. 引起突发性睡眠
9. 一名 60 岁男性帕金森病患者服用左旋多巴期间，出现了幻听、幻视，选用下列哪一种药物缓解症状？（　　）
   A. 苯海索　　B. 氯丙嗪　　C. 司来吉兰　　D. 卡比多巴　　E. 氯氮平
10. 一名 20 岁男性精神分裂症患者服用氯丙嗪期间，出现了右手震颤，选用下列哪一种药物缓解症状？（　　）
    A. 苯海索　　B. 氯丙嗪　　C. 司来吉兰　　D. 卡比多巴　　E. 氯氮平

Case study

Key points:
(1) Principles of levodopa treatment.
(2) Combination drug therapy for Parkinson disease.

Key words: Parkinson disease; levodopa; Trihexyphenidyl; MAO-B inhibitor

Case

Patient Wang, 68 years old, developed tremor and inflexibility in his left hand two years ago, which did not affect his daily life. In the last six months, the patient's left foot developed uncontrollable shaking. In addition, he felt weak, walked slowly and with a limp, and his mobility was significantly reduced. The patient went to the hospital and reported that he had lost his sense of smell for many years and denied medical history such as poisoning and family history. Physical examination revealed poor facial expression and slightly increased muscle tone in the left upper limb; a slight tremor was observed when the left hand was horizontally extended; walking was slightly lame and unnatural; and the swing of the arm was reduced. No obvious abnormalities were found in various biochemical tests. The patient was diagnosed with Parkinson disease and was treated with levodopa. Due to the lack of efficacy, the patient doubled the dose on his own. After increasing the dose, the patient developed uncomfortable symptoms including nausea, vomiting, dizziness and weakness when standing, involuntary abnormal movements of arms and legs, difficulty in urination, and so on. The patient went to the hospital for follow-up.

◎ **Essay questions**

1. Why did the patient experience abnormalities?
2. Is the patient eligible for sinemet (carbidopa/levodopa combination)? Can the patient be treated with additional trihexyphenidyl (anticholinergic) or MAO-B inhibitors?

Multiple-choice questions

1. Which of the following drugs increases the efficacy of levodopa and reduces adverse effects? (   )
    A. Chlorpromazine   B. Vitamin B_6 C. Atropine
    D. Carbidopa   E. Trihexyphenidyl
2. Which of the following descriptions of carbidopa is correct? (   )
    A. Carbidopa cannot pass the blood-brain barrier
    B. Carbidopa increases central dopamine release
    C. Carbidopa has a strong antitumor effect when used alone
    D. Carbidopa inhibits aromatic L-amino acid decarboxylase activity
    E. Carbidopa activates dopamine receptors
3. Which of the following descriptions of trihexyphenidyl is false? (   )
    A. Trihexyphenidyl has weaker anticholinergic effects than atropine
    B. Trihexyphenidyl passes the blood-brain barrier
    C. Trihexyphenidyl promotes dopamine release
    D. Trihexyphenidyl has good capability to reduce tremors
    E. Trihexyphenidyl aggravates dementia symptoms
4. Which of the following descriptions of levodopa is false? (   )
    A. Levodopa is a prodrug
    B. Levodopa is effective in elderly patients
    C. Levodopa is ineffective in Parkinsonism

D. Levodopa is effective in mildly ill patients

E. Levodopa has low bioavailability

5. Which of the following drugs can enhance the efficacy of levodopa? (　　)

    A. Trihexyphenidyl　　　B. Chlorpromazine　　　C. Selegiline

    D. Carbidopa　　　　　　E. Clozapine

6. Which of the following drugs should not be combined with levodopa? (　　)

    A. Benserazide　　　　　B. Vitamin B_6　　　　C. Selegiline

    D. Carbidopa　　　　　　E. Tolcapone

7. Which of the following drugs cannot cross the blood-brain barrier? (　　)

    A. Chlorpromazine　　　B. Vitamin E　　　　　C. Selegiline

    D. Benserazide　　　　　E. Tolcapone

8. Which of the following descriptions about the adverse effects of levodopa is false? (　　)

    A. Levodopa irritates the gastrointestinal tract

    B. Levodopa dilates blood vessels

    C. Levodopa causes involuntary abnormal movements

    D. Levodopa causes an on-off response

    E. Levodopa causes sudden sleep attack

9. Which of the following drugs would be used to relieve the symptoms of a 60-year-old male with Parkinson disease who develops auditory hallucinations and visual hallucinations while taking levodopa? (　　)

    A. Trihexyphenidyl　　　B. Chlorpromazine　　　C. Selegiline

    D. Carbidopa　　　　　　E. Clozapine

10. Which of the following drugs is chosen to relieve symptoms in a 20-year-old male schizophrenic who develops a tremor in his right hand while taking chlorpromazine? (　　)

    A. Benzhexol　　　　　　B. Chlorpromazine　　　C. Selegiline

    D. Carbidopa　　　　　　E. Clozapine

第十六章案例学习和选择题答案

第十七章　抗精神失常药

知识要点

一、抗精神分裂症药

1. 药品分类
(1) 第一代经典抗精神分裂症药：如氯丙嗪(chlorpromazine)。
(2) 第二代非经典抗精神分裂症药：如氯氮平(clozapine)。

2. 作用机制
氯丙嗪又名冬眠灵，药理作用广泛：①拮抗中脑-边缘系统和中脑-皮质系统多巴胺(dopamine，DA)受体产生抗精神分裂症作用，拮抗黑质-纹状体通路 DA 受体导致锥体外系运动失调，拮抗结节-漏斗通路 DA 受体导致内分泌失调；②阻断了延髓催吐化学感受区 DA 受体，发挥镇吐作用；③抑制下丘脑体温调节中枢，使得体温随环境温度变化；④拮抗 α 受体可致血管扩张、血压下降，拮抗 M 胆碱受体，引起口干、便秘、视物模糊。

氯氮平特异性拮抗中脑-边缘系统和中脑-皮质系统 DA 受体的 D_4 亚型，对黑质-纹状体通路和结节-漏斗通路 DA 受体无亲和力，药理作用机制还涉及阻断 5-羟色胺受体 $5-HT_{2A}$，协调 5-HT 与 DA 系统之间的相互作用和平衡，也被称为 5-羟色胺和多巴胺受体阻断药。

3. 药理作用
1) 氯丙嗪
(1) 抗精神分裂症作用：又称神经安定作用(neuroleptic effect)，迅速控制患者兴奋躁动状态，大剂量连续用药能消除患者的幻觉和妄想等症状。对阴性症状无效，甚至加重 II 型精神分裂症病情。

(2) 镇吐作用：可对抗 DA 受体激动剂阿扑吗啡引起的呕吐反应，但不能对抗前庭刺激引起的呕吐，抑制位于延髓与催吐化学感受区旁呃逆的中枢调节部位，对顽固性呃逆有效。

(3) 体温调节作用：降温作用随外界环境温度而变化，亦可干扰散热机制，升高体温。

(4) 对自主神经系统的作用：降压、口干、便秘、视物模糊。

(5) 对内分泌系统的影响：增加催乳素的分泌，抑制促性腺激素和糖皮质激素的分泌。

2）氯氮平

抗精神分裂症作用：疗效与氯丙嗪相当，且阴性和阳性症状均有效，起效迅速。

4. 临床应用

1）氯丙嗪

(1) I 型精神分裂症。

(2) 呕吐和顽固性呃逆。

(3) 低温麻醉与人工冬眠：辅助治疗严重创伤、感染性休克、高热惊厥、中枢性高热及甲状腺危象等，配合物理降温，降低心、脑等生命器官的耗氧量，用于脑手术和心血管手术。

2）氯氮平

仅适用于对至少 2 种不同抗精神病药足量足疗程治疗无效的难治性精神分裂症患者的治疗。

5. 不良反应

1）氯丙嗪

最常见的不良反应包括中枢抑制症状（嗜睡等）、M 胆碱受体拮抗症状（口干、便秘、视物模糊等）和 α 肾上腺素受体拮抗症状（直立性低血压等）。

锥体外系不良反应：①帕金森综合征；②静坐不能；③急性肌张力障碍；④迟发性运动障碍。前三种可用抗胆碱药缓解，第四种用抗胆碱药反而使症状加重。

氯丙嗪可以引起精神异常，一旦发生应立即减量或停药；诱发惊厥与癫痫，有惊厥或癫病史者慎用；引发过敏反应，可出现肝损害、黄疸、粒细胞减少、溶血性贫血和再生障碍性贫血等；引起内分泌系统紊乱，如高催乳素血症、乳腺增大、抑制儿童生长等。

一次吞服大剂量氯丙嗪可导致急性中毒，患者出现昏睡、血压下降至休克水平，并出现心肌损害，应立即对症治疗。必要时可使用去甲肾上腺素，禁用肾上腺素，慎用多巴胺，因可加重低血压。

2）氯氮平

最常见的不良反应包括中枢抑制症状（嗜睡等）、M 胆碱受体拮抗症状（口干、便秘、视物模糊等）和 α 肾上腺素受体拮抗症状（直立性低血压等）。

严重的不良反应包括粒细胞缺乏症（高风险）、癫痫发作（剂量越高越易发生），以及体位性低血压、心肌炎等心血管系统和呼吸系统的不良反应。流行病学研究表明，使用氯氮平的患者出现高血糖、高血脂和体重增加，增加心血管和脑血管不良事件风险。

二、抗躁狂症药

1. 药品

抗躁狂症药有碳酸锂（lithium carbonate）。

2. 作用机制

确切机制不清楚，属于中枢非特异性药物。目前认为其治疗机制主要包括抑制去甲肾上腺素（norepinephrine，NA）和 DA 释放；加速 NA 和 DA 灭活；抑制腺苷酸环化酶和磷脂酶 C 所介导的反应；影响 Na^+、Ca^{2+}、Mg^{2+} 分布和葡萄糖代谢。

3. 药理作用

对急性躁狂和轻度躁狂疗效显著；对抑郁症也有效，但弱于抗躁狂作用；可以减少躁狂和抑郁复发。

4. 临床应用

临床应用于躁狂症和躁狂抑郁症。

5. 不良反应

安全范围窄，需要监测血药浓度。

轻度的毒性症状包括恶心、呕吐、腹痛、腹泻和细微震颤；较严重的毒性反应涉及神经系统，包括精神紊乱、反射亢进、明显震颤、惊厥，直至昏迷死亡。

三、抗抑郁药

1. 药品分类

(1) 三环类：丙米嗪(imipramine)。

(2) 5-HT再摄取抑制药：氟西汀(fluoxetine)。

2. 作用机制

丙米嗪阻断中枢神经系统NA和5-HT在神经末梢的再摄取，增高突触间隙的递质浓度，振奋精神；阻断M胆碱受体（口干、便秘、视物模糊）；阻断α_1肾上腺素受体降低血压；阻断组胺H_1受体过度镇静；阻断外周单胺类再摄取，使得心肌中NA浓度增高，引发心动过速等不良反应。

氟西汀选择性抑制5-HT再摄取，对肾上腺素受体、组胺受体、$GABA_B$受体、M受体、5-HT受体几乎没有亲和力。

3. 药理作用

1) 丙米嗪

(1) 中枢神经系统作用：丙米嗪使抑郁症患者振奋精神，情绪高涨。

(2) 自主神经系统作用：阻断M受体，引起口干、视力模糊等。

(3) 心血管系统作用：阻断α_1受体，减低血压；增加NA再摄取，引起心律失常。

2) 氟西汀

抗抑郁疗效与丙米嗪相当，但安全性明显优于丙米嗪。

4. 临床应用

1) 丙米嗪

(1) 抑郁症：对内源性抑郁症、更年期抑郁症效果较好，对反应性抑郁症效果一般，对精神分裂症伴发的抑郁状态效果差。

(2) 遗尿症：6岁以上儿童遗尿可以使用丙米嗪，疗程以3个月为限。

(3) 焦虑和恐惧症：具有抗焦虑作用，对伴有焦虑状态的抑郁症患者疗效显著，对疾病恐惧症有效。

2) 氟西汀

(1) 抑郁症：疗效与三环类抗抑郁药相当，但不良反应少。

(2) 强迫症：有效且安全性好，属于一线用药，但起效时间慢。

(3) 神经性贪食症：氟西汀显著改善抑郁以及对碳水化合物的渴望，改变病态的饮食行为。

5. 不良反应

1) 丙米嗪

常见的不良反应包括口干、便秘、视物模糊、直立性低血压、心动过速等。前列腺肥大、青光眼患者禁用。

2) 氟西汀

常见的不良反应包括食欲减退、性功能下降。肝、肾功能不全者须减量，延长服药间隔时间。心血管疾病、糖尿病者应慎用。

丙米嗪或氟西汀与单胺氧化酶 MAO 抑制剂合用时，须警惕"血清素综合征"，表现为不安、激越、高热、强直、意识障碍，甚至昏迷死亡。

案例学习

学习要点：
(1) 治疗精神分裂症的药物分类。
(2) 锥体外系不良反应。
(3) 治疗抑郁药物分类。
(4) 抗精神病药物相互作用。

关键词：多巴胺受体阻断剂；多巴胺神经通路；5-羟色胺

案例一

李某，男，22 岁，就读某高校计算机专业二年级。一年多以前，他感觉总是能听见同学背后议论他，怀疑自己被人监视。李某认为同学通过监视器知道了自己的想法。他经常旷课，多数时间躺在床上看电脑，有时自言自语，有时嚎啕大哭，甚至半夜高歌。他没有烟酒嗜好，没有接触过毒品，没有重大疾病史，近期也没有感染或吸毒史。体格检查、常规生化检查、肝肾功能、心电图和脑电图均正常。李某被诊断为精神分裂症。

李某接受氯丙嗪治疗 2 周后，体重增加了 3 千克，总是想睡觉，没有力气，双手臂常常抖动且不受控制。医生与李某交谈后得知，他不再认为同学通过监视器监视他，但还是能听到一些奇怪的声音。体格检查发现，肌张力增加，双上肢震颤。医生决定给李某换药，询问家族遗传史后得知，其祖母患有糖尿病。

◎ **问答题**

1. 目前治疗精神分裂症的药物有哪几类？患者选用氯丙嗪治疗是否合适？
2. 患者出现手臂不自主抖动的原因是什么？应如何治疗？
3. 患者能否换用氯氮平进行治疗？

案例二

患者王某，男，47 岁，因反复发作胸痛伴有双侧手部麻痹，到急诊科就诊。他出现持续性胸痛 10 分钟，双手感觉异常。医生紧急对王某进行了心电图和血清肌钙蛋白检查。心电图检查结果显示，正常心电图，窦性心动过速。血清肌钙蛋白检查结果，发现肌钙蛋白 I 阴性，肌钙蛋白 T 在正常范围内。病人疼痛缓解后，医生要求王某进行心电图运动负荷试验，但实验结果未发现异常。医生询问既往病史和家族遗传史，得知王某以往身心健康，未发现心血管疾病。医生建议他不适随诊。

王某因胸痛反复发作，自觉体力欠佳，难以集中精力工作，经常失眠，体重明显下降。王某再次前往医院就诊。医生与王某交谈中，得知其开有一家实体服装店，但生意惨淡。王某的儿子就读于一所私立学校，学费昂贵。王某告诉医生，最近总是感觉心情不好，非常担心自己的身体健康状况，也感到经济压力很大。交谈过程中，王某表示自己对什么都没兴趣，但否认出现幻觉、妄想等精神障碍。体格检查未见明显异常，血液常规检测、肝肾功能和甲状腺功能均正常。心电图和脑电图均属正常。王某被诊断为抑郁症，他否认有家族遗传史。

王某接受药物治疗 3 周后复诊，自述未发生胸痛，但仍然对事物提不起兴趣。复诊前 2 天，王某在听说服装店的房屋租金要上涨后出现失眠，并开始使用阿普唑仑。王某否认有自杀的意图。

王某接受药物治疗 1 年后复诊。王某告诉医生，已无胸痛、失眠等症状。王某自述心情和食欲都比以前好，服装店已转让，儿子已经顺利毕业，目前就职于一家国有大型企业。

◎ 问答题

1. 在王某被确诊为抑郁症后，医生可以选择何种抗抑郁药物进行治疗？病人是否需要治疗疼痛？

2. 王某被确诊为抑郁症，使用氟西汀进行治疗。他在接受催眠药物治疗时，是否需要调整药物使用方案？

◎ 选择题

1. 氯丙嗪引起乳房肿大与乳漏，是由于（　　）。
   A. 阻断结节-漏斗通路的 D_2 受体　　B. 阻断黑质-纹状体通路的 D_2 受体
   C. 阻断中脑-皮质通路 M 受体　　D. 激活中脑边缘系统 M 胆碱受体
   E. 激活中枢 β_2 受体

2. 氯丙嗪引起低血压状态时，应使用哪种药物？（　　）
   A. 多巴胺　　B. 肾上腺素　　C. 去甲肾上腺素　　D. 异丙肾上腺素　　E. 阿托品

3. 下列哪种药物可拮抗 D_2 和 $5-HT_2$ 受体？（　　）
   A. 利培酮　　B. 丙米嗪　　C. 氟奋乃静　　D. 氯丙嗪　　E. 碳酸锂

4. 下列哪一药物属于 5-HT 再摄取抑制药？（　　）
   A. 马普替林　　B. 氟西汀　　C. 利醅酮　　D. 阿米替林　　E. 碳酸锂

5. 丙米嗪引起体位性低血压是由于（　　）。
   A. 阻断 M 型胆碱受体　　B. 阻断 α 肾上腺素受体　　C. 阻断 β 肾上腺素受体
   D. 阻断 N 型胆碱受体　　E. 阻断 H_1 型胆碱受体

6. 下列关于治疗情感障碍药物的说法哪一项是准确的？（　　）
   A. 碳酸锂治疗浓度范围宽　　　　　　B. 碳酸锂不穿越胎盘屏障
   C. 过量摄入氯化钠会增强碳酸锂的毒性　D. 丙米嗪缓解双相情感障碍
   E. 碳酸锂缓解双相情感障碍

7. 氯丙嗪降低体温作用的特点是（　　）。
   A. 产热减少，散热增加　　B. 产热减少，散热减少　　C. 产热不变，散热增加
   D. 只降低发热者体温　　　E. 体温随环境温度变化而变化

8. 一位35岁男性病人情绪低落，时常感觉生活无趣，正在接受药物治疗。他抱怨服药后，总是口渴，小便次数增加。当移动双手时，他会出现轻微的颤抖。他最可能服用的药物是下面哪种药物？（　　）
   A. 碳酸锂　　B. 利醅酮　　C. 阿米替林　　D. 丙米嗪　　E. 氟西汀

9. 一位20岁年轻病人服用抗精神病药物两个月后出现发烧，自述疲劳乏力。体检发现四肢有明显瘀点，实验室检查显示白细胞和血小板减少。病人被诊断为药物性粒细胞缺乏症，他很可能使用了下列哪一种药物？（　　）
   A. 碳酸锂　　B. 丙米嗪　　C. 氟哌啶醇　　D. 氯氮平　　E. 氟西汀

10. 一位老年男性病人服用司来吉兰治疗帕金森病。大约半年后，他因情绪低落口服氟西汀，突然出现全身肌肉僵硬、流汗、高烧。出现上述症状最可能的原因是（　　）。
    A. 药物性粒细胞缺乏症　　B. 合并严重的细菌感染　　C. 多巴胺失调综合征
    D. 5-羟色胺综合征　　　　E. 药物间的拮抗作用

Case study

Key points：
(1) Classification of drugs for schizophrenia.
(2) Extrapyramidal side effects.
(3) Classification of anti-depressants.
(4) Interactions of antipsychotic drugs.

Key words： dopamine receptor antagonists; dopaminergic pathways; 5-hydroxytryptamine

Case 1

Patient Li, male, 22 years old, is in the second year of computer science at a university. More than a year ago, he felt that he could always hear his classmates talking about him behind his back and suspected that he was being watched. He thought that his classmates knew his thoughts through the monitor. He often missed classes and spent most of his time lying in bed looking at his computer, sometimes talking to himself, sometimes bawling, and even singing in the middle of the night. He has no tobacco or alcohol habit, no drug exposure, no history of major illness, and no recent history of infection or drug use. Physical examination, routine biochemical tests, liver and kidney functions, electrocardiogram, and electroencephalogram were normal. He was diagnosed with schizophrenia.

After being treated with chlorpromazine for 2 weeks, Li gained 3 kilograms. He always wanted to sleep and had no energy. His arms often shook and were out of control. The physician spoke with Li and learned that he no longer thought that his classmates were watching him through a monitor, but he could still hear strange noises. Physical examination revealed increased muscle tone and tremors in both upper extremities. The doctor decided to change the medication and learned that his grandmother had diabetes after asking about the family genetic history.

◎ **Essay questions**

1. What types of medications are currently available for the treatment of schizophrenia? Is it appropriate for the patient to be treated with chlorpromazine?
2. What is the cause of the patient's involuntary arm shaking? How should the patient be treated?
3. Can the patient switch to clozapine for the treatment?

Case 2

Patient Wang, male, 47 years old, went to the Emergency Department with recurrent chest pain accompanied by paralysis of both hands. He experienced persistent chest pain for 10 minutes and had abnormal sensations in both hands. Wang Ping received the emergency examinations for electrocardiogram (ECG) and serum troponin. The evaluation indicated the normal ECG with sinus tachycardia, and both troponin I and troponin T in the normal range. The doctor asked him to conduct an exercise electrocardiogram after pain relief, but no abnormal repolarization was found in the test. The doctor collected his medical records and family health history and knew that he was physically and mentally healthy in the past without cardiovascular disease. The doctor advised him to follow up once he felt uncomfortable.

After that, Wang suffered from recurrent chest pain, poor physical strength, difficulty concentrating on work, frequent insomnia and significant weight loss. Wang Ping made a follow-up appointment. He told the doctor that he ran a clothes entity store, but business was dismal. Wang's son was enrolled in a private school with expensive tuition. Wang told the doctor that recently he always felt bad, was very worried about his physical health, and also felt a lot of financial pressure. During the conversation, Wang said he was not interested in anything, but denied having mental disorders such as hallucinations and delusions. Physical examination showed no obvious abnormalities, and routine blood tests, liver and kidney function, and thyroid function were all normal. The electrocardiogram and electroencephalogram were normal. Wang was diagnosed with depression, and he denied having a family genetic history.

Wang received medication for 3 weeks and then returned for a follow-up visit. Wang reported no chest pain but still had no interest in things. Two days before the follow-up visit, Wang developed insomnia and began using alprazolam after hearing that the housing rent for his clothes store was going to rise again. Wang denied suicidal intent.

Wang received medication for 1 year and then returned for a follow-up visit. He told the doctor no chest pain and insomnia anymore. He reported that his mood and appetite were better than before, that his clothes store had been transferred, and that his son successfully graduated and worked in a large state-owned enterprise.

◎ **Essay questions**
1. What antidepressant medication could the doctor have chosen for the treatment after Wang was diagnosed with depression? Does the patient need treatment for pain?
2. Wang was diagnosed with depression and treated with fluoxetine. Does the medication regimen need to be adjusted while receiving hypnotics?

Multiple-choice questions

1. Chlorpromazine causes breast enlargement with milk leakage due to (   ).
   A. blockade of D_2 receptors in the tuberoinfundibular pathway
   B. blockade of D_2 receptors in the nigrostriatal pathway
   C. blockade of M receptors in the mesocortical pathway
   D. activation of M cholinergic receptors in the mesolimbic pathway
   E. activation of central β_2 receptors
2. Which drug should be used when chlorpromazine causes a hypotensive state (   ).
   A. Dopamine   B. Epinephrine   C. Norepinephrine
   D. Isoprenaline   E. Atropine
3. Which of the following drugs antagonizes D_2 and $5-HT_2$ receptors? (   )
   A. Risperidone   B. Imipramine   C. Fluphenazine
   D. Chlorpromazine   E. Lithium carbonate
4. Which of the following drugs is a 5-HT reuptake inhibitor? (   )
   A. Maprotiline   B. Fluoxetine   C. Risperidone
   D. Amitriptyline   E. Lithium carbonate
5. Promethazine causes postural hypotension due to (   ).
   A. blockade of M cholinergic receptors   B. blockade of α adrenergic receptors
   C. blockade of β adrenergic receptors   D. blockade of N cholinergic receptors
   E. blockade of H_1 cholinergic receptors
6. Which statement is correct regarding the treatment of affective disorders? (   )
   A. Lithium carbonate has a wide range of therapeutic concentrations
   B. Lithium carbonate does not cross the placental barrier
   C. Excessive intake of sodium chloride enhances the toxicity of lithium carbonate
   D. Imipramine relieves bipolar disorder
   E. Lithium carbonate relieves bipolar disorder
7. The hypothermic effect of chlorpromazine is characterized by (   ).
   A. decreased heat production and increased heat dissipation
   B. decreased heat production and decreased heat dissipation

C. unchanged heat production and increased heat dissipation

D. lowering the body temperature only in the febrile person

E. changes in body temperature in response to ambient temperature

8. A 35-year-old male patient who suffers from depression and often feels uninterested in life is currently receiving medication. He complains of persistent thirst and increased urination after taking the medication. A slight tremor occurs when he moves his hands. Which of the following medications is he most likely taking? (　　)

   A. Lithium carbonate　　B. Risperidone　　C. Amitriptyline
   D. Imipramine　　E. Fluoxetine

9. A young 20-year-old patient who had received antipsychotics for several weeks developed periodic fevers and felt fatigued. Physical examination revealed significant petechiae on the extremities, and laboratory tests indicated leukopenia and thrombocytopenia. The patient was diagnosed with drug-induced granulocyte deficiency, and he was likely on which of the following medications? (　　)

   A. Lithium carbonate　　B. Lithizone　　C. Haloperidol
   D. Clozapine　　E. Fluoxetine

10. An elderly male patient received selegiline for the treatment of Parkinson's disease. About six months later, he orally took fluoxetine for depression and suddenly developed generalized muscle stiffness, sweating and high fever. The most likely cause of these symptoms is (　　).

    A. drug-induced granulocyte deficiency　　B. severe bacterial infection
    C. dopamine dysregulation syndrome　　D. 5-Hydroxytryptamine syndrome
    E. antagonism between two drugs

第十七章案例学习和选择题答案

第十八章 镇痛药

知识要点

一、阿片受体激动药

1. 药品分类

(1) 阿片生物碱类镇痛药：如吗啡（morphine）。

(2) 人工合成类镇痛药：如哌替啶（pethidine）。

2. 作用机制

吗啡作用于脊髓胶质区、丘脑内侧、脑室及导水管周围灰质等部位的阿片受体，包括 μ、κ、δ 受体，模拟内源性阿片肽兴奋阿片受体，激活机体抗痛系统，抑制痛觉传导通路上行传入大脑皮层，以及激活中脑的痛觉下行控制环路，发挥中枢性镇痛作用。

3. 药理作用

1) 吗啡

(1) 中枢神经系统作用如下：①镇痛作用：吗啡镇痛作用强，对大部分疼痛有效，对持续性钝痛的效果大于间歇性锐痛，对神经痛效果不明显。②镇静、致欣快作用：吗啡对情绪的影响可能与激活边缘系统和蓝斑核的阿片受体有关，以及中脑腹侧背盖区-伏隔核多巴胺能神经通路与阿片受体的相互作用有关。吗啡可缓解疼痛引起的焦虑、紧张、恐惧等反应，提升机体对疼痛的耐受力。吗啡致欣快作用是导致药物成瘾的原因。③抑制呼吸作用：该抑制作用可能与吗啡降低脑干呼吸中枢对 CO_2 的敏感性以及抑制脑桥呼吸调节中枢有关。不同于麻醉药或其他中枢抑制药，吗啡对延髓心血管中枢无明显抑制作用。④镇咳作用：吗啡镇咳作用可能与其激动延髓孤束核的阿片受体有关。吗啡抑制延髓咳嗽中枢，减少咳嗽反射，从而发挥镇咳作用。⑤缩瞳作用：吗啡激动阿片受体使得支配瞳孔的副交感神经兴奋，瞳孔括约肌收缩，瞳孔缩小。⑥其他中枢作用：吗啡激动阿片受体使得延髓催吐化学感受器兴奋，引起恶心、呕吐等。

(2) 对平滑肌的作用如下：①胃肠道平滑肌：吗啡能提高胃肠道平滑肌张力，减慢胃蠕动和胃排空，延缓肠内容物通过，可引起便秘。②胆道平滑肌：吗啡能引起胆道括约肌痉挛性收缩，使胆总管压和胆囊内压升高，可致上腹不适甚至胆绞痛，可用阿托品缓解。③其他平滑肌：降低子宫平滑肌张力、收缩幅度和频率，延长产妇产程；提高膀胱括约肌张力，易引起尿潴留；大剂量吗啡使得支气管平滑肌兴奋，诱发或加重哮喘。

(3)心血管系统：吗啡能扩张血管，使外周阻力降低，易引起直立性低血压；吗啡能模拟缺血性预适应(ischemic preconditioning，IPC)，对心肌缺血性损伤具有保护作用；吗啡能抑制呼吸使体内 CO_2 增加，脑血管扩张，颅内压增高。

(4)免疫系统：吗啡抑制免疫，与其激动 μ 受体有关。

2)哌替啶

(1)中枢神经系统：哌替啶的镇痛作用弱于吗啡；镇静、致欣快、呼吸抑制作用与吗啡相当；无明显的中枢性镇咳作用。

(2)对平滑肌的作用：大剂量哌替啶引起支气管平滑肌收缩，有轻微子宫兴奋作用，但对妊娠末期子宫收缩无影响，不延长产程。

(3)扩血管作用：哌替啶扩血管作用与吗啡相当。

4. 临床应用

1)吗啡

(1)疼痛：吗啡用于评分为 7 分以上的剧烈疼痛，如创伤、烧伤、晚期癌痛，对神经疼痛效果差；胆绞痛和肾绞痛患者需合用阿托品；吗啡可减轻心肌梗死患者疼痛、焦虑以及心脏负荷。

(2)心源性哮喘：心源性哮喘是指左心衰竭突发急性肺水肿引起呼吸困难、气喘。吗啡治疗心源性哮喘的机制如下：①扩张外周血管，使外周阻力降低，减轻心脏负荷；②消除患者紧张、焦虑、恐惧的情绪；③降低呼吸中枢对 CO_2 的敏感性，缓解浅表急促的呼吸。吗啡对尿毒症等其他原因引起的肺水肿也有效。休克、昏迷和严重肺部疾病患者禁用。

(3)腹泻：吗啡可以缓解急、慢性消耗性腹泻症状，如伴有细菌感染，应加用抗菌药。

2)哌替啶

(1)镇痛：哌替啶取代吗啡用于手术、创伤、癌痛等。胆绞痛和肾绞痛患者需合用阿托品。产妇临产前 2~4 小时不宜使用，易引发新生儿呼吸抑制。

(2)心源性哮喘：哌替啶取代吗啡用于治疗心源性哮喘。

(3)麻醉前给药和人工冬眠：哌替啶可缓解患者紧张、焦虑的情绪，减少麻醉药物用量。哌替啶、氯丙嗪、异丙嗪三者组成冬眠合剂。

5. 不良反应

1)吗啡

(1)治疗量吗啡可引起恶心、呕吐、便秘、呼吸抑制、排尿困难、胆绞痛、直立性低血压、免疫抑制等。

(2)长期使用吗啡易产生耐受性(tolerance)和成瘾性(addiction)。耐受性是指长期用药导致中枢神经系统对药物敏感性降低，需加大药物剂量才能达到原来的药效。成瘾性是指出现病态人格，有强迫性觅药行为。

(3)吗啡急性中毒表现为昏迷、深度呼吸抑制以及针尖样瞳孔，伴有缺氧，血压降低和尿潴留。吗啡急性中毒致死的主要原因是呼吸抑制，应立即人工呼吸、给氧以及静脉注射纳洛酮。吗啡合用麻醉药、镇静催眠药或酒精等会加重呼吸抑制。

2）哌替啶

哌替啶可引起吗啡类似的不良反应，如恶心、呕吐、直立性低血压等不良反应。大剂量哌替啶可明显抑制呼吸，长期应用易发生耐受性和成瘾性。

二、阿片受体拮抗药

1. 药品

阿片受体拮抗药有纳洛酮（naloxone）。

2. 药理作用

竞争性拮抗各型阿片受体。

3. 临床应用

（1）阿片类药物的急性中毒：首选用于已知或疑为阿片类药物中毒，可对抗阿片类药物引起的各种效应，使意识恢复清醒。

（2）解除阿片类药物所致麻醉术后呼吸抑制：纳洛酮可用于解救阿片类药物辅助麻醉后出现的术后呼吸抑制。当纳洛酮用药剂量过大或给药过快时，可减弱阿片类药物的镇痛效果，故应控制纳洛酮的给药剂量和给药速度。

（3）鉴别阿片类药物成瘾：纳洛酮可诱发阿片类药物成瘾者出现戒断症状，结合用药史和尿检结果进行鉴别。纳洛酮鉴别为阴性时，也不能排除阿片类药物成瘾。

（4）适用于治疗急性酒精中毒、脊髓损伤、脑卒中和脑外伤等。

（5）作为工具药用于研究疼痛与镇痛。

案例学习

学习要点：

（1）心源性哮喘药物治疗原则。

（2）药物成瘾。

关键词：吗啡；戒断症状；药物成瘾

案例一

一名53岁的男性患者，急诊入院。患者自述4个月前发生心肌梗死，经治疗后好转，近半个月未服用任何药物。3小时前，突然剧烈咳嗽，咳出粉红色泡沫样痰，不能平卧，患者烦躁不安，大汗淋漓。体格检查，患者心率120次/分钟，呼吸38次/分钟，血压165/96 mmHg，两肺可闻及湿啰音。该患者被诊断为心源性哮喘。

◎ 问答题

患者是否可以选用吗啡治疗，如果选用需要注意防范哪些风险？

案例二

一名26岁的男性患者来到医院急诊室。他自称海洛因成瘾，焦虑不安，伴有呕吐、腹泻和肌肉疼痛。体格检查，患者体温38.5℃，呼吸急促，瞳孔扩大。

◎ 问答题

患者出现这些体征和症状最可能的原因是什么？哪种药物可减轻患者的症状？

◎ 选择题

1. 关于阿片类镇痛药的药理学作用，以下描述正确的是（　　）。
   A. 有解热镇痛作用　　　B. 有抗炎作用　　　C. 有抗炎作用
   D. 镇痛作用强，无成瘾性　E. 镇痛作用强，反复使用易成瘾

2. 吗啡发挥镇痛作用的机制是（　　）。
   A. 激动中枢阿片受体　　B. 阻断中枢阿片受体　C. 抑制中枢PG的合成
   D. 抑制外周PG的合成　　E. 激动环氧化酶

3. 以下不属于吗啡药理作用的是（　　）。
   A. 镇痛　　B. 镇静　　C. 致欣快　　D. 呼吸抑制　　E. 泻下

4. 常用哌替啶替代吗啡的原因是（　　）。
   A. 镇痛作用强　　　　B. 呼吸抑制作用轻　　C. 对支气管平滑肌无影响
   D. 作用维持时间长　　E. 成瘾性轻

5. 以下不属于哌替啶临床应用的是（　　）。
   A. 手术镇痛　　　　B. 心源性哮喘　　　　C. 胆绞痛
   D. 镇咳　　　　　　E. 晚期癌症疼痛

6. 人工冬眠合剂的药物组成是（　　）。
   A. 哌替啶、氯丙嗪、异丙嗪　B. 哌替啶、氯丙嗪、丙咪嗪　C. 吗啡、氯丙嗪、异丙嗪
   D. 吗啡、氯丙嗪、丙咪嗪　　E. 芬太尼、哌替啶、氯丙嗪

7. 以下哪一种药物可以诱发吗啡成瘾者的戒断症状？（　　）
   A. 哌替啶　　B. 纳洛酮　　C. 美沙酮　　D. 芬太尼　　E. 阿托品

8. 以下哪一种药物可用于分娩止痛？（　　）
   A. 吗啡　　B. 甲基吗啡　　C. 哌替啶　　D. 可待因　　E. 纳洛酮

9. 一名42岁女性患者，右上腹部持续性疼痛，并阵发性加剧，且伴有恶心、呕吐，被诊断为胆绞痛，该患者宜用下列哪种药物治疗？（　　）
   A. 阿托品　　B. 阿司匹林　　C. 哌替啶　　D. 哌替啶与阿托品合用
   E. 阿司匹林与阿托品合用

10. 一名60岁男性患者，因严重癌痛服用吗啡缓释片，未经医生允许擅自缩短服药间隔，一周后出现了嗜睡、呼吸浅慢、瞳孔缩小和血压下降等症状。患者应立即使用下列哪种药物解救？（　　）
    A. 普萘洛尔　　B. 纳洛酮　　C. 去甲肾上腺素　　D. 肾上腺素　　E. 阿托品

📖 Case study

Key points：

(1) Principles of cardiac asthma pharmacotherapy.

(2) Drug addiction.

Key words: morphine; withdrawal symptoms; drug addiction

Case 1

A 53-year-old male patient was admitted to the hospital in an emergency. The patient reported that he had a myocardial infarction 4 months ago, which was treated and improved, and he had not taken any medication for the past half month. 3 hours ago, he suddenly coughed violently and coughed up pink foamy sputum, could not lie down, and was irritable and sweating profusely. Physical examination revealed that the patient's heart rate was 120 beats per minute, respiratory rate was 38 breaths per minute, blood pressure was 165/96 mmHg, and wet rhonchi could be heard in both lungs. The patient was diagnosed with cardiogenic asthma.

◎ **Essay questions**

Is morphine therapy an option for the patient and what are the current risks to guard against?

Case 2

A 26-year-old male patient presented to the hospital emergency room. He reported heroin addiction and anxiety with vomiting, diarrhea and muscle pain. Physical examination revealed that the patient had a temperature of 38.5℃, shortness of breath and greater pupil size than normal.

◎ **Essay questions**

What is the most likely cause for the patient's signs and symptoms? Which medication would alleviate the patient's symptoms?

Multiple-choice question

1. Which following statement about the pharmacological effect of opioid analgesics is correct? (　　)
   A. Have antipyretic and analgesic effects
   B. Have an anti-inflammatory effect
   C. Have anti-inflammatory effects
   D. They are powerful analgesics and non-addictive
   E. They are powerful analgesics and addictive when used repeatedly
2. The mechanism by which morphine exerts its analgesic effect is (　　).
   A. by activating central opioid receptors　　B. by blocking central opioid receptors
   C. by inhibiting central PG synthesis　　D. by inhibiting peripheral PG synthesis
   E. by activating cyclooxygenase
3. Which of the following is not a pharmacologic effect of morphine? (　　)
   A. Analgesia　　　B. Sedation　　　C. Euphoria
   D. Respiratory depression　　E. Diarrhea

4. What is the reason pethidine is commonly used as a substitute for morphine? (   )
   A. Pethidine has strong analgesic effects
   B. Pethidine has mild respiratory depression
   C. Pethidine does not affect bronchial smooth muscle
   D. Pethidine has a long duration of action
   E. Pethidine causes mild addiction
5. Which of the following is not a clinical application of pethidine? (   )
   A. Analgesia for surgery   B. Cardiogenic asthma
   C. Biliary colic   D. Cough suppression
   E. Advanced cancer pain
6. What is the drug composition of artificial hibernation compounds? (   )
   A. Pethidine, chlorpromazine, promethazine   B. Pethidine, chlorpromazine, imipramine
   C. Morphine, chlorpromazine, promethazine   D. Morphine, chlorpromazine, imipramine
   E. Fentanyl, pethidine, chlorpromazine
7. Which of the following drugs can induce withdrawal symptoms in morphine addicts? (   )
   A. Pethidine   B. Naloxone   C. Methadone
   D. Fentanyl   E. Atropine
8. Which of the following drugs can be used for labor pain relief? (   )
   A. Morphine   B. Methylmorphine C. Pethidine
   D. Codeine   E. Naloxone
9. A 42-year-old female patient with persistent pain in the right upper abdomen that worsened in paroxysms, accompanied by nausea and vomiting, was diagnosed with biliary colic. Which of the following treatments would be appropriate for her? (   )
   A. Atropine   B. Aspirin   C. Pethidine
   D. Pethidine and atropine   E. Aspirin and atropine
10. A 60-year-old male patient, who took morphine extended-release tablets for severe cancer pain, developed drowsiness, shallow and slowed respiration, miosis, and decreased blood pressure after he shortened the intervals without his physician's permission for a week. Which of the following drugs should he use immediately? (   )
    A. Propranolol   B. Naloxone   C. Norepinephrine
    D. Epinephrine   E. Atropine

第十八章案例学习和选择题答案

第十九章 解热镇痛抗炎药

知识要点

一、非选择性环氧化酶抑制药

1. 药品分类

(1) 水杨酸类：如阿司匹林(aspirin)。

(2) 苯胺类：如对乙酰氨基酚(acetaminophen)。

(3) 芳基丙酸类：如布洛芬(ibuprofen)。

2. 作用机制

解热镇痛抗炎药又名非甾体抗炎药(nonsteroidal anti-inflammatory drugs, NSAIDs)，发挥解热、镇痛、抗炎作用的主要机制是通过抑制环氧合酶(cyclooxygenase, COX)的活性，减少局部组织或者中枢部位的前列腺素(prostaglandin, PG)的合成。

COX 分为 COX-1、COX-2 等多种同工酶。COX-1 具有生理学功能，保护胃肠黏膜，调节血小板聚集、外周血管阻力和肾血流量分布。COX-2 为诱导型，可被损伤性因子或多种细胞因子诱导表达。NSAIDs 抑制 COX-1 引发药物不良反应，抑制 COX-2 可以减轻炎症。

1) 解热机制

在病理情况下，大量产生的细胞因子如 IL-1β、TNF-α、IFN-α 等，触发下丘脑视前区附近合成和释放前列腺素 E_2(PGE$_2$)，经环磷酸腺苷(cAMP)作用于体温调节中枢，使体温调定点上移，体温升高。NSAIDs 通过抑制下丘脑 COX，减少 PG 的合成，使体温调定点恢复正常。

2) 镇痛机制

NSAIDs 抑制 COX，减少 PG 的合成，阻断信号传导，降低局部痛觉感受器对致痛物质的敏感性。部分 NSAIDs 能作用脊髓，可阻碍中枢神经系统 PG 合成或干扰伤害感受系统的介质和调质的产生，产生镇痛作用。

3) 抗炎机制

在炎症反应过程中，组织产生的 PG 可致血管扩张和组织水肿，与缓激肽等协同致炎。NSAIDs 通过抑制 COX，减少 PG 的合成，以及抑制某些细胞黏附分子的活性表达，发挥抗炎作用。

4）其他

部分 NSAIDs 可使得血小板中的 COX 失活，不可逆性抑制血小板聚集。

3. 药理作用

1）阿司匹林

（1）解热镇痛及抗风湿：阿司匹林使发热者的体温恢复正常，对正常人的体温无明显影响；可用于轻度疼痛治疗，如头痛、牙痛、痛经等；减轻炎症引起的红、肿、热、痛等症状，可作为急性风湿热的鉴别诊断依据，迅速缓解风湿性关节炎的症状。

（2）影响血小板的功能：小剂量阿司匹林不可逆地抑制血小板 COX，减少血栓素（TXA_2）生成，从而抑制血小板的聚集，发挥抗血栓和抗凝血作用。注意：大剂量阿司匹林抑制血管壁内皮细胞的 COX，使前列环素（PGI_2）合成减少，促进血小板的聚集和血栓的形成。

（3）儿科用于皮肤黏膜淋巴结综合征（川崎病）的治疗。

2）对乙酰氨基酚

对乙酰氨基酚（扑热息痛）抑制中枢神经系统 COX，发挥解热镇痛作用，而对外周组织 COX 无明显作用，故无抗炎作用。

3）布洛芬

布洛芬有抗炎、解热、镇痛的作用。

4. 临床应用

1）阿司匹林

（1）阿司匹林（0.3~0.6 g/d）用于治疗感冒发热，以及疼痛评分为 1~3 分的头痛、牙痛、肌肉痛、痛经等。

（2）采用大剂量阿司匹林（3~5 g/d）抗风湿。

（3）采用小剂量阿司匹林（50~100 mg/d）预防和治疗缺血性心脏病、脑缺血病、房颤、人工心脏瓣膜、动静脉瘘或其他手术后的血栓形成。

（4）儿科治疗皮肤黏膜淋巴结综合征（川崎病）。

2）对乙酰氨基酚

用于解热和轻度疼痛治疗，同阿司匹林。对不适宜使用阿司匹林的发热或疼痛患者可使用该药。

3）布洛芬

用于风湿性关节炎、骨关节炎、强直性关节炎、急性肌腱炎、滑液囊炎等，也可用于感冒发热和轻度疼痛，如痛经等。

5. 不良反应

1）阿司匹林

（1）胃肠道反应：药物直接刺激胃黏膜和延髓催吐化学感应区，引发恶心呕吐；大剂量可抑制胃壁细胞 COX 减少 PGE_2 合成，导致胃溃疡、胃出血。合用 PGE_1 衍生物米索前列醇（misoprostol）可降低溃疡发生率。

（2）加重出血倾向：大剂量或长期使用阿司匹林可抑制凝血酶原的形成，导致凝血障碍，可用维生素 K 预防。严重肝功能不全、血友病、产妇、孕妇、凝血酶原合成功能低下者禁用。术前1周停用。

（3）水杨酸反应：阿司匹林（5 g/d）引发眩晕、恶心、呕吐、耳鸣、听力减退，严重者出现高热、脱水、酸碱平衡失调，甚至精神错乱。一旦出现中毒症状应立即停药，静脉滴注碳酸氢钠，碱化尿液，加速排泄。

（4）过敏反应：药物抑制PG合成，导致花生四烯酸生成白三烯以及其他脂氧酶代谢产物增加，引起支气管痉挛，诱发哮喘。"阿司匹林哮喘"不是基于抗原-抗体反应引发的过敏反应，肾上腺素对其无效。采用抗组胺药和糖皮质激素进行治疗。哮喘、鼻息肉及慢性荨麻疹患者禁用。

（5）瑞夷综合征（Reye syndrome）：急性肝脂肪变性-脑病综合征，表现为肝衰竭合并脑病。儿童病毒感染时应慎用阿司匹林退热。

（6）对肾脏的影响：阿司匹林抑制PG合成，损害了其对肾脏的保护作用，引起水肿、多尿等症状。

2）对乙酰氨基酚

过量中毒导致肝损伤，长期大量用药可造成肾毒性，如肾绞痛、肾衰竭等。

3）布洛芬

胃肠道反应、头痛、耳鸣、眩晕、支气管哮喘等。

二、选择性环氧化酶-2抑制药

1. 药品名称

二芳基吡唑类：塞来昔布（celecoxib）。

2. 药理作用

塞来昔布对COX-2的抑制作用较COX-1高375倍。在治疗剂量时，塞来昔布对COX-1无明显作用，对TXA_2的合成也无影响，但抑制PGI_2的合成。塞来昔布有抗炎、解热、镇痛的作用。

3. 临床应用

塞来昔布可用于风湿性、类风湿关节炎、骨关节炎、术后镇痛、牙痛、痛经、家族性腺瘤性息肉等。

4. 不良反应

塞来昔布引起胃肠道反应、出血和溃疡的概率较低。塞来昔布长期使用可出现较严重的心血管系统不良反应，如心肌梗死和卒中，有血栓形成倾向者慎用。磺胺类药物过敏者禁用。

案例学习

学习要点：

（1）阿司匹林的不良反应。

（2）花生四烯酸代谢通路。

关键词： 非甾体抗炎药；阿司匹林；对乙酰氨基酚

案例

一名45岁的女性患者，出现发热、头痛、鼻塞，前往医院就诊。患者自述因气候骤降受寒。体格检查显示体温为39℃，实验室检查显示外周血白细胞计数降低，流感病毒抗原检测阳性。医生诊断为流感，使用布洛芬退热。患者回家后，按医嘱服药。服药半小时后，患者胸口发闷、呼吸急促、喘息，进而出现紫绀、呼吸困难、大汗。患者被紧急送往医院急诊室。

◎ 问答题
1. 患者服药后出现异常的最可能原因是什么？
2. 患者应立即使用哪些药物治疗？

选择题

1. 非甾体抗炎药的退热机制是(   )。
   A. 抑制血栓素TXA_2合成　B. 抑制前列腺素PG合成　C. 抑制花生四烯酸合成
   D. 抑制白三烯合成　　　　 E. 抑制前列环素PGI_2合成

2. 解热镇痛抗炎药的镇痛机制是(   )。
   A. 抑制传入神经冲动传导　B. 激动阿片受体　　　C. 抑制PG的合成
   D. 抑制TXA_2的合成　　　E. 抑制白三烯合成

3. 关于非甾体抗炎药的药理学特征描述正确的是(   )。
   A. 具有解热和镇痛作用　B. 具有较强抗炎作用　C. 抑制脂加氧酶
   D. 促进血栓形成　　　　E. 可降低正常体温

4. 关于非甾体抗炎药的临床应用和不良反应，以下描述不正确的是(   )。
   A. 阿司匹林可用于预防术后血栓形成
   B. 布洛芬可用于骨关节炎的治疗
   C. 阿司匹林可与阿片样物质联用，降低术后疼痛
   D. 塞来昔布的胃溃疡发生率较高
   E. 肾功能低下患者长期使用对乙酰氨基酚可导致肾衰竭

5. 以下不属于阿司匹林不良反应的是(   )。
   A. 凝血障碍　B. 水杨酸反应　C. 瑞夷综合征　D. 过敏反应　E. 直立性低血压

6. 消化性溃疡患者可选用的退热药物是(   )。
   A. 阿司匹林　B. 吡罗昔康　C. 吲哚美辛　D. 对乙酰氨基酚　E. 布洛芬

7. 下列哪一种属于非选择性COX抑制剂的药物？(   )
   A. 丙磺舒　B. 罗非昔布　C. 塞来昔布　D. 布洛芬　E. 别嘌醇

8. 一名60岁女性，表现出早期类风湿关节炎的体征和症状，决定使用非甾体抗炎药治疗。如果患者有如下哪一种既往病史，不适宜使用塞来昔布控制她的关节炎症状？
   (   )
   A. 心肌梗死　B. 痛风　C. 哮喘　D. 骨质疏松　E. 消化性溃疡

9. 70岁老年男性患者因缺血性心脏病长期服用阿司匹林肠溶片，现需排期做胆结石手

术。已知阿司匹林半衰期为20分钟。患者停用阿司匹林多久后，可以进行手术？
（　　）

  A. 约2小时 B. 约24小时 C. 约72小时 D. 约5天 E. 约7天

10. 一名58岁的男性患者，因双膝关节疼痛一个月，前往就诊。医生诊断为风湿性关节炎。该患者可以使用以下哪些药物？（　　）

  A. 阿司匹林 B. 布洛芬 C. 对乙酰氨基酚 D. 双氯芬酸钠 E. 塞来昔布

Case study

Key points：

(1) Side effects of aspirin.

(2) Arachidonic acid metabolic pathway.

Key words：nonsteroidal anti-inflammatory drugs；aspirin；acetaminophen

Case

A 45-year-old female patient presented to the hospital with fever, headache and nasal congestion. The patient reported that she caught a cold due to the sudden drop in temperature. Physical examination revealed a temperature of 39℃. Laboratory tests showed a decreased peripheral blood leukocyte count and a positive test for influenza virus antigen. The doctor diagnosed influenza and used ibuprofen to treat fever. The patient went home and took the medication following the prescription. Half an hour after taking the medication, she developed chest tightness, shortness of breath, wheezing and then cyanosis, dyspnea and sweating. The patient went urgently to the hospital emergency room.

Essay questions

1. What is the most likely cause of the patient's abnormality after taking the medication?
2. What medications should the patient be treated with immediately?

Multiple-choice questions

1. What is the antipyretic mechanism of NSAIDs? (　　)

  A. Inhibition of thromboxane TXA_2 synthesis

  B. Inhibition of prostaglandin PG synthesis

  C. Inhibition of arachidonic acid synthesis

  D. Inhibition of leukotriene synthesis

  E. Inhibition of prostacyclin PGI_2 synthesis

2. What is the mechanism of analgesia with NSAIDs? (　　)

  A. NSAIDs inhibit afferent nerve impulse conduction

  B. NSAIDs agonize the opioid receptors

  C. NSAIDs inhibit PG synthesis

D. NSAIDs inhibit TXA$_2$ synthesis

E. NSAIDs inhibit leukotriene synthesis

3. Which following statement about the pharmacological characteristics of NSAIDs is accurate? (　　)

   A. All have antipyretic and analgesic effects

   B. All have strong anti-inflammatory effects

   C. All inhibit lipoxygenase

   D. All promote thrombosis

   E. All reduce normal body temperature

4. Which following statement about the clinical applications and adverse reactions of NSAIDs is incorrect? (　　)

   A. Aspirin can be used to prevent thrombosis after surgery

   B. Ibuprofen can be used for osteoarthritis treatment

   C. Aspirin and opioids can be combined to reduce postoperative pain

   D. Celecoxib has a higher incidence of gastric ulcer

   E. Long-term treatment of acetaminophen in patients with low kidney function can lead to kidney failure

5. Which of the following is not an adverse effect of aspirin? (　　)

   A. Coagulation disorder   B. Salicylic acid reaction

   C. Reye's syndrome   D. Allergic reaction

   E. Orthostatic hypotension

6. Which of the following drugs can be used by a patient with peptic ulcer? (　　)

   A. Aspirin   B. Piroxicam   C. Indomethacin

   D. Acetaminophen   E. Ibuprofen

7. Which of the following is a non-selective COX inhibitor? (　　)

   A. Probenecid   B. Rofecoxib   C. Celecoxib

   D. Ibuprofen   E. Allopurinol

8. A 60-year-old woman who exhibits signs and symptoms of early rheumatoid arthritis decides to be treated with an NSAID. The use of celecoxib to control the patient's arthritic symptoms is not appropriate if she has which of the following past medical history? (　　)

   A. Myocardial infarction   B. Gout   C. Asthma

   D. Osteoporosis   E. Peptic ulcer

9. A 70-year-old elderly male patient who has been taking aspirin enteric-coated tablets for a long time for ischemic heart disease has been scheduled for gallstone surgery. The half-life of aspirin is known to be 20 minutes. How long after discontinuing aspirin can this patient undergo surgery? (　　)

   A. About 2 hours   B. About 24 hours   C. About 72 hours

   D. About 5 days   E. About 7 days

10. A 58-year-old male patient went to the hospital with a month-long history of pain in both knees. The doctor diagnosed rheumatoid arthritis. Which of the following drugs could be used for this patient? (   )

   A. Aspirin
   B. Ibuprofen
   C. Acetaminophen
   D. Diclofenac sodium
   E. Celecoxib

第十九章案例学习和选择题答案

第二十章　离子通道概论及钙通道阻滞药

知识要点

一、钙通道阻滞药分类和代表药物

1. 选择性钙通道阻滞药

(1) 二氢吡啶类：硝苯地平、尼群地平、尼卡地平、氨氯地平、尼莫地平等。
(2) 苯并噻氮䓬类：地尔硫䓬、克仑硫䓬、二氯呋利等。
(3) 苯烷胺类：维拉帕米、加洛帕米、噻帕米等。

2. 非选择性钙通道阻滞药

非选择性钙通道阻滞药有普尼拉明、苄普地尔、卡罗维林、氟桂利嗪等。

二、药理作用

1. 对心肌的作用

(1) 负性肌力作用：减少心肌细胞内 Ca^{2+} 量，呈现负性肌力作用，并降低心肌耗氧量。同时，钙通道阻滞药的降压作用可使交感神经活性反射性增高，抵消部分负性肌力作用。

(2) 负性频率和负性传导作用：降低窦房结自律性，减慢房室结传导，减慢心率。此作用以维拉帕米和地尔硫䓬的作用最强。

2. 对平滑肌的作用

(1) 血管平滑肌：舒张血管，主要舒张动脉，又以冠状血管和脑血管较为敏感，也可舒张外周血管。

(2) 其他平滑肌：对支气管平滑肌的松弛作用较为明显，较大剂量也可松弛胃肠道、输尿管和子宫平滑肌。

(3) 抗动脉粥样硬化：①减少 Ca^{2+} 内流，减轻 Ca^{2+} 超载所致的动脉壁损害。②抑制平滑肌增殖和动脉基质蛋白质合成，增加血管壁顺应性。③抑制脂质过氧化，保护内皮细胞。④硝苯地平提高溶酶体酶和胆固醇酯的水解活性，降低细胞内胆固醇水平。

(4) 对红细胞和血小板结构和功能的影响：①红细胞：抑制 Ca^{2+} 内流，减轻 Ca^{2+} 超载对红细胞的损伤。②对血小板活化的抑制作用：地尔硫䓬抑制血栓素的产生和由 ADP、肾上腺素及 5-HT 等所引起的血小板聚集。

(5) 对肾功能的影响：钙通道阻滞药舒张血管的同时，不伴有水钠潴留作用。二氢吡啶类药物还能明显增加肾血流，排钠利尿。钙通道阻滞药对肾脏的保护作用，在伴有肾功能障碍的高血压病和心功能不全的治疗中都有重要意义。

三、临床应用

1. 高血压

二氢吡啶类药物扩张外周血管作用强，是控制高血压的常用药物。高血压兼有冠心病，选用硝苯地平；兼有脑血管病，选用尼莫地平；伴有快速性心律失常，选用维拉帕米。钙通道阻滞药可与β受体阻断药合用，消除反射性心动过速；也可与利尿药合用，消除扩管药引起的水钠潴留。

2. 心绞痛

（1）变异性心绞痛：硝苯地平疗效最佳。

（2）稳定型心绞痛：三类钙通道阻滞药均适用。

（3）不稳定型心绞痛：维拉帕米和地尔硫䓬疗效较好。

3. 心律失常

钙通道阻滞药治疗室上性心动过速及后除极触发活动所致心律失常效果良好。维拉帕米和地尔硫䓬减慢心率效果较明显。

4. 脑血管疾病

尼莫地平、氟桂利嗪可预防蛛网膜下腔出血引起的脑血管痉挛及脑栓塞。

5. 其他

钙通道阻滞药还可用于外周血管痉挛性疾病、雷诺病、预防动脉粥样硬化、支气管哮喘、偏头痛。

四、不良反应

面部潮红、头痛、眩晕、恶心、便秘等。维拉帕米和地尔硫䓬的严重不良反应有低血压及心功能抑制等。

案例学习

学习要点：

（1）掌握钙通道阻滞药抗高血压的作用机制、临床应用和降压特点。

（2）熟悉钙通道阻滞药的药物相互作用。

关键词：硝苯地平；高血压；心衰；地高辛

案例

男性，68岁，高血压患者，因有支气管哮喘和慢性肾小球肾炎病史，一直服用硝苯地平缓释片 20 mg，口服，1次/天治疗。一周前出现心衰症状，医嘱予以加服地高辛 0.25 mg，口服，1次/天。第5天出现恶心、呕吐、心律失常。

◎ 问答题

1. 结合二氢吡啶类钙通道阻滞药抗高血压的作用机制、临床应用和降压特点，谈谈本案例中选择硝苯地平缓释片抗高血压的原因。
2. 分析加用地高辛后出现上述症状的原因。
3. 上述患者的用药可以如何调整？

◎ 选择题

1. 能抑制血栓烷 A_2（TXA_2）的产生而抗血小板聚集的钙通道阻滞药是(　　)。
   A. 硝苯地平　　B. 地尔硫䓬　　C. 维拉帕米　　D. 普尼拉明　　E. 尼卡地平
2. 钙通道阻滞药不具有下列哪项作用？(　　)
   A. 负性肌力作用　　　B. 负性频率作用　　　C. 扩张血管作用
   D. 改善组织血流量　　E. 加快传导作用
3. 下列哪个药物属于非选择性钙通道阻滞药？(　　)
   A. 加洛帕米　　B. 尼莫地平　　C. 氟桂利嗪　　D. 地尔硫䓬　　E. 二氯呋利
4. 钙通道阻滞药的主要临床用途是(　　)。
   A. 高血压、心绞痛、心律失常
   B. 高血压、心衰、外周血管痉挛性疾病
   C. 心绞痛、哮喘、心衰
   D. 心衰、冠状动脉粥样硬化、心律失常
   E. 肝硬化、心衰、肾功能障碍
5. 钙通道阻滞药可能引起以下哪项不良反应？(　　)
   A. 心悸　　　　　　　B. 糖脂代谢紊乱　　　C. 肾功能损害
   D. 水和电解质紊乱　　E. 体位性低血压
6. 下列药物对心动频率抑制作用最强的是(　　)。
   A. 硝苯地平　　B. 地尔硫䓬　　C. 维拉帕米　　D. 普尼拉明　　E. 氟桂利嗪
7. 对脑血管有选择性扩张作用的钙通道阻滞药是(　　)。
   A. 硝苯地平　　B. 尼莫地平　　C. 氨氯地平　　D. 尼群地平　　E. 尼索地平
8. 患者，女，23 岁，受寒后手指会突然变白，局部发凉、麻木，有针刺感，持续几分钟后皮肤会变潮红，热饮后发作减缓。诊断为雷诺氏综合征，该患者可服用的治疗药物是(　　)。
   A. 地塞米松　　B. 维生素 E　　C. 维拉帕米　　D. 硝苯地平　　E. 氟桂利嗪
9. 患者，女，45 岁，长期从事脑力劳动，近一个月来出现旋转性头晕，伴有恶心呕吐、耳鸣等症状，头部有麻木感和持续胀痛，诊断为脑血管痉挛，该患者宜服用的药物为(　　)。
   A. 硝苯地平　　B. 地尔硫䓬　　C. 维拉帕米　　4. 尼群地平　　E. 氟桂利嗪
10. 患者，男，36 岁，经常熬夜。近期常感到心悸、无力、头晕。发作时 ECG 显示，心率 200 次/分，QRS 波呈室上性，且后无 P 波，诊断为阵发性室上性心动过速。患者可选用的治疗药物为(　　)。

A. 硝苯地平　　B. 地尔硫䓬　　C. 维拉帕米　　D. 普萘洛尔　　E. 地高辛

Case study

Key points:

(1) Master the mechanism of action, clinical application and antihypertensive characteristics of calcium channel blockers.

(2) Be familiar with the drug interaction of calcium channel blockers.

Key words: nifedipine; high blood pressure; heart failure; digoxin

Case

A 68-year-old man with hypertension and a history of bronchial asthma and chronic glomerulonephritis was treated with sustained release tabletof nifedipine 20 mg. po. qd. He developed symptoms of heart failure a week ago and was prescribed digoxin 0.25 mg. po. qd. Five days later, the symptoms of nausea, vomiting and arrhythmia occurred.

◎ **Essay questions**

1. Please explain the reason to choose sustained release tablet of nifedipine to treat hypertension in this case based on the mechanism, clinical use and antihypertensive character.
2. Please explain the reason of the symptom after the addition of digoxin.
3. What modification should be taken for this patient?

Multiple-choice questions

1. Which calcium channel blocker can inhibit the production of TXA_2 and has anti-platelet aggregation effect? (　　)
   A. Nifedipine　　　　B. Diltiazem　　　　C. Verapamil
   D. Prenylamine　　　E. Nicardipine
2. Which is not the action of calcium channel blockers? (　　)
   A. Negative inotropic action　　　B. Negative chronotropic action
   C. Vessel dilation effect　　　　　D. Improvement to tissue blood flow
   E. Acceleration to conduction
3. Which drug is non-selective calcium channel blocker? (　　)
   A. Gallopamil　　　　B. Nimodipine　　　　C. Flunarizine
   D. Diltiazem　　　　　E. Diclofurime
4. The main clinical uses of calcium channel blockers are (　　)
   A. hypertension, angina, arrhythmia
   B. hypertension, heart failure, peripheral vascular spasmodic disease
   C. angina, asthma, heart failure
   D. heart failure, atherosclerosis of coronary artery, arrhythmia

E. liver cirrhosis, heart failure, kidney dysfunction

5. Which adverse effect can be caused by calcium channel blockers? (   )
   A. Palpitation
   B. Glucose and lipid metabolism disorder
   C. Kidney dysfunction
   D. Water and electrolyte disturbance
   E. Postural hypotension

6. Which drug has the strongest negative chronotropic action to the heart? (   )
   A. Nifedipine
   B. Diltiazem
   C. Verapamil
   D. Prenylamine
   E. Flunarizine

7. Which calcium channel blocker has selective cerebrodilatation effect? (   )
   A. Nifedipine
   B. Nimodipine
   C. Amlodipine
   D. Nitrendipine
   E. Nisoldipine

8. Patient, female, 23 years old, her finger will suddenly become white, chilled, numb and tinging when catching cold, and several minutes later, the skin become flushed. The symptoms subsides after a hot drink. She is diagnosed as symmetrical asphyxia. Which drug can be used to treat this disease? (   )
   A. Dexamethasone
   B. Vitmin E
   C. Verapamil
   D. Nifedipine
   E. Flunarizine

9. A 45-year-old female patient, who is engaged in mental work for a long time, feels rotational dizziness, nausea, vomiting, tinnitus, numbness and persistent swelling pain in the head this month. She is diagnosed as cerebral angiospasm. Which drug can be used to treat this disease? (   )
   A. Nipedipine
   B. Diltiazem
   C. Verapamil
   D. Nitrendipine
   E. Flunarizine

10. A 36-year-old male patient, who often stays up late at night, feels palpitation, fatigue and swirled these days. ECG indicates that his heart beating rate is 200 bpm, QRS wave is supraventricular, without P save behind it. He is diagnosed as paroxysmal supraventricular tachycardia. Which drug can be used to treat this patient? (   )
    A. Nipedipine
    B. Diltiazem
    C. Verapamil
    D. Propranolol
    E. Digoxin

第二十章案例学习和选择题答案

第二十一章　抗心律失常药

知识要点

一、抗心律失常药的基本作用机制

抗心律失常药通过降低自律性、减少后除极、消除折返来发挥作用。

1. 降低自律性

可通过降低动作电位 4 相斜率、提高动作电位发生阈值、增加静息膜电位绝对值、延长动作电位时程等方式降低异常自律性。

2. 减少后除极

钙通道阻滞药通过抑制细胞内钙超载减少迟后除极；钠通道阻滞药抑制迟后除极 0 相去极化。缩短动作电位时程的药物可减少早后除极。

3. 消除折返

药物改变传导性或延长有效不应期可消除折返。

二、抗心律失常药的分类

1. Ⅰ类

钠通道阻滞药：根据作用强度，分为 Ia、Ib、Ic 三个亚类。Ia 类适度阻滞钠通道，降低动作电位 0 相上升速率，不同程度抑制心肌细胞膜 K^+、Ca^{2+} 通透性，延长复极过程，以延长有效不应期最为显著。本类药有奎尼丁、普鲁卡因胺等。Ib 类轻度阻滞钠通道，轻度减慢动作电位 0 相上升速率，降低自律性，缩短或不影响动作电位时程，本类药有利多卡因、苯妥英钠等。Ic 类明显阻滞钠通道，显著减低动作电位 0 相上升速率和幅度，减慢传导作用最明显，代表药为普罗帕酮、氟卡尼等。

2. Ⅱ类

β 受体阻断药：阻断心肌 β 受体，减慢 4 相自动除极而降低自律性，降低动作电位 0 相上升速率，减慢传导，代表药为普萘洛尔等。

3. Ⅲ类

延长动作电位时程药：阻滞多种钾通道，抑制钾电流，延长动作电位时程和有效不应期，但对动作电位幅度和去极化速率影响很小，代表药为胺碘酮。

4. Ⅳ类

钙通道阻滞药：抑制 L 型 Ca^{2+} 内流，降低窦房结自律性，减慢房室传导，抑制细胞内钙超载，代表药为维拉帕米、地尔硫䓬等。

三、常用抗心律失常药

1. 奎尼丁

（1）药理作用及机制：阻滞激活状态的钠通道，并使通道复活减慢，抑制异位起搏和除极化组织的兴奋性和传导性，延长除极化组织的不应期。抑制钾外流而延长心房、心室细胞及浦肯野纤维的动作电位时程和有效不应期，消除折返，产生抗心律失常作用。还有抗胆碱和阻滞外周血管 α 受体作用。

（2）临床应用：广谱抗心律失常药，适用于房颤、房扑、室上性和室性心动过速转复和预防，也可用于频发室上性和室性早搏的治疗。

（3）不良反应：腹泻、金鸡纳反应、房室及室内传导阻滞、Q-T 间期延长、尖端扭转型室性心动过速、血管扩张、血压下降、增加窦性心率、加快房室传导。

2. 利多卡因

（1）药理作用及机制：抑制阻滞钠通道的激活和失活状态，对除极化心室组织作用强（如缺血区）；阻止 2 相钠内流，缩短浦氏纤维和心室肌 APD；减少动作电位 4 相去极斜率，降低自律性。对正常心肌细胞的电生理特性影响小。

（2）临床应用：室性心律失常，如心脏手术、心导管术、急性心肌梗死或强心苷中毒所致室性心动过速或室颤。

（3）不良反应：头晕、嗜睡、感觉异常；心率减慢、房室传导阻滞和低血压，二、三度房室传导阻滞者禁用。眼球震颤是利多卡因中毒的早期信号。

3. 普罗帕酮

（1）药理作用及机制：明显阻滞心肌 Na^+ 通道开放态和失活态；减慢心房、心室和浦氏纤维的传导速度；抑制钾通道，绝对延长 ERP。

（2）临床应用：维持室上性心动过速（包括房颤）的窦性心律，也用于治疗室性心律失常。

（3）不良反应：折返性室性心动过速，充血性心衰；消化道不良反应，如恶心、呕吐、味觉改变等；窦性心动过缓、支气管痉挛。肝肾功能不全，心电图 QRS 延长超过 20% 或 Q-T 间期明显延长者宜减量或停药。

4. 普萘洛尔

（1）药理作用及机制：阻断 β 受体而发挥作用。抑制窦房结、心房、浦氏纤维自律性；降低儿茶酚胺所致的迟后除极而防止触发活动；减慢房室传导；延长房室交界细胞的有效不应期。

（2）临床应用：主要用于室上性心律失常，尤其是交感神经兴奋性过高、甲亢及嗜铬细胞瘤引起的窦性心动过速，也可用于运动、情绪变动所致室性心律失常。

（3）不良反应：窦性心动过缓、房室传导阻滞、低血压；精神抑郁、记忆力减退；诱发心衰和哮喘。长期应用可引起糖脂代谢异常。突然停药可致反跳现象。

5. 胺碘酮

（1）药理作用及机制：阻滞 K^+、Na^+、Ca^{2+} 通道；降低窦房结和浦氏纤维自律性和传导性；明显延长心肌 APD、ERP；非竞争性阻断 α、β 受体，扩张冠脉。

(2)临床应用：广谱，对房扑、房颤、室上性、室性心动过速均有效。

(3)不良反应：窦性心动过缓、房室传导阻滞以及 Q-T 间期延长，静脉给药可能引起低血压，长期应用可见角膜褐色微粒沉着、甲状腺功能障碍、间质性肺炎、肝坏死。

6. 维拉帕米

(1)药理作用及机制：阻滞激活、失活状态的 L 型钙通道。降低窦房结和缺血时的异位自律性，减少或消除后除极所引发的触发活动；减慢房室传导，终止房室结折返，防止心房扑动、心房颤动引起的心室率加快；延长窦房结、房室结的有效不应期。

(2)临床应用：室上性和房室结折返性心律失常，是阵发性室上性心动过速的首选用药。

(3)不良反应：口服安全，静脉给药可引起血压降低、暂时窦性停搏。二、三度房室传导阻滞、心功能不全、心源性休克病人禁用。老年人、肾功能低下者慎用。

案例学习

学习要点：

(1)掌握抗心律失常药物分类、经典抗心律失常药物作用机制、临床应用和不良反应。

(2)熟悉不同抗心律失常药物的作用特点、注意事项。

(3)了解不同类型心律失常如何选择治疗药物。

关键词：抗心律失常药物；奎尼丁；利多卡因；普罗帕酮；普萘洛尔；胺碘酮；维拉帕米

案例

张先生，56 岁，公司部门经理。某天的部门会议中，他感到心脏跳动不规则，伴有恶心感。坚持开完会议后，他仍然感到气短和不适，因而到医院就医。医生检查发现患者心率 120~150 次/分，心律不齐；血压 130/75 mmHg，血氧饱和度 100%。ECG 提示心房纤颤，没有明显缺血表现。医生予以静滴地尔硫䓬治疗后，患者心律降到 75~90 次/分，但心律仍然不齐。用药 12 小时后，房颤仍然持续，患者仍有心悸感。因此，在 ECG 监护下，医生予以患者静滴伊布利特治疗，30 分钟后患者恢复窦性心律。随后，患者出院，予以口服阿司匹林治疗。

患者出院 3 周后，再次出现心悸表现。医生建议在阿司匹林基础上，加服胺碘酮 400 mg/kg。用药后患者心悸症状明显缓解，但用药 4 周后，患者无明显诱因出现干咳、呼吸困难、乏力、厌食、胸痛等表现，X 线胸片表现为双侧弥漫性间质改变及广泛斑片状肺泡浸润。停用胺碘酮并予以泼尼松治疗后肺部症状明显缓解。出院后予以胺碘酮 200 mg/kg 维持治疗，患者耐受良好。

◎ 问答题

1. 为什么地尔硫䓬减慢患者心率但不能改善房颤？
2. 为什么伊布利特必须在 ECG 监护下才能用药？

3. 为什么伊布利特和胺碘酮对房颤治疗有效？
4. 胺碘酮大剂量应用后可能导致哪些不良反应？
5. 阿司匹林用于房颤治疗的用药目的和作用机制是什么？

选择题

1. 治疗阵发性室上性心动过速的首选药物是（　　）。
   A. 利多卡因　　B. 阿托品　　C. 地高辛　　D. 普萘洛尔　　E. 维拉帕米
2. 关于胺碘酮的药理作用，下列哪种说法正确？（　　）
   A. α受体激动剂　B. β受体激动剂　C. 激活钙通道　D. 抑制钾通道　E. 激活钠通道
3. 利多卡因对哪种心律失常无效（　　）。
   A. 心梗致室性心律失常　　B. 强心苷中毒致室性心律失常　　C. 心室纤颤
   D. 室上性心律失常　　　　E. 室性早搏
4. 治疗强心苷中毒引起的窦性心动过缓和轻度房室传导阻滞宜选用（　　）。
   A. 异丙肾上腺素　B. 苯妥英钠　C. 肾上腺素　D. 利多卡因　E. 阿托品
5. 下列关于奎尼丁抗心律失常作用的叙述，错误的是（　　）。
   A. 降低浦肯野纤维自律性
   B. 对钠通道、钾通道都有抑制作用
   C. 延长心房、心室和浦肯野纤维的动作电位时程和有效不应期
   D. 轻度阻滞钠通道，缩短浦氏纤维和心室肌的动作电位时程
   E. 减慢心房、心室和浦肯野纤维传导性
6. 长期应用会导致角膜褐色颗粒沉着的抗心律失常药是（　　）。
   A. 奎尼丁　　B. 普萘洛尔　　C. 利多卡因　　D. 胺碘酮　　E. 普罗帕酮
7. 患者，男性，突发心前区剧痛，急诊诊断为急性心肌梗死，并伴室性心动过速，应首选的抗心律失常药物是（　　）。
   A. 奎尼丁　　B. 维拉帕米　　C. 普罗帕酮　　D. 利多卡因　　E. 地高辛
8. 患者，男性，70岁，活动后气短进行性加重3年，突发心悸伴喘憋2小时。既往陈旧性前壁心肌梗死4年。查体：BP 160/70 mmHg，P 96次/分，端坐位，双肺可闻及湿啰音，心率125次/分，心律绝对不齐，第一心音强弱不等。诊断为陈旧性前壁心肌梗死、慢性心功能不全合并房颤。控制该患者心律失常的首选药物是（　　）。
   A. 地尔硫䓬　　B. 利多卡因　　C. 普罗帕酮　　D. 维拉帕米　　E. 胺碘酮
9. 患者服用某抗心律失常药一段时间后感觉畏寒和疲倦，体检显示其促甲状腺激素水平升高。以下哪种药物最有可能引起上述不良反应？（　　）
   A. 普鲁卡因胺　　B. 索他洛尔　　C. 多非利特　　D. 维拉帕米　　E. 胺碘酮
10. 患者，女性，45岁，服用苯妥英钠和奎尼丁治疗以控制房颤，还服用小剂量的安定治疗失眠以及接受雌激素替代疗法。近期，因尿路感染在接受环丙沙星治疗。近几个月来出现耳鸣、听力减退、头痛、恶心和视力模糊等现象。可能引起上述不良反应的药物是（　　）。
    A. 环丙沙星　　B. 雌激素　　C. 苯妥英钠　　D. 安定　　E. 奎尼丁

Case study

Key points:

(1) Master the classification of antiarrhythmic drugs, mechanism of action, clinical application and adverse reactions of classical antiarrhythmic drugs.

(2) Be familiar with the action characteristics and precautions of different antiarrhythmic drugs.

(3) Understand how to choose treatment drugs for different types of arrhythmia.

Key words: antiarrhythmic drugs; quinidine; lidocaine; propafenone; propranolol; amiodarone; verapamil

Case

Mr. Zhang, 56 years old, department manager. One day during a department meeting, he felt his heart beat irregularly, accompanied by nausea. He still felt short of breath and uncomfortable after the meeting, so he went to the hospital for medical treatment. His heart rate was 120-150 beats/min and arrhythmia, blood pressure was 130/75 mmHg, oxyhemoglobin saturation was 100%. ECG showed atrial fibrillation without obvious ischemia. After treatment with diltiazem, his heart rate dropped to 75-90 beats/min, but the rhythm remained uneven. After 12 hours of medication, atrial fibrillation continued and the patient still had palpitations. Therefore, the patient was treated with intravenous ibutilide under ECG monitoring and returned to sinus rhythm 30 minutes later. The patient was subsequently discharged and given oral aspirin.

The patient's palpitations recurred 3 weeks after discharge. Doctors recommended amiodarone 400 mg/kg in addition to aspirin. Palpitation symptoms were significantly relieved after medication, but 4 week later, the patient had no obvious causes of dry cough, dyspnea, fatigue, anorexia, chest pain and other manifestations, and X-ray chest films showed bilateral diffuse interstitial changes and extensive patchy alveolar infiltration. The pulmonary symptoms were relieved after amiodarone was discontinued and prednisone was given. After discharge, amiodarone was given 200 mg/kg maintenance therapy, which was well tolerated by the patient.

◎ **Essay questions**

1. Why does diltiazem slow patients' heart rate but not improve atrial fibrillation?
2. Why should ibutilide be administered under ECG monitoring?
3. Why are ibutilide and amiodarone effective for AF treatment?
4. What adverse reactions may be caused by large doses of amiodarone?
5. What are the purpose and the mechanism of aspirin in the treatment of atrial fibrillation?

Multiple-choice questions

1. The first choice for the treatment of paroxysmal supraventricular tachycardia is (   ).

A. lidocaine B. atropine C. digoxin
   D. propranolol E. verapamil
2. Which of the following is right about the pharmacological effects of amiodarone ( ).
   A. α-receptor agonists B. β-receptor agonists
   C. activate calcium channels D. inhibit potassium channels
   E. activate sodium channels
3. Which arrhythmias do not respond to lidocaine? ( )
   A. Ventricular arrhythmias caused by myocardial infarction
   B. Ventricular arrhythmias caused by cardiac glycoside poisoning
   C. Ventricular fibrillation
   D. Supraventricular arrhythmia
   E. Premature ventricular beats
4. Sinus bradycardia and mild atrioventricular block caused by cardiac glycoside poisoning should be treated with ( ).
   A. isoproterenol B. phenytoin sodium C. adrenaline
   D. lidocaine E. atropine
5. Which of the following statements is incorrect about the antiarrhythmic effects of quinidine? ( )
   A. Reduces the autorhythmicity of Purkinje fibers
   B. Inhibits both sodium channel and potassium channels
   C. Prolongs the action potential duration and effective refractory period of atrial, ventricular and Purkinje fibers
   D. Mildly blocks sodium channels and shortens the action potential duration of the Purkinje fibers and ventricular muscles
   E. Decreases atrial, ventricular, and Purkinje fiber conductivity
6. Which antiarrhythmic drugs can cause corneal brown granules after long-term use? ( )
   A. Quinidine B. Propranolol C. Lidocaine
   D. Amiodarone E. Propafenone
7. The patient, male, has acute precardiac pain and is diagnosed as acute myocardial infarction with ventricular tachycardia. The first choice of antiarrhythmic drug is ( ).
   A. quinidine B. verapamil C. propafenone
   D. lidocaine E. digoxin
8. Patient, male, 70 years old. His shortness of breath after the activity increased progressively for 3 years. Today, he has sudden heart palpitation accompanied by gasping for 2 hours. He has had previous old anterior wall myocardial infarction for 4 years. Physical examination: BP 160/70mmHg, P 96 times/min, sitting position, moist rales can be heard in both lungs, heart rate 125 times/min, absolute arrhythmia, the first heart sound intensity is different. The diagnosis is old anterior myocardial infarction, chronic cardiac insufficiency combined with

atrial fibrillation. The preferred drug for controlling arrhythmia in this patient is ( ).

    A. diltiazem   B. lidocaine   C. propafenone

    D. verapamil   E. amiodarone

9. The patient felt chills and fatigue after taking an antiarrhythmic drug for a period of time, and physical examination revealed elevated levels of thyrotropin. Which of the following drugs is most likely to cause these adverse reactions? ( )

    A. Procainamine   B. Sotalol   C. Dofilide

    D. Verapamil   E. Amiodarone

10. Patient, female, 45 years old. Sheis treated with phenytoin and quinidine to control atrial fibrillation, small doses of diazepam for insomnia and estrogen replacement therapy. She is recently treated with ciprofloxacin for a urinary tract infection. Tinnitus, hearing loss, headache, nausea and blurred vision occur in recent months. The drugs that may cause the above adverse reactions is ( ).

    A. ciprofloxacin   B. estrogen   C. phenytoin sodium

    D. diazepam   E. quinidine

第二十一章案例学习和选择题答案

第二十二章 作用于肾素-血管紧张素系统的药物

知识要点

一、肾素抑制药

通过结合肾素作用于肾素-血管紧张素系统，阻止血管紧张素原转化为血管紧张素I，降低血浆肾素、血管紧张素I和血管紧张素II水平，抑制RAS功能。代表药物为阿利吉仑。

二、血管紧张素转化酶抑制药(ACEI)

1. 药理作用

抑制AngII生成；保存缓激肽活性；保护血管内皮细胞功能；保护心肌细胞功能；增敏胰岛素受体。

2. 临床应用

高血压；充血性心力衰竭与心肌梗死；糖尿病肾病和其他肾病。

3. 不良反应

首剂低血压；咳嗽；高血钾；低血糖；肾功能损伤；引起胎儿畸形、发育不良或死胎；血管神经性水肿；含-SH结构的ACEI可产生味觉障碍、皮疹、白细胞减少等青霉胺样反应。

4. 常用ACEI

(1)卡托普利：第一个应用于临床的ACEI。结构含有-SH基团，直接抑制ACE。临床主要用于治疗高血压、充血性心力衰竭、心肌梗死、糖尿病肾病。不良反应除了咳嗽等不良反应外，因含-SH基团，可有青霉胺样反应。禁用于双侧肾动脉狭窄患者和孕妇。

(2)其他ACEI：依那普利、耐诺普利、贝那普利、福辛普利。

三、血管紧张素II受体阻断药(ARB)

1. 基本药理作用与应用

AT_1受体被阻滞后，AngII收缩血管和刺激肾上腺皮质释放醛固酮的作用被抑制，导致血压下降。AT_1受体阻断药能通过减轻心脏后负荷治疗充血性心力衰竭，也可通过抑制AngII所介导的心血管细胞增殖肥大作用防治心血管重构。

2. 常用AT_1受体阻断药

(1)氯沙坦：对AT_1受体有选择性阻断作用，可用于高血压的治疗。不良反应少，较少发生干咳，少数患者用药后出现眩晕。禁用于孕妇、哺乳期妇女和肾动脉狭窄者。

（2）其他常用药物：如缬沙坦、厄贝沙坦、坎地沙坦。

案例学习

学习要点：
（1）掌握血管紧张素转化酶抑制药的药理作用和适应证。
（2）掌握血管紧张素转化酶抑制药的不良反应和处理措施。
（3）掌握血管紧张素转化酶抑制药与 AT_1 受体阻断药的异同点。
关键词： 血管紧张素转化酶抑制药；高血压；心衰；利尿药；AT_1 受体阻断药

案例

王先生，50岁，体检时发现高血压。因患者有肝炎和严重的肝功能不良，医生予以卡托普利治疗，并嘱咐首剂减半。患者服药1月后血压控制良好，但抱怨不明原因的干咳。医生停用卡托普利，换成缬沙坦继续治疗，患者自述干咳的现象得到缓解。5年后患者因肝硬化水肿就医，医生加用螺内酯治疗。一周后查血电解质发现血钾浓度为 6.5 mmol/L，换用氢氯噻嗪后血钾降至正常。

问答题

1. 患者有严重的肝功能不良，在选择血管紧张素转化酶抑制药或 AT_1 受体阻断药时需要注意哪些问题？
2. 为什么卡托普利首剂要减半？
3. 请解释本案例中缬沙坦替代卡托普利治疗高血压的机制。
4. 请解释本案例中用氢氯噻嗪替代螺内酯的原因。

选择题

1. 有关血管紧张素转化酶抑制药的叙述，错误的是（　　）。
   A. 减少血管紧张素Ⅱ的生成　　B. 减少缓激肽降解　　C. 减轻心室扩张
   D. 增加醛固酮的生成　　E. 降低心脏前、后负荷
2. 血管紧张素转化酶抑制药的禁忌证不包括（　　）。
   A. 孕妇　　B. 高血钾　　C. 糖尿病　　D. 哺乳期妇女　E. 双侧肾动脉狭窄
3. 可特异性抑制肾素-血管紧张素转化酶的药物是（　　）。
   A. 可乐定　　B. 氢氯噻嗪　　C. 利血平　　D. 依那普利　　E. 呋塞米
4. 对于高血压合并2型糖尿病患者，下列药物有利于延缓糖尿病肾病进展的是（　　）。
   A. 普萘洛尔　　B. 吲达帕胺　　C. 缬沙坦　　D. 硝苯地平　　E. 氢氯噻嗪
5. 患者，男性，55岁，高血压病史5年，头痛频繁发作1周，嗜烟酒，肥胖，血糖轻度升高，超声心动图示左心室壁轻度增厚。降压宜首选的药物是（　　）。
   A. 硝苯地平　　B. 普萘洛尔　　C. 氢氯噻嗪　　D. 依那普利　　E. 哌唑嗪
6. 患者，男性，30岁，间断水肿3年，血压升高4个月。查体：BP 165/95 mmHg，双下

肢轻度水肿。尿沉渣镜检：RBC30~35/HP，尿蛋白定量 1.5g/24h。血肌酐 135 μmol/L，血清白蛋白 42 g/L。患者降压治疗首选的药物是（　　）。

　　A. 血管紧张素转换酶抑制药　　B. α 受体拮抗药　　C. β 受体拮抗药

　　D. 钙通道阻滞药　　E. 利尿药

7. 最易引起干咳的降压药是（　　）。

　　A. 美托洛尔　　B. 卡托普利　　C. 哌唑嗪　　D. 硝苯地平　　E. 氢氯噻嗪

8. 患者，女性，67 岁，双下肢水肿 1 个月，既往高血压病史 15 年，未规范用药治疗。查体：BP 160/100 mmHg，双下肢轻度凹陷性水肿。实验室检查：血肌酐 107 μmol/L，血钾 3.4 mmol/L，尿蛋白（++）。应首选的降压药物是（　　）。

　　A. 钙通道阻滞药　　B. α 受体阻滞药　　C. 噻嗪类利尿药

　　D. 血管紧张素转换酶抑制药　　E. β 受体阻滞药

9. 关于 AT_1 受体阻断药的叙述，正确的是（　　）。

　　A. 反馈性增加血浆肾素，导致血浆 AngII 浓度升高

　　B. 与血管紧张素转换酶抑制药比较，作用更广泛

　　C. 不会引起高血钾

　　D. AT_1 受体被阻滞后醛固酮产生增加

　　E. 促进心肌细胞增殖肥大

10. 血管紧张素转换酶抑制药与其他降压药相比，特点中不包括（　　）。

　　A. 长期应用不易引起脂质代谢紊乱

　　B. 能防止或逆转心肌肥大和血管增生

　　C. 适用于各型高血压

　　D. 改善高血压患者的生活质量

　　E. 降压作用强大，可伴有明显的反射性心率加快

📖 Case study

Key points：

(1) Master the pharmacological effects and indications of angiotensin-converting enzyme inhibitors.

(2) Master the adverse reactions and treatment measures of angiotensin converting enzyme inhibitors.

(3) Master the similarities and differences between angiotensin converting enzyme inhibitors and AT_1 receptor blockers.

Key words：angiotensin converting enzyme inhibitor; high blood pressure; heart failure; diuretic; AT_1 receptor blocker

Case

Mr. Wang, 50-year-old, was found hypertension in the physical exam. Since he had hepatitis and serous hepatic insufficiency, he was given captopril, with the first dose halved, to treat hypertension. Mr. Wang's blood pressure was well controlled, but he complained cough with unknown reason. Then he was asked to take valsartan instead of captopril. Several days later, the symptom of cough was relieved. Five years later, he was hospitalized due to cirrhotic edema, and spirolactone was added for his treatment. One week later, the electrolyte exam found that the serum potassium level was 6.5 mmol/L. His serum potassium reduced to normal after spirolactone was switched to hydrochlorothiazide.

◎ **Essay questions**

1. What is the caution when an ACEI or AT_1 receptor blocker is chosen to treat the patient with severe hepatic dysfunction?
2. Why should captopril be initiated with half dose?
3. Please explain the mechanism that the replacement of valsartan for captopril in this case?
4. Why was hydrochlorothiazide administered as the replacement of spirolactone in this case?

Multiple-choice questions

1. Which is incorrect about the statement of angiotensin conversing enzyme inhibitor? (   )
    A. Reduce the formation of angiotensinII   B. Reduce the degradation of bradykinin
    C. Relieve ventricular dilatation   D. Increase the production of aldosterone
    E. Reduce the preload and afterload of the heart
2. The contraindication of ACEI does not include (   ).
    A. pregnant women   B. hyperkalemia   C. diabetes
    D. nursing mother   E. bilateral renal artery stenosis
3. Which drug specifically inhibits ACE? (   )
    A. Clonidine   B. Hydrochlorothiazide   C. Reserpine
    D. Enalapril   E. Furosemide
4. Which drug is helpful to delay the progression of diabetic nephropathy to the patient who has hypertension and type 2 diabetes? (   )
    A. Propranolol   B. Indapamide   C. Valsartan
    D. Nifedipine   E. Hydrochlorothiazide
5. Patient, male, 55-year-old, has had hypertension for 5 years and headache for 1 week. He is fat and addicted to tobacco and wine. His blood glucose is mildly increased. The ultrasonic cardiogram reveals slight thickening of the left ventricular wall. The first choice for the treatment of hypertension is (   ).
    A. nifedipine   B. propranolol   C. hydrochlorothiazide
    D. enalapril   E. prazosin
6. Patient, male, 30-year-old, has had edema for 3 years and hypertension for 4 months. The physical exam finds the blood pressure of 165/95 mmHg and mild edema of both lower legs. Urine sediment microscopy reveals that the red blood cell is 30-35/HP, urine protein

1.5 g/24h. Scr 135 μmol/L, ALB 42 g/L. The first choice for his hypertension is (   ).
   A. ACEI
   B. α-receptor blocker
   C. β-receptor blocker
   D. calcium channel blocker
   E. diuretics

7. The antihypertensive drug that can cause cough is (   ).
   A. metoprolol
   B. captopril
   C. prazosin
   D. nifedipine
   E. hydrochlorothiazide

8. A 67-year-old female has had hypertension for 15 years and edema of both lower legs for one month, she has not regular pharmacological treatment. Physical exam indicates the blood pressure of 160/100 mmHg and mild edema of both lower legs. Scr is 107 μmol/L, potassium is 3.4 mmol/L, urine protein (++). The first choice of antihypertensive drug is (   ).
   A. calcium channel blocker
   B. α-receptor blocker
   C. thiazide diuretic
   D. ACEI
   E. β-receptor blocker

9. Which is the right description about AT_1 receptor blockers? (   )
   A. Increases plasma renin and AngII level
   B. Has more indications than ACEI
   C. Does not cause hyperkalemia
   D. Increases the production of aldosterone
   E. Induces the cardiac hypertrophy.

10. The character of ACEIs compared with other antihypertensive drug does not include (   ).
    A. long-term application does cause lipid metabolism disorders
    B. prevent or reverse myocardial hypertrophy and vascular hyperplasia
    C. are indicated to all types of hypertension
    D. improve the quality of life of hypertensive patients
    E. the antihypertensive effect is powerful and can be accompanied by a significant reflexive heart rate increase

第二十二章案例学习和选择题答案

第二十三章 利 尿 药

知识要点

一、利尿药的分类

按其作用靶点或作用机制分为以下七类：

（1）钠钾二氯共转运体抑制药，也称袢利尿药，为高效能利尿药，主要作用于髓袢升支粗段，抑制 Na^+-K^+-$2Cl^-$ 共转运体，利尿作用强，代表药为呋塞米。

（2）钠氯共转运体抑制药，包括噻嗪类及类噻嗪类利尿药，为中效能利尿药，主要作用于远曲小管近端，抑制 Na^+-Cl^- 共转运体，如氢氯噻嗪、吲达帕胺等。

（3）醛固酮受体阻断药，属于保钾利尿药，为低效能利尿药，主要作用于远曲小管远端和集合管，拮抗醛固酮作用，利尿作用弱，减少 K^+ 排出，如螺内酯、依普利酮等。

（4）上皮钠通道阻滞药，属于保钾利尿药和低效能利尿药，主要抑制远曲小管远端和集合管上皮细胞表达的 Na^+ 通道，利尿作用弱，减少 K^+ 排出，如氨苯蝶啶、阿米洛利等。

（5）碳酸酐酶抑制药，主要作用于近曲小管，抑制碳酸酐酶活性，利尿作用弱，代表药为乙酰唑胺。

（6）精氨酸升压素受体阻断药，单纯抑制集合管水的重吸收发挥利尿作用，其对电解质的排泄影响较小，代表药为托伐普坦。

（7）渗透性利尿药，也称为脱水药，主要通过提高血浆渗透压，产生组织脱水作用，并作用于髓袢及肾小管其他部位产生渗透性利尿作用，代表药为甘露醇。

二、常用利尿药

1. 呋塞米

呋塞米又名速尿，是钠钾二氯共转运体抑制药中最先应用于临床、最具代表性的药物，其利尿作用迅速、强大、短暂。

1）药理作用

（1）利尿。呋塞米可逆地结合髓袢升支粗段的钠钾二氯共转运体，减少 Na^+、K^+ 和 Cl^- 的重吸收，降低肾的稀释功能和浓缩功能，排出大量等渗尿，利尿作用快而强。

（2）扩张血管。抑制前列腺素（PG）分解酶的活性，使 PGE_2 含量增加，还可以降低血管对血管收缩因子的反应性，以及开放阻力血管钾离子通道，起扩张血管作用。扩张肾血管，增加肾血流量尤其是肾皮质血流量，可预防急性肾衰竭。扩张肺部容量静脉，增加全身静脉血容量使回心血量减少，心室舒张末期压力降低，有助于急性左心衰竭和肺淤血的治疗。

2）临床应用

（1）水肿性疾病。治疗心脏、肝、肾等病变引起的各类水肿，与其他药物合用治疗急性肺水肿和急性脑水肿等。

（2）高血压危象。不作为治疗原发性高血压的首选药物，但当钠氯共转运体抑制药疗效不佳，尤其当伴有肾功能不全或出现高血压危象时，呋塞米尤为适用。

（3）预防急性肾衰竭。可用于各种原因导致肾脏血流灌注不足，在纠正血容量不足的同时及时应用，可减少急性肾小管坏死的机会。

（4）高钾血症、高钙血症、稀释性低钠血症（尤其是当血钠浓度低于 120 mmol/L 时，勿用大剂量）、抗利尿激素分泌失调综合征、急性药物/毒物中毒。

（5）放射性核素检查。卡托普利加呋塞米介入肾动态显像，是诊断肾动脉狭窄的无创性方法，但有一定假阳性和假阴性，临床应结合患者病情综合判定。

3）不良反应

（1）碱中毒。过度利尿会导致细胞外液体积减少，出现浓缩型碱中毒，在老年患者、慢性肾脏病患者及服用非甾体抗炎药时更为常见。

（2）水、电解质紊乱。大剂量或长期应用时可出现低钾血症、低氯血症、低氯性碱中毒、低钠血症及相关的口渴、乏力、肌肉酸痛、心律失常等。

（3）过敏反应。作为磺胺类药物，可引起过敏反应，如皮疹、急性间质性肾炎等，对本药过敏患者应改用依他尼酸。

（4）耳毒性。可引起可逆性的耳毒性，耳鸣、听力障碍多见于大剂量静脉快速注射时，在肾功能不全状态或同时应用氨基苷类药物时，低剂量呋塞米也可引起耳毒性。

（5）其他少见不良反应，有视物模糊、黄视症、光敏感、头晕、头痛、纳差、恶心、呕吐、腹痛、腹泻、胰腺炎、肌肉强直等。

2. 氢氯噻嗪

氢氯噻嗪是钠氯共转运体抑制药。

1）药理作用

（1）利尿。抑制远曲小管近端的钠氯共转运体，减少 NaCl 的重吸收，降低肾的稀释功能，而对浓缩功能没有影响。可以抑制碳酸酐酶，增加尿中 HCO_3^- 排出。还可以抑制磷酸二酯酶活性，减少肾小管脂肪酸摄取，降低线粒体耗氧量，抑制肾小管对 Na^+ 和 Cl^- 的重吸收。

（2）降压。用药早期通过利尿作用，降低血容量降压；长期用药则通过扩张血管降压。减少对 Na^+ 和 Cl^- 的重吸收，增加远曲小管尿液中的水和 Na^+，激活致密斑的管-球反射，使肾素、血管紧张素分泌增多，收缩肾脏入球小动脉和出球小动脉，使肾血流量和肾小球滤过率下降。

2）临床应用

治疗各种水肿性疾病、原发性高血压、中枢性或肾性尿崩症。

3）不良反应

（1）电解质紊乱。较为常见的是低钾血症，长期缺钾可以损伤肾小管，严重时可引起肾小管上皮的空泡样变，以及严重快速型心律失常等。

（2）肾衰竭。脱水会引起血容量和肾血流量减少，引起肾小球滤过率降低，可加重氮质血症，肾功能严重损害患者可诱发肾衰竭。

（3）肝性脑病。长期应用时，H^+排出减少，血氨升高，可诱发肝病患者肝性脑病。

（4）胰岛素抵抗。引起糖耐量降低，血糖升高，产生胰岛素抵抗。对糖耐量正常的患者影响不大，但加重糖尿病患者的病情。

（5）代谢紊乱。可引起血清总胆固醇和甘油三酯中度升高，低密度脂蛋白和极低密度脂蛋白升高，高密度脂蛋白降低，影响脂代谢。氢氯噻嗪可以竞争性抑制尿酸的分泌，血尿酸升高，诱发痛风。

（6）其他不良反应：可能引起过敏反应、血白细胞减少、血小板减少性紫癜、胆囊炎、胰腺炎、性功能减退、光敏感、色觉障碍等。

3. 螺内酯

螺内酯是非选择性醛固酮受体阻断药。

1）药理作用

螺内酯是醛固酮的竞争性拮抗药，结合到胞质中的醛固酮受体，阻止醛固酮-受体复合物的核转位，拮抗醛固酮作用，减少钠和水的重吸收，表现出排钠保钾和利尿作用。螺内酯还通过减轻去甲肾上腺素的升压作用，减缓心血管重构；阻断醛固酮刺激产生胶原物质，减轻心肌纤维化；改善血管内皮细胞功能和平滑肌张力，缓解心肌缺血；提高血钾水平，发挥抗心律失常作用。上述药理学机制共同发挥保护心脏作用，适用于治疗充血性心力衰竭。

2）临床应用

（1）与醛固酮升高有关的顽固性水肿。螺内酯对肝硬化和肾病综合征水肿患者较为有效。

（2）充血性心力衰竭。螺内酯改善充血性心力衰竭患者的状况。

3）不良反应

不良反应较轻，少数患者可引起头痛、困倦与精神紊乱等。久用可引起高钾血症，尤其当肾功能不良时，故肾功能不全者禁用。此外，还有性激素样副作用，可引起男性乳房女性化和性功能障碍、妇女多毛症等，停药可消失。

4. 氨苯蝶啶

1）药理作用

作用于远曲小管末端和集合管，通过阻滞管腔上皮钠通道而减少Na^+的重吸收。由于减少Na^+的重吸收，使管腔的负电位降低，驱动K^+分泌的动力减少，抑制了K^+分泌，产生排Na^+、利尿、保K^+的作用。

2）临床应用

氨苯蝶啶常与排钾利尿药合用治疗顽固性水肿。

3）不良反应

不良反应少。长期服用可致高钾血症，严重肝、肾功能不全及有高钾血症倾向者禁用。偶见嗜睡、恶心、呕吐、腹泻等症状。氨苯蝶啶和吲哚美辛合用可能引起急性肾衰竭。

5. 乙酰唑胺

乙酰唑胺是碳酸酐酶抑制药的原形药。

1）药理作用

乙酰唑胺通过抑制碳酸酐酶的活性而抑制 HCO_3^- 的重吸收。由于 Na^+ 在近曲小管可与 HCO_3^- 结合排出，近曲小管 Na^+ 重吸收会减少，水的重吸收减少。但集合管 Na^+ 重吸收会增加，使 K^+ 的分泌相应增多（Na^+-K^+ 交换增多）。因而碳酸酐酶抑制药主要造成尿中 HCO_3^-、K^+ 和水的排出增多。由于碳酸酐酶还参与集合管酸的分泌，因此集合管也是这类药物利尿的次要部位。乙酰唑胺还抑制肾脏以外部位碳酸酐酶依赖的 HCO_3^- 的转运，减少房水和脑脊液的生成量和 pH 值。

2）临床应用

（1）青光眼。减少房水的生成，降低眼内压，对多种类型的青光眼有效。

（2）急性高山病。乙酰唑胺可减少脑脊液的生成和降低脑脊液及脑组织的 pH，减轻症状，改善机体功能。在开始攀登前 24 小时口服乙酰唑胺可起到预防作用。

（3）碱化尿液。采用乙酰唑胺碱化尿液可促进尿酸、胱氨酸和弱酸性物质的排泄，但只在使用初期有效，长时间服用乙酰唑胺要注意补充碳酸氢盐。

（4）代谢性碱中毒。当心力衰竭患者在使用过多利尿药造成代谢性碱中毒时，由于补盐可能会增加心室充盈压，因而可使用乙酰唑胺。此外乙酰唑胺在纠正碱中毒的同时，其微弱的利尿作用也对心力衰竭有益。还可用于迅速纠正呼吸性酸中毒继发的代谢性碱中毒。

（5）其他临床应用：用于癫痫的辅助治疗、伴有低钾血症的周期性瘫痪，以及严重高磷酸盐血症，以增加磷酸盐的尿排泄等。

3）不良反应

（1）过敏反应。作为磺胺的衍生物，可能会造成骨髓抑制、皮肤毒性、磺胺样肾损害。

（2）代谢性酸中毒。长时间用药后，体内贮存的 HCO_3^- 减少可导致高氯性酸中毒，继而引起其他肾小管节段对 Na^+ 重吸收增加，因此乙酰唑胺有效利尿作用仅维持 2~3 天。

（3）尿结石。其减少 HCO_3^- 的作用会导致磷酸盐尿和高钙尿症。长期用药也会引起肾脏排泄可溶性物质的能力下降，而且钙盐在碱性 pH 条件下相对难溶，易形成肾结石。

（4）失钾。同时补充 KCl 可以纠正。

（5）其他毒性。较大剂量可引起嗜睡和感觉异常；肾衰竭患者使用该类药物可引起蓄积而造成中枢神经系统毒性。

6. 托伐普坦

托伐普坦是精氨酸升压素受体阻断药。

1）药理作用

特异性拮抗精氨酸升压素，减少肾集合管主细胞囊泡内水通道 AQP2 向腔面膜的运输和调控 AQP2 基因表达，提高自由水的清除和尿液排泄，降低尿液的渗透压，促使血钠浓度提高。

2）临床应用

治疗高容量性和正常容量性低钠血症，包括伴有心力衰竭、肝硬化以及抗利尿激素分泌失调综合征的患者。也可用于治疗常染色体显性遗传多囊肾病。

3）不良反应

口渴、口干、乏力、便秘、尿频或多尿以及高血糖。

7. 甘露醇

甘露醇是脱水药，临床主要用 20% 的高渗溶液静脉注射或静脉滴注。其特点为：①静脉给药后不易通过毛细血管进入组织；②易经肾小球滤过；③不易被肾小管再吸收。

1）药理作用与临床应用

（1）脱水。静脉注射后能迅速提高血浆渗透压，使组织间液向血浆转移而产生组织脱水作用，可降低颅内压和眼内压。甘露醇是治疗脑水肿、降低颅内压的首选药物，也可用于青光眼急性发作和患者术前降低眼内压。

（2）利尿。静脉注射甘露醇后，血浆渗透压升高，血容量增加，稀释血液，增加循环血容量及肾小球滤过率。该药在肾小球滤过后不被重吸收，导致肾小管和集合管内渗透压升高，水在近曲小管、髓袢降支和集合管的重吸收减少，产生利尿作用。可用于预防急性肾衰竭。改善急性肾衰竭早期的血流动力学变化，对肾衰竭伴有低血压者效果较好。

2）不良反应

注射过快时可引起一过性头痛、眩晕、畏寒和视物模糊。因可增加循环血量而增加心脏负荷，慢性心功能不全者禁用。活动性颅内出血者禁用。

案例学习

学习要点：
(1) 掌握袢利尿药和噻嗪类利尿药的药理作用、不良反应。
(2) 熟悉利尿药与其他药物联用的药物相互作用。

关键词： 袢利尿药；噻嗪类；药理作用；适应证；不良反应；药物相互作用

案例

王大爷，72 岁，因连续 4 晚夜间呼吸困难就医。自述感觉胸部有压迫感，无法呼吸，坐起后呼吸困难可稍微缓解。这几天的尿量也比平时减少。查体发现王大爷有心动过速，中度高血压，双下肢凹陷性水肿，双肺湿啰音。血肌钙蛋白 T 水平正常，血肌酐和尿素氮水平升高。心电图显示陈旧性心肌梗死。心脏 B 超显示左室射血分数降低，心室大小正常。王大爷被诊断为急性心衰、肾功能不全。医生予以毛花苷丙、硝酸甘油、依那普利和呋塞米治疗。3 天后急性心衰症状有所缓解。但 1 天后王大爷再次出现胸闷心慌症状，心电图检查示频发的室性早搏，血钾浓度 2.5 mmol/L。停用毛花苷丙和呋塞米，并予以补钾、利多卡因治疗后缓解。因冠脉造影显示冠脉左前降支狭窄，行球囊扩张术并安装支架。术后心脏 B 超显示左室射血分数为 35%，予以 ACEI 和氢氯噻嗪治疗。

◎ 问答题

1. 王大爷呼吸困难和双下肢水肿的原因是什么？
2. 为什么给王大爷予以呋塞米治疗？
3. 王大爷再次出现心慌胸闷的原因是什么？
4. 术后为什么选择 ACEI 和氢氯噻嗪？

◎ 选择题

1. 易引起听力减退或暂时耳聋的药物是（　　）。
   A. 氢氯噻嗪　　B. 螺内酯　　C. 阿米洛利　　D. 依他尼酸　　E. 乙酰唑胺
2. 吲哚美辛会干扰以下哪种利尿药的作用？（　　）
   A. 螺内酯　　B. 氨苯蝶啶　　C. 甘露醇　　D. 呋塞米　　E. 乙酰唑胺
3. 对切除肾上腺的动物无利尿作用的药物是（　　）。
   A. 呋塞米　　B. 氢氯噻嗪　　C. 氨苯蝶啶　　D. 螺内酯　　E. 阿米洛利
4. 下列联合用药不合理的是（　　）。
   A. 氢氯噻嗪+螺内酯　　B. 呋塞米+氯化钾　　C. 呋塞米+氢氯噻嗪
   D. 氢氯噻嗪+氯化钾　　E. 呋塞米+氨苯蝶啶
5. 糖尿病患者伴发高血压和高血脂，适宜选择下列哪种利尿剂治疗？（　　）
   A. 氢氯噻嗪　　B. 呋塞米　　C. 乙酰唑胺　　D. 依他尼酸　　E. 阿米洛利
6. 下列哪种药物可用于治疗青光眼？（　　）
   A. 乙酰唑胺　　B. 呋塞米　　C. 吲达帕胺　　D. 依他尼酸　　E. 布美他尼
7. 患儿，6 岁，水肿 1 周，加重 3 日。开始为眼睑，逐渐波及全身，第二日出现尿量明显减少，一日 150~200 ml。尿常规：蛋白（+），红细胞 20/HP，血压 120/75 mmHg。治疗应选择下列哪个药物（　　）。
   A. 口服双氢克尿噻　　B. 静注呋塞米　　C. 静注 50%葡萄糖
   D. 静注 20%甘露醇　　E. 静注硝普钠
8. 患者，男性，35 岁，体检发现血压 150/120 mmHg，血钾 2.8 mmol/L（血钾正常值 3.5~5.5 mmol/L）。腹部 CT 检查发现右肾上腺 1.0 cm 的低密度占位性病变，拟行手术治疗。术前准备首选的药物是（　　）。
   A. 托拉塞米　　B. 呋塞米　　C. 氨苯蝶啶　　D. 螺内酯　　E. 氢氯噻嗪
9. 患者，男，45 岁，患高血压 20 年，一直服用缬沙坦治疗。一周前感冒，昨日夜间突然出现头晕、胸闷、气喘、咳粉红色泡沫样痰。查体：血压 170/90 mmHg，心率 95 次/分。急诊入院，适用下列哪种利尿药治疗（　　）。
   A. 口服氢氯噻嗪　　B. 静注呋塞米　　C. 静注甘露醇
   D. 静注乙酰唑胺　　E. 口服螺内酯
10. 患者，男，40 岁。近日去西藏旅游，3 小时前出现头痛、呕吐、嗜睡、共济失调和昏迷的症状。查体：血压 160/90 mmHg，心率 90 次/分。急诊入院，诊断为高原脑水肿。适宜用哪种药物治疗（　　）。

A. 静注呋塞米　　B. 静注肾上腺素　　C. 静注硝普钠
D. 静注乙酰唑胺　　E. 静注螺内酯

Case study

Key points:
(1) Master the pharmacological effects and adverse reactions of loop diuretics and thiazide diuretics.
(2) Be familiar with drug interactions between diuretics and other drugs.

Key words: loop diuretics; thiazines; pharmacological action; indication; adverse reaction; drug interaction

Case

Mr. Wang, a 72-year-old male, was taken to the emergency department due to waking up with shortness of breath for 4 nights. He felt tight in the chest and could not get a breath, this discomfort was relieved somewhat by sitting up in bed. His urine volume these days was less than before. Physical exam revealed tachycardia, mild hypertension, pitting edema of the feet and lower legs, and bilateral pulmonary crackles on inspiration. Serum troponin T level is normal, but serum creatinine and blood urea nitrogen are mildly elevated. The electrocardiogram showed evidence of an old myocardial infarction. Echocardiography reveals diminished left ventricular ejection fraction without ventricular dilatation. Mr. Wang was diagnosed with acute heart failure and renal insufficiency. Pharmacologic therapy was started, including lanatoside, nitroglycerin, enalapril and furosemide. Mr. Wang's condition stabilized over the course of 3 days. But 1 day later, he felt chest distress and palpitation again, the electrocardiogram showed frequent premature ventricular beats, serum potassium was 2.5 mmol/L. Lanatoside and furosemide were discontinued, after the treatment of potassium and lidocaine, his symptom was controlled. Elective coronary angiography revealed significant stenosis of the left anterior descending coronary artery. Mr. Wang underwent balloon angioplasty and stent placement and remains stable. An echocardiogram demonstrated an ejection fraction of 35%, he was discharged on a regimen that includes an ACEI and hydrochlorothiazide.

◎ **Essay questions**
1. What mechanisms led to Mr. Wang's pulmonary congestion and pedal edema?
2. Why was Mr. Wang given furosemide?
3. What was the reason that Mr. Wang felt chest distress and palpitation again?
4. Why was Mr. Wang prescribed ACEI and hydrochlorothiazide after surgery?

Multiple-choice questions

1. Which drug is easy to cause dysacusis or temporary deafness? (　　)

A. Hydrochlorothiazide B. Spirolactone C. Amiloride
D. Ethacrynic acid E. Acetazolamide

2. Indomethacin interferes with the action of which of the following diuretics?（　）
   A. Spirolactone B. Aminopteridine C. Mannitol
   D. Furosemide E. Acetazolamide

3. Which drug is ineffective to the animal that the adrenal was resected?（　）
   A. Furosemide B. Hydrochlorothiazide C. Aminopteridine
   D. Spirolactone E. Amiloride

4. Which combination drug therapy is unreasonable?（　）
   A. Hydrochlorothiazide+spirolactone B. Furosemide+potassium chloride
   C. Furosemide+hydrochlorothiazide D. Hydrochlorothiazide+potassium chloride
   E. Furosemide+aminopteridine

5. Which diuretic is suitable to treat the diabetic patient accompanied with hypertension and hyperlipidemia?（　）
   A. Hydrochlorothiazide B. Furosemide C. Indapamide
   D. Ethacrynic acid E. Amiloride

6. Which drug can be used to treat glaucoma?（　）
   A. Acetazolamide B. Furosemide C. Acetazolamide
   D. Ethacrynic acid E. Bumetanide

7. A six-year-old boy has had edema for 1 week, which become more serous these 3 days. The edema begin from eyelid, then spread to the whole body. In these 2 days, the urine volume become less obviously, which is 150-200 ml per day. Urine protein (+), red cells in the urine is 20/HP, blood pressure is 120/75 mmHg. Which pharmacological therapy should be given?（　）
   A. Hydrochlorothiazide orally B. Furosemide intravenously
   C. 50% glucose intravenously D. 20% mannitol intravenously
   E. Nitropuna intravenously

8. A 35-year-old male patient has the blood pressure of 150/120 mmHg, his serum potassium is 2.8 mmol/L (normal level is 3.5-5.5 mmol/L). CT reveals a 1.0 cm size of low density space occupying lesion at his right adrenal, which is planned to be resected by a surgery. Which drug should be given before surgery?（　）
   A. Torasemide B. Furosemide C. Aminopteridine
   D. Spirolactone E. Hydrochlorothiazide

9. A 45-year-old male patient having hypertension for 20 years, is treated with valsartan. One week ago, he suddenly felt swirled, chest distress, short of breath, and coughed with pink frothy sputum. Physical exam found that his blood pressure is 170/90 mmHg, heart beating rate is 95 bpm. He was sent to the emergency department, which pharmacological therapy should be given?（　）

A. Hydrochlorothiazide orally B. Furosemide intravenously

C. Mannitol intravenously D. Acetazolamide intravenously

E. Spirolactone orally

10. Male, 40-year-old, travels in Xizang these days. He suffered headache, vomiting, drowsiness, dystaxia and coma 3 hours ago. His blood pressure is 160/90 mmHg, heart beating rate is 90 bpm. He is diagnosed as high altitude cerebral edema, which pharmacological therapy should be given? (   )

A. Furosemide intravenously B. Epinephrine intravenously

C. Nitropuna intravenously D. Acetazolamide intravenously

E. Spirolactone intravenously

第二十三章案例学习和选择题答案

第二十四章 抗高血压药

知识要点

一、常用抗高血压药（一线用药）

1. 利尿药

利尿药主要有：氢氯噻嗪（hydrochlorothiazide）、呋塞米（furosemide）、吲达帕胺（indapamide）。

（1）药理作用：噻嗪类利尿药是利尿降压药中最常用的一类。用药初期，利尿药可减少细胞外液容量及心输出量，长期使用可降低血管阻力。

（2）临床应用：大规模临床试验表明，噻嗪类利尿药可降低高血压并发症如脑卒中和心力衰竭的发病率和死亡率。单独使用噻嗪类作降压治疗时，剂量不宜超过 25 mg。对合并有氮质血症或尿毒症的高血压患者、高血压危象患者可选用呋塞米。吲达帕胺不引起血脂改变，伴有高脂血症的患者可用吲达帕胺代替噻嗪类利尿药。

（3）不良反应：长期大量使用噻嗪类除引起电解质改变外，还会对脂质代谢、糖代谢产生不良影响。

2. 钙通道阻滞药

钙通道阻滞药主要有：硝苯地平（nifedipine）、氨氯地平（amlodipine）、尼群地平（nitrendipine）、拉西地平（lacidipine）。

（1）药理作用：血管平滑肌细胞的收缩有赖于细胞内游离钙，若抑制了钙离子的跨膜转运，则可使细胞内游离钙浓度下降。钙通道阻滞药通过减少细胞内钙离子含量而松弛血管平滑肌，进而降低血压。

（2）临床应用：硝苯地平对轻、中、重度高血压均有降压作用，目前多推荐使用缓释片剂，以减轻迅速降压造成的反射性交感活性增加。氨氯地平作用与硝苯地平相似，但降压作用较为平缓，持续时间显著延长，每日口服一次，为长效药。

（3）不良反应：钙通道阻滞药相对比较安全，不良反应与其阻滞钙通道扩张血管有关，常见颜面潮红、头痛、眩晕、恶心、便秘等。

3. β肾上腺素受体阻断药

β肾上腺素受体阻断药主要有：普萘洛尔（propranolol）、阿替洛尔（atenolol）、拉贝洛尔（labetalol）、卡维地洛（carvedilol）。

（1）药理作用：可通过多种机制产生降压作用，即减少心输出量、抑制肾素释放、在不同水平抑制交感神经系统活性和增加前列环素合成等。

(2)临床应用：用于各种程度原发性高血压。可作为抗高血压的首选药单独应用，也可与其他抗高血压药合用。对心输出量及肾素活性偏高者疗效较好。

(3)不良反应：心功能抑制，如窦性心动过缓和房室传导阻滞；诱发加重哮喘；停药反跳现象。

4. 血管紧张素转化酶抑制药(ACEI)

血管紧张素转化酶抑制药（ACEI）主要有：卡托普利（captopril）、依那普利（enalapril）、赖诺普利（lisinopril）、贝那普利（benazepril）、福辛普利（fosinopril）。

(1)药理作用：抑制血管紧张素转化酶（ACE），使血管紧张素Ⅱ生成减少，从而产生血管舒张；同时减少醛固酮分泌，以利于排钠；特异性肾血管扩张亦加强排钠作用；由于抑制缓激肽的水解，使缓激肽增多；抑制交感神经系统活性。

(2)临床应用：适用于各型高血压。尤其是合并有糖尿病及胰岛素抵抗、左心室肥厚、心力衰竭、急性心肌梗死的高血压患者，可明显改善生活质量且无耐受性，停药不反跳。

(3)不良反应：首剂低血压；刺激性咳嗽；高血钾；低血糖；肾功能损伤；对妊娠与哺乳的影响；血管神经性水肿。

5. AT_1 受体阻断药(ARB)

AT_1 受体阻断药（ARB）主要有：氯沙坦（losartan）、缬沙坦（valsartan）。

(1)药理作用：竞争性阻断 AT_1 受体，对抗血管紧张素Ⅱ绝大多数药理学作用，从而产生降压作用。

(2)临床应用：适用于各型高血压，与ACEI适应证类似。

(3)不良反应：首剂低血压；高血钾；低血糖；肾功能损伤；对妊娠与哺乳的影响。

二、其他抗高血压药物

1. 中枢性降压药

(1)第一代中枢性降压药：可乐定。本类药物通过兴奋延髓背侧孤束核突触后膜的 α_2 受体，也作用于延髓腹外侧区的咪唑啉 I_1 受体从而抑制交感神经中枢的传出冲动，使外周血管扩张、血压下降。

(2)第二代中枢性降压药：莫索尼定。本类药物作用与可乐定相似，但对咪唑啉 I_1 受体的选择性比可乐定高，不良反应少。

2. 血管平滑肌扩张药

本类药物通过直接扩张血管而产生降压作用，如肼屈嗪、硝普钠。

3. 神经节阻断药

由于交感神经对血管的支配占优势，本类药物可使血管特别是小动脉扩张，血压下降，如樟磺咪芬。

4. α_1 肾上腺受体阻断药

本类药物可降低动脉血管阻力，增加静脉容量，增加血浆肾素活性，不易引起反射性心率增加，并对血脂代谢有良好作用，如哌唑嗪。

5. 去甲肾上腺素能神经末梢阻断药

本类药物通过影响儿茶酚胺的储存及释放产生降压作用，如利血平、胍乙啶。

6. 钾通道开放药

本类药物使钾离子外流增多，细胞膜超极化，膜兴奋性降低，钙离子内流减少，血管平滑肌舒张，血压下降，如米诺地尔、吡那地尔。

7. 肾素抑制药

本类药物通过抑制肾素活性，使血管紧张素原生成血管紧张素Ⅰ减少，进而血管紧张素Ⅱ降低，血压下降，如阿利吉仑。

案例学习

学习要点：
（1）高血压病血压水平分类及易患病因素。
（2）抗高血压一线用药的作用机制和用药原则。
（3）长期大剂量应用利尿药引起的不良反应及相关机制。
关键词：高血压；利尿药；钙通道阻滞药；不良反应

案例

患者，女，60岁，反复头晕18年，曾确诊为原发性高血压病，间断服用抗高血压药物，近1周不断加重，伴头疼，无视物旋转，无胸痛、胸闷，无肢体活动障碍。患者近7年有支气管哮喘、肾小球肾炎病史。体格检查：血压180/110 mmHg，神清烦躁，自动体位，眼球无震颤，双眼睑轻度水肿，嘴唇无紫绀，口角无歪斜，颈软，两肺呼吸音粗糙并闻及哮鸣音，心界向左扩大，心率80次/分，律齐，肌张力正常，生理反射存在，病理反射未引出。心电图检查：左室肥厚伴劳损，头颅CT均正常。尿常规检查：尿蛋白（+），红细胞3个。诊断：①原发性高血压病（3级重度）；②支气管哮喘；③慢性肾小球肾炎。

◎ **问答题**

1. 该病人该如何选用抗高血压药？为什么？
2. 该病人禁止使用哪些药物？
3. 利尿药在治疗原发性高血压病中的优缺点有哪些？
4. 高血压与哪些因素有关？除了药物治疗之外，还有哪些方法对原发性高血压病有缓解作用？

选择题

1. 以下哪种药物最适合治疗中度糖尿病高血压伴轻度蛋白尿患者（　　）。
   A. 依那普利　　B. 普萘洛尔　　C. 氢氯噻嗪　　D. 硝苯地平　　E. 可乐定
2. 氯沙坦的作用（　　）。
   A. 降低AT_1受体活性　　B. 减少缓激肽生成　　C. 减少血管紧张素Ⅱ的生成

D. 减少肾素生成　　　　E. 减少血管紧张素Ⅰ的生成

3. 在选择噻嗪类利尿药治疗糖尿病高血压伴轻度蛋白尿患者时加用螺内酯的原因是?（　　）
   A. 减少高尿酸血症　　B. 减少 Mg^{2+} 损失　　C. 减少 Na^+ 损失
   D. 减少 K^+ 损失　　E. 减少 Ca^+ 损失

4. 对于正在用胰岛素治疗的糖尿病伴高血压患者，以下哪种药物建议谨慎服用？（　　）
   A. 肼屈嗪　　B. 哌唑嗪　　C. 胍乙啶　　D. 普萘洛尔　　E. 可乐定

5. 下列哪项不是 ACEI 的药理作用？（　　）
   A. 阻止 AngⅡ 的生成　　B. 保护血管内皮细胞　　C. 促进缓激肽降解
   D. 抑制心血管重构　　E. 抗动脉粥样硬化

6. 高血压伴有血浆肾素偏高者宜选用（　　）。
   A. 可乐定　　B. 硝苯地平　　C. 氢氯噻嗪　　D. 硝普钠　　E. 普萘洛尔

7. 高血压伴阵发性室上性心动过速患者宜选用（　　）。
   A. 普鲁卡因胺　　B. 奎尼丁　　C. 维拉帕米　　D. 胺碘酮　　E. 普罗帕酮

8. 关于卡托普利，下列哪种说法是错误的？（　　）
   A. 降低外周血管阻力
   B. 可用于其他药物治疗无效的高血压病人
   C. 增加醛固酮释放
   D. 可与噻嗪类利尿药联用
   E. 食物影响其吸收，宜在进餐前一小时服用

9. 高血压合并消化性溃疡者宜选用（　　）。
   A. 可乐定　　B. 甲基多巴　　C. 肼屈嗪　　D. 利血平　　E. 胍乙啶

10. 普萘洛尔不适用于下列何种高血压？（　　）
    A. 高血压伴心绞痛　　B. 高血压伴支气管哮喘　　C. 高血压伴心动过速
    D. 高血压伴心输出量偏高者　　E. 高血压伴肾素活性偏高者

Case study

Key points:
(1) Classification of blood pressure levels and susceptibility factors for hypertension.
(2) The mechanism of action and medication principles of first-line antihypertensive drugs.
(3) Adverse reactions and related mechanisms caused by long-term high-dose use of diuretics.

Key words: hypertension; diuretics; calcium channel blocker; adverse reactions

Case

The patient, female, 60 years old. She has repeated dizziness for 18 years and has been diagnosed with essential hypertension, intermittent taking antihypertensive drugs. The state of illness has got worse in the past 1 week, with headache, no object rotation, no chest pain and chest tightness, no physical activity disorders. The patient has the history of bronchial asthma, glomerulonephritis for nearly 7 years. Physical examination: blood pressure 180/110 mmHg, sober, irritability, active posture, no nystagmus, mild edema in the eyelids, no cyanosis in the lips, nodistortion of commissure, softness of the neck. The two lungs have rough breathing sounds, and wheezing sound can be heard. Heart border is expanded to the left, heart rate 80 times/min, regular rate, normal muscle tension, physiological reflection exists, no pathological reflex. ECG examination: left ventricular hypertrophy with strain, normal head CT. Urine routine examination: urine protein (+), three red blood cells. Diagnosis: ① essential hypertension (grade 3 severe); ② bronchial asthma; ③ chronic glomerulonephritis.

◎ **Essay questions**

1. How to choose the antihypertensive drugs for the patient? Why?
2. Which drugs are prohibited for the patient?
3. What are the advantages and disadvantages of diuretic drugs in the treatment of essential hypertension?
4. Which factors have relationship with hypertension? In addition to drug treatment, which methods should we consider for alleviating essential hypertension?

Multiple-choice questions

1. Which of the following drugs would be the best to treat moderate hypertension in a diabetic patient with mild proteinuria? (   )
    A. Enalapril B. Propranolol C. Hydrochlorothiazide
    D. Nifedipine E. Clonidine
2. Losartan acts to (   ).
    A. decrease AT_1 receptor activity
    B. decrease bradykinin production
    C. decrease production of angiotension II
    D. decrease rennin production
    E. decrease production of angiotension I
3. What is the reason for the addition of spironolactone when choosing thiazide diuretics to treat diabetic hypertensive patients with mild proteinuria? (   )
    A. reduce hyperuricemia
    B. reduce Mg^{2+} loss
    C. reduce Na^+ loss
    D. reduce K^+ loss
    E. reduce Ca^+ loss
4. In a hypertensive patient who is taking insulin to treat diabetes, which of the following drugs is to be used with extra caution and advice to the patient? (   )
    A. Hydralazine B. Prazosin C. Guanethidine
    D. Propranolol E. Clonidine
5. Which of the following is not the pharmacological effect of ACEI? (   )
    A. Blocking the production of Ang II B. Protecting vascular endothelial cell

C. Promoting degradation of bradykinin   D. Inhibiting cardiovascular remodeling

   E. Anti-atherosclerosis

6. Which is suitable drug for patients with hypertension accompanied by high plasma renin level? (   )

   A. Clonidine   B. Nifedipine   C. Hydrochlorothiazide

   D. Sodium nitroprusside   E. Propranolol

7. Which is suitable drug for patients with hypertension accompanied by paroxysmal supraventricular tachycardia? (   )

   A. Procainamide   B. Quinidine   C. Verapamil

   D. Amiodarone   E. Propafenone

8. Which of the following statements about captopril is incorrect? (   )

   A. Reduces peripheral vascular resistance

   B. Can be used for hypertensive patients who are ineffective in other medications

   C. Increases aldosterone release

   D. Can take combined with thiazide diuretics

   E. Food interferes with its absorption and we should take it one hour before meals

9. Patients with hypertension and peptic ulcer is recommended (   ).

   A. clonidine   B. methyldopa   C. hydrazine

   D. reserpine   E. guanethidine

10. Propranolol is not indicated for which of the following types of hypertension? (   )

    A. Hypertension with angina pectoris   B. Hypertension with bronchial asthma

    C. Hypertension with tachycardia   D. Hypertension with high cardiac output

    E. Hypertension with high renin activity

第二十四章案例学习和选择题答案

第二十五章 治疗心力衰竭的药物

知识要点

一、充血性心力衰竭(CHF)的病理生理学

1. 心肌功能及结构变化

各种心脏疾病导致心肌细胞肥大或凋亡、心肌细胞外基质堆积,胶原结构紊乱,心肌组织纤维化,表现为心肌肥厚、心腔扩大等心肌重构现象。可产生左心、右心或全心功能障碍,多以收缩性心力衰竭为主,少数以舒张功能障碍为主。

2. 神经内分泌变化

(1)交感神经系统因心衰被反射性激活。
(2)肾素血管紧张素醛固酮系统(RAAS)激活。
(3)其他包括精氨酸加压素、内皮素、心房钠尿肽和脑钠肽等增多。

3. 心肌肾上腺素 β 受体信号转导的变化

(1)$β_1$ 受体下调。
(2)$β_1$ 受体与兴奋性 Gs 蛋白脱偶联或减敏导致细胞内钙降低。
(3)G 蛋白偶联受体激酶活性增加与受体减敏有关。

二、常用治疗 CHF 药物

1. 血管紧张素转化酶抑制药(ACEI)

常用药物有卡托普利(captopril)、依那普利(enalapril)、福辛普利(fosinopril)等。

(1)抗 CHF 作用及机制:ACEI 通过抑制血管紧张素转化酶(ACE),抑制血管紧张素 Ⅰ 转化为血管紧张素 Ⅱ(AngⅡ),降低血液及组织中 AngⅡ 含量;ACEI 还抑制缓激肽降解。①减弱 AngⅡ 收缩血管作用,降低外周阻力减轻心脏后负荷;②减少醛固酮生成,减轻水钠潴留降低心脏前负荷;③降低交感神经活性;④抑制并逆转 AngⅡ 及醛固酮导致的心肌和血管重构,改善心功能;⑤增多的缓激肽可促进 NO 和内源性 PGI_2 等物质合成和释放,进一步扩张血管降低心脏负荷。

(2)临床应用:可用于各阶段心衰治疗。

(3)不良反应:此类药物不良反应轻微,患者一般耐受良好。可有如下反应:①干咳,20%~30%患者用药后会出现无痰性干咳并因此停药,与缓激肽等在肺部聚集过多有关;②可引起胎儿发育障碍,故一旦证实妊娠应立即停药;③其他不良反应,如首剂低血

压、高血钾、低血糖、血管神经性水肿及含巯基的卡托普利产生的味觉障碍等。

2. 血管紧张素Ⅱ受体（AT_1）阻断药（ARBs）和醛固酮受体阻断药

常用 ARBs 有氯沙坦（losartan）、缬沙坦（valsartan）等，可从受体水平阻断血管紧张素Ⅱ的各种效应，对 CHF 患者可减轻心脏前、后负荷，改善心功能；可抑制和逆转心血管重构。对缓激肽系统无明显影响，无干咳不良反应。近年来血管紧张素受体-脑啡肽酶抑制药沙库巴曲缬沙坦也用于 CHF 治疗。

螺内酯可竞争性拮抗醛固酮受体，抑制其水钠潴留作用，减轻心脏前负荷；可抑制醛固酮导致的心血管重构。

3. β肾上腺素受体阻断药

常用于治疗 CHF 的 β 肾上腺素受体阻断药（β adrenoceptor antagonists）：如卡维地洛（carvedilol）、美托洛尔（metoprolol）、比索洛尔（bisoprolol）等。

（1）治疗 CHF 作用：①拮抗交感神经活性：β 肾上腺素受体阻断药通过拮抗过量儿茶酚胺对心脏的毒性作用，避免能量过度消耗和心肌受损，改善心肌重构；减少肾素释放，抑制 RAAS 过度激活对心肌的毒性作用。②β 肾上腺素受体阻断药的抗心律失常与抗心肌缺血作用，降压作用等均有利于 CHF 治疗。

（2）临床应用：对扩张型心肌病及缺血性早期 CHF，长期使用可阻止临床症状恶化、改善心功能及降低猝死发生率。宜从小剂量开始，可与强心苷类合用。

（3）注意事项及不良反应：①应从小剂量开始，长期应用，平均用药 3 个月可见心功能改善；②适应证以扩张性心肌病 CHF 疗效最好；③应合并应用其他抗 CHF 药；④长期应用可能引起血脂异常，可能导致心功能严重减弱，支气管哮喘患者慎用。

4. 利尿药

常用于治疗 CHF 的利尿药：噻嗪类如氢氯噻嗪、袢利尿药如呋塞米、保钾利尿药螺内酯等。

（1）抗 CHF 作用及机制：①呋塞米可抑制髓袢升枝粗段上皮细胞膜上的 Na^+-K^+-$2Cl^-$ 共同转运体，抑制钠和氯离子重吸收，降低髓质高渗透压，抑制集合管尿液的最终浓缩过程，促进钠水排泄并降低血容量及心脏前负荷；②利尿可降低静脉压，消除或缓解静脉淤血及其引起的肺水肿和外周水肿；③螺内酯还可抑制心肌重构。

（2）临床应用：噻嗪类适用于伴有水肿或有明显淤血表现的轻度 CHF 患者。对中重度或单用噻嗪类疗效不佳者可用呋塞米等袢利尿药。

（3）大剂量利尿药特别是呋塞米等高效利尿药对治疗 CHF 不利：①循环血量降低继而降低心输出量加重心衰；②血容量迅速减少可反射性兴奋交感神经，加重心衰；③易引起电解质紊乱如低钾血症，所以使用呋塞米时应注意补钾或与保钾利尿药合用。

5. 强心苷类正性肌力药物

常用药物有地高辛（digoxin）和毛花苷 C（cedilanid，西地兰）等。

（1）抗 CHF 作用及机制（强心苷类可抑制心肌细胞膜上的钠钾泵功能，间接增高细胞内钙浓度）：①有正性肌力作用，显著增强心肌收缩力，增加心输出量，改善心衰症状；②心输出量增加可反射性兴奋迷走神经，强心苷还增加心肌对迷走神经的敏感性，对心脏产生负性频率作用，减慢心率；③可抑制肾小管钠钾泵减少钠重吸收，产生利尿效果从而缓解 CHF 症状。

（2）临床应用：地高辛常用于治疗以收缩功能障碍为主的 CHF 和治疗某些心律失常（如房颤、房扑及阵发性室上性心动过速）。

（3）地高辛安全范围较小，剂量过大或长期使用可能产生以下不良反应：心脏反应主要有快速性心律失常、房室传导阻滞或窦性心动过缓；胃肠道出现厌食、恶心呕吐等反应；中枢神经系统可产生色觉障碍及眩晕、头痛失眠等反应。

6. 其他药物

非苷类正性肌力药，如儿茶酚胺类多巴酚丁胺与异布帕明、磷酸二酯酶抑制剂米力农及匹莫苯、扩血管药硝酸酯类和硝普钠、钙增敏药等。钠-葡萄糖共转运体 2 抑制药达格列净等近年来被发现对心血管系统有保护作用，可降低 CHF 死亡率和再住院率。

案例学习

学习要点：
（1）血管紧张素转化酶抑制药治疗 CHF 的机制。
（2）β 受体阻断药治疗 CHF 的作用与临床应用。
（3）呋塞米的药理作用与临床应用。
（4）地高辛的药理作用、临床应用及不良反应。

关键词： 充血性心衰；血管紧张素转化酶抑制药；β 受体拮抗药；利尿药；地高辛

案例

李先生 65 岁，因为呼吸急促和恶心来到医院就诊。他有过两次心肌梗死发作史，第二次发作一年后被诊断为充血性心衰（CHF），第二次发作后运动能力明显降低。心脏 B 超显示其左心室射血分数仅为 25%（正常>55%），并有轻度二尖瓣关闭不全。入院前他用过阿司匹林、卡维地洛、卡托普利、地高辛、呋塞米和螺内酯等药物治疗。他体内装有内置心室除颤器以防治持续性室性心律失常和心源性猝死。

在急诊室体检发现其血压为 90/50 mmHg，心率 120 次/分，心电图显示房颤。给予胺碘酮治疗后，他的心率降到了约 80 次/分。实验室检查发现血钠 148 mmol/L（正常为 135~145 mmol/L），血钾为 2.9 mmol/L（正常为 3.5~5.1 mmol/L），尿素氮 56 mg/dL（正常为 7~19 mg/dL），肌酐为 4.8 mg/dL（正常为 0.6~1.2 mg/dL）。血浆中地高辛浓度为 3.2 ng/mL（治疗浓度约 1 ng/mL）。

李先生被送进心脏重症监护室（ICU）。他被静脉缓慢给予钾盐以改善低血钾。基于他严重的临床心功能失代偿表现，对他进行了肺动脉插管以监测心室压，然后开始静脉给予多巴酚丁胺。他的尿量逐渐增加，症状开始好转。他在 ICU 住了 7 天，血浆地高辛浓度降低到了治疗范围。

◎ 问答题

1. 请解释卡托普利和螺内酯治疗 CHF 的作用。
2. 为什么李先生患有 CHF 还被给予卡维地洛治疗？
3. 为什么李先生有低血钾？
4. 地高辛对心脏正性肌力作用的机制是什么？

◎ 选择题

1. 李先生用阿司匹林的治疗目的是（　　）。
   A. 止痛　　　B. 升高血压　　　C. 抗血小板　　　D. 改善心功能　　E. 预防炎症
2. 以下哪项不是地高辛的不良反应？（　　）
   A. 胃肠道反应　　　　　B. 神经精神系统反应　　　C. 心律失常
   D. 粒细胞减少　　　　　E. 色觉障碍
3. 氯沙坦拮抗的受体是（　　）。
   A. 肾素受体　　　　　B. $β_1$ 肾上腺素受体　　　C. 血管紧张素 II 的 AT_1 受体
   D. 醛固酮受体　　　　E. 血管紧张素 II 的 AT_2 受体
4. 能防止和逆转 CHF 时心肌重构并降低病死率的药物是（　　）。
   A. 地高辛　　　B. 卡托普利　　　C. 硝普钠　　　D. 氢氯噻嗪　　E. 米力农
5. 强心苷与下列哪种药物合用时易引起低血钾？（　　）
   A. 氢氯噻嗪　　B. 螺内酯　　　C. 乙酰唑胺　　　D. 甘露醇　　　E. 缬沙坦
6. 地高辛加强心肌收缩力的机制是（　　）。
   A. 兴奋 $β_1$ 受体　　　　B. 阻断心肌迷走神经　　　C. 促进交感神经递质的释放
   D. 抑制心肌细胞膜的 Na^+-K^+-ATP 酶　　　E. 直接加强心肌肌纤蛋白收缩力
7. 美托洛尔治疗 CHF 的作用机制是（　　）。
   A. 抑制交感神经活性　　　　B. 上调心肌 β 受体　　　C. 减少肾素释放，抑制 RAAS
   D. 抗心律失常及心肌缺血作用　　E. 以上都是
8. β 受体阻断药治疗 CHF 病人的潜在缺点是（　　）。
   A. 限制地高辛与钠钾泵的结合
   B. 减弱交感张力增高在维持肾血流量方面的益处
   C. 进一步降低心输出量并诱发肺水肿
   D. 减慢心率并与产后抑郁发生有关
   E. 在产后心肌病恢复期间使用不可预防左心室重构
9. 为什么患 CHF 的李先生同时服用 β 受体阻滞药和地高辛？（　　）
   A. 这种联合用药可以使两种药剂量都低于中毒剂量
   B. 这样联用可以防止缺血性心衰病人心肌梗死复发
   C. 联合用药可降低死亡率并改善病人功能状态
   D. 这样联用后 CHF 病人就不需使用利尿药

E. 联合用药可引起心肌重构并恢复左心室射血分数，从而治愈心衰

10. 易引起顽固性干咳的抗 CHF 药物是( )。
    A. 卡维地洛　B. 福辛普利　　C. 氯沙坦　　D. 氢氯噻嗪　　E. 地高辛

Case study

Key points:
(1) The mechanisms of ACEI treating CHF.
(2) The effects and clinical uses of β blockers for the treatment of CHF.
(3) The pharmacological effects and clinical uses of furosemide.
(4) The pharmacological effects, clinical uses and adverse reactions of digoxin.

Key words: congestive heart failure (CHF); angiotension converting enzyme inhibitor (ACEI); β blocker; diuretic; digoxin

Case

Mr. Li, a 65 year old man came to hospital with shortness of breath and nausea. He had been diagnosed as congestive heart failure and systolic dysfunction one year after his second myocardial infarctions. Since the second infarction, he has had significant limitation of exercise capacity. A two dimensional echocardiogram is notable for a left ventricular ejection fraction of 25% (normal >55%) and moderate mitral valve regurgitation. He has been treated with aspirin, carvedilol, captopril, digoxin, furosemide and spironolactone. He also had an automatic internal cardiac defibrillator placed to prevent sustained ventricular arrhythmia and sudden cardiac death.

Physical examination in the emergency room found a blood pressure of 90/50 mmHg and a heart rate of 120 bpm. ECG indicates atrial fibrillation. He was started on amiodarone, and his HR decreases to approximately 80 bpm. Laboratory tests show serum Na^+ of 148 mmol/L (normal 135-145 mmol/L), K^+ 2.9 mmol/L (normal 3.5-5.1 mmol/L), BUN 56 mg/dL (normal 7-19 mg/dL), and creatinine 4.8 mg/dL (normal 0.6-1.2 mg/dL). The serum digoxin level is 3.2 ng/mL (therapeutic concentration about 1ng/mL).

Mr. Li was admitted to the cardiology intensive care unit. He was given intravenous K^+ to increase serum K^+ concentration. Based on the severity of his clinical decompensation, a pulmonary artery catheter is placed to monitor cardiac pressures, then he was started on dobutamine intravenously, his urine output increased and feel symptomatically improved. He was monitored for 7 days, and his digoxin level decreases to the therapeutic range.

◎ **Essay questions**

1. Please explain the effects of captopril and spironolactone in the treatment of CHF.
2. Why was Mr. Li given carvedilol even though he had CHF?
3. Why does Mr. Li have hypokalemia?
4. What is the mechanism of digoxin's positive inotrope effects on the heart?

Ⅲ Multiple-choice questions

1. Mr. Lee's therapeutic goal with aspirin is (   ).
   A. pain relief   B. elevate blood pressure   C. antiplatelet
   D. improve cardiac function   E. prevent inflammation
2. Which of the following is not an adverse reaction to digoxin (   ).
   A. gastrointestinal reactions   B. neuropsychiatric reactions   C. cardiac arrhythmias
   D. granulocytopenia   E. color vision disorders
3. The receptor antagonized by losartan is (   ).
   A. renin receptors   B. $β_1$-adrenergic receptors   C. angiotensin Ⅱ AT_1 receptor
   D. aldosterone receptors   E. angiotensin Ⅱ AT_2 receptors
4. The drug that prevents and reverses myocardial remodeling in CHF and reduces mortality is (   ).
   A. digoxin   B. captopril   C. sodium nitroprusside
   D. hydrochlorothiazide   E. milrinone
5. Cardiac glycosides tends to cause hypokalemia when combined with which of the following drugs (   ).
   A. hydrochlorothiazide   B. spironolactone   C. acetazolamide
   D. mannitol   E. valsartan
6. The mechanism by which digoxin enhances myocardial contractility is (   ).
   A. excitation of $β_1$ receptors
   B. blocking the myocardial vagus nerve
   C. promoting the release of sympathetic neurotransmitters
   D. inhibiting the Na^+-K^+-ATPase of myocardial cell membrane
   E. directly enhance myocardial contractility of myofibrillar proteins
7. The mechanism of action of metoprolol in the treatment of CHF is (   ).
   A. inhibition of sympathetic nerve activity   B. upregulation of myocardial β-receptors
   C. reduce renin release and inhibit RAAS   D. antiarrhythmic and ischemic effects
   E. all of the above
8. A potential disadvantage of beta-blockers in the treatment of patients with CHF is (   ).
   A. limiting digoxin binding to the sodium-potassium pump
   B. attenuating the benefits of increased sympathetic tone in maintaining renal blood flow
   C. further decreasing cardiac output and inducing pulmonary edema
   D. slows heart rate and is associated with the development of postpartum depression
   E. cannot be used during recovery from postpartum cardiomyopathy to prevent left ventricular remodeling
9. Why is Mr. Li, who has CHF, taking both beta-blockers and digoxin? (   )
   A. This combination keeps the dose of both drugs below the toxic dose

B. This combination can prevent recurrence of myocardial infarction in patients with ischemic heart failure
C. The combination reduces mortality and improves functional status of the patient
D. The combination eliminates the need for diuretics in patients with CHF
E. The combination induces myocardial remodeling and restores left ventricular ejection fraction, thereby curing the heart failure.

10. The anti-CHF drug that tends to cause a persistent dry cough is (　　).
    A. carvedilol　　　　B. fosinopril　　　　C. losartan
    D. hydrochlorothiazide　　E. digoxin

第二十五章案例学习和选择题答案

第二十六章 调血脂药与抗动脉粥样硬化药

知识要点

一、调血脂药

1. 主要降低总胆固醇(TC)和低密度脂蛋白(LDL)的药物

1)他汀类

他汀类主要有:洛伐他汀(lovastatin)、辛伐他汀(simvastatin)、普伐他汀(pravastatin)、阿托伐他汀(atorvastatin)。

(1)药理作用:①调血脂作用。明显降低血浆低密度脂蛋白(LDL)及总胆固醇(TC)水平,也可使极低密度脂蛋白(VLDL)和甘油三酯(TG)水平降低,高密度脂蛋白(HDL)升高。机制:特异性和竞争性地抑制羟甲基戊二酸单酰辅酶A(HMG-CoA)还原酶,使肝胆固醇合成减少。由于胆固醇减少,通过负反馈调节促使肝细胞表面LDL受体合成增加,使血浆中的LDL大量被摄入肝脏,经LDL受体途径代谢为胆汁酸排出体外。②非调血脂作用(多效性作用)。③肾保护作用。

(2)临床应用:①调节血脂,主要用于杂合子家族性和非家族性Ⅱa、Ⅱb和Ⅲ型高脂蛋白血症,也可用于2型糖尿病和肾病综合征引起的高胆固醇血症。②肾病综合征。③预防心脑血管急性事件。

(3)不良反应:不良反应少而轻,大剂量应用时患者偶可出现胃肠反应、皮肤潮红、头痛失眠等暂时性反应。需注意本类药物可引起肌肉不良反应,表现为肌痛、肌炎和横纹肌溶解症,有肌肉不适或无力应检测肌酸激酶(CK),必要时减量或停药。孕妇、儿童、哺乳期妇女及肝肾功能异常者不宜应用。

2)胆固醇吸收抑制剂

(1)胆汁酸结合树脂(胆酸螯合剂),如考来烯胺(cholestyramine)、考来替泊(colestipol)。此药口服不吸收,在肠道通过离子交换与胆汁酸结合后使胆汁酸失去活性,减少食物中脂类(包括胆固醇)的吸收并阻止胆汁酸在肠道内重吸收。由于大量胆汁酸丢失,肝内胆固醇经7α-羟化酶的作用转化为胆汁酸,导致肝细胞表面LDL受体增加或活性增强,低密度脂蛋白胆固醇(LDL-C)经受体进入肝细胞,使血浆TC和LDL-C水平降低。若与他汀类合同,有协同作用。

(2)胆固醇吸收抑制药:依折麦布(ezetimibe),通过与小肠上皮刷状缘上的NPC1L1蛋白特异性结合,抑制饮食及胆汁中胆固醇的吸收,而不影响胆汁酸和其他物质的吸收。

2. 主要降低甘油三酯(TG)及极低密度脂蛋白(VLDL)的药物

1) 贝特类

贝特类主要有：吉非贝齐(gemfibrozil)、非诺贝特(fenofibrate)、苯扎贝特(bezafibrate)。

(1) 药理作用：①激活过氧化物酶体增殖物激活受体(PPAR-α，是一种调节基因表达的转录因子)，增加脂蛋白酯酶(LPL)、载脂蛋白(Apo)A I 表达。②增加 LPL 活化，加速 TG 的分解；减少肝合成和分泌 VLDL，增加 HDL。

(2) 临床应用：主要用于以 TG 或 VLDL 升高为主的原发性高脂血症，如Ⅱb、Ⅲ、Ⅳ型高脂血症，亦可用于低 HDL 和高动脉硬化性疾病风险(如 2 型糖尿病)的高脂蛋白血症患者。

(3) 不良反应：主要为消化道反应，如食欲减退、恶心、腹胀等，其次为乏力、头痛、失眠、皮疹、阳痿等。肌炎不常见，但一旦发生则可能导致横纹肌溶解症。一般不与他汀类合用以减少横纹肌溶解的风险。患肝胆疾病、孕妇、儿童及肾功能不全者禁用。

2) 烟酸(nicotinic acid)

烟酸可降低细胞环磷酸腺苷(cAMP)的水平，使激素敏感脂肪酶的活性降低，脂肪组织中的 TG 不易分解出游离脂肪酸(FFA)，肝脏合成 TG 的原料不足，VLDL 的合成和释放减少，LDL 的来源也减少。烟酸属广谱调血脂药，对Ⅱb 和Ⅳ型高脂血症作用最好。

二、抗氧化剂

抗氧化剂防止氧自由基对脂蛋白的氧化修饰，阻止动脉粥样硬化发生和发展。如普罗布考和维生素 E。

三、多烯脂肪酸

多烯脂肪酸有调血脂和抗动脉粥样硬化的效应，适用于高 TG 性高脂血症，如 n-3 型多烯脂肪酸和 n-6 型多烯脂肪酸。

四、黏多糖和多糖类

黏多糖和多糖类有保护血管内皮免受各种因子损伤的效应，如低分子量肝素和天然类肝素。

案例学习

学习要点：

(1) 高脂血症的分型和治疗原则。

(2) 调血脂药的分类及其作用机制。

(3) 贝特类药物药理作用、临床应用及用药注意事项。

关键词：高脂血症；调血脂药；贝特类；甘油三酯

案例

患者，男，58岁，10年前在例行体检时发现血压升高，最高达170/110 mmHg，一直规则服用氨氯地平及美托洛尔治疗，血压控制在130/80 mmHg左右。10天前，他出现头昏、心前区不适就诊。体检：静息心电图(ECG)正常，胸痛发作时，ECG胸前导联ST段明显压低；心脏超声提示：左室壁增厚，左室舒张功能降低；冠状动脉造影提示：左冠状动脉前降支中段狭窄达55%。服用单硝酸异山梨片(20 mg 口服，一日3次)和阿司匹林肠溶片(100 mg 口服，一日1次)，数天后症状缓解。实验室检查：总胆固醇(TC)4.8 mmol/L，低密度脂蛋白胆固醇(LDL-C)2.95 mmol/L，甘油三酯(TG)5.65 mmol/L，高密度脂蛋白胆固醇(HDL-C)1.04 mmol/L。谷丙转移酶(GPT)、肌酸激酶(CK)、尿素氮(BUN)、肌酐(CREA)均正常。

◎ 问答题

1. 该患者患有什么疾病？
2. 本例中选用阿司匹林的目的及用药依据是什么？
3. 该患者该如何用药调节血脂异常？有什么注意事项？

选择题

1. 下列药物中主要降低胆固醇合成的是(　　)。
   A. 考来烯胺　　B. 烟酸　　C. 洛伐他汀　　D. 亚油酸　　E. 吉非贝齐
2. 一名33岁的男性患者服用了治疗高脂血症的药物后出现牙龈出血，且易瘀血，凝血酶原时间也延长了。他最可能服用了下列哪种药物？(　　)
   A. 阿托伐他汀　　B. 考来烯胺　　C. 吉非贝齐　　D. 烟酸　　E. 普罗布考
3. 降低总胆固醇和低密度脂蛋白最明显的药物是(　　)。
   A. 烟酸　　B. 多烯脂肪酸　　C. 普罗布考　　D. 洛伐他汀　　E. 非诺贝特
4. HMG-CoA还原酶抑制药药理作用为(　　)。
   A. 抑制体内胆固醇氧化酶　　　B. 阻断HMG-CoA转化为甲羟戊酸
   C. 使肝脏LDL受体表达减弱　　D. 具有促进细胞分裂作用
   E. 具有增强细胞免疫作用
5. 下列关于贝特类药物的作用错误的是(　　)。
   A. 降低TG和VLDL　　B. 可增加HDL　　C. 抗血栓形成
   D. 降低血液黏度　　E. 降低血压
6. 以下哪一项是抗高血脂药物治疗最常见的副作用？(　　)
   A. 血压升高　　B. 胃肠道紊乱　　C. 神经系统异常　　D. 心悸　　E. 偏头痛
7. 通过发挥抗氧化作用而用于防止高胆固醇血症的药物是(　　)。
   A. 普罗布考　　B. 考来烯胺　　C. 普伐他汀　　D. 依折麦布　　E. 烟酸
8. 非诺贝特的不良反应中哪一项是错误的？(　　)
   A. 食欲减退　　B. 乏力　　C. 头痛　　D. 皮疹　　E. 皮肤潮红
9. 能明显提高HDL的药物是(　　)。

A. 依折麦布　　B. 烟酸　　　C. 考来烯胺　　D. 多烯脂肪酸　　E. 硫酸软骨素

10. 能明显降低血浆甘油三酯的药物是(　　)。

A. 胆汁酸结合树脂　　B. 抗氧化剂　　C. 他汀类　　D. 多烯脂肪酸　　E. 贝特类

Case study

Key points:

(1) Classification and treatment principles of hyperlipidemia.

(2) Classification and mechanism of action of lipid-lowering drugs.

(3) Pharmacological effects, clinical applications, and medication precautions of fibrates.

Key words: hyperlipidemia; lipid-lowering drugs; fibrates; triglyceride

Case

The patient, male, 58 years old, was found to have elevated blood pressure, up to 170/110 mmHg, during a routine physical examination 10 years ago, and had been taking amlodipine and metoprolol regularly, with his blood pressure controlled at about 130/80 mmHg. 10 days ago, he presented to the doctor with dizziness and precordial discomfort. Physical examination: the resting electrocardiogram (ECG) was normal, and during chest pain episodes, the ST segment of the ECG precordial lead was obviously depressed. Cardiac ultrasound suggested that the left ventricular wall thickened and the left ventricular diastolic function decreased. Coronary artery angiography suggested that the middle stenosis of the anterior descending branch of the left coronary artery was up to 55%. Symptoms resolved after several days of isosorbide mononitrate tablets (20 mg orally, 3 times a day) and aspirin enteric-coated tablets (100 mg orally, once a day). Laboratory tests: total cholesterol (TC) 4.8 mmol/L, low-density lipoprotein cholesterol (LDL-C) 2.95 mmol/L, triglycerides (TG) 5.65 mmol/L, and high-density lipoprotein cholesterol (HDL-C) 1.04 mmol/L. Glutamyltransferase (GPT), creatine kinase (CK), urea nitrogen (BUN), and creatinine (CREA) were normal.

◎ Essay questions

1. What disease is the patient suffering from?
2. What is the purpose and rationale for the use of aspirin in this case?
3. How should the patient take medication to regulate dyslipidemia? What are the precautions?

Multiple-choice questions

1. Which of the following drugs mainly reduce cholesterol synthesis(　　).

A. cholestyramine　　B. niacin　　C. lovastatin

D. linoleic acid　　E. gemfibrozil

2. A 33-year-old man has been prescribed medication for hyperlipidemia. He has been noted to have bleeding from his gums and easy bruisability. His prothrombin time is elevated. Which of

the following agents is most likely to be involved? (　　)
   A. Atorvastatin　　B. Cholestyramine　　C. Gemfibrozil
   D. Niacin　　E. Probucol
3. The drug that lowers total cholesterol and LDL most significantly is (　　).
   A. niacin　　B. polyenoic fatty acids　　C. probucol
   D. lovastatin　　E. fenofibrate
4. The pharmacological effect of HMG-CoA reductase inhibitors is (　　).
   A. inhibit cholesterol oxidase in vivo
   B. block the conversion of HMG-CoA to mevalonate
   C. decrease hepatic LDL receptor expression
   D. promote cell division
   E. enhance cellular immunity
5. What is incorrect about fibrates? (　　)
   A. Decrease TG and VLDL　　B. Increase HDL
   C. Anti-thrombotic formation　　D. Reduce blood viscosity
   E. Reduce blood pressure
6. Which one of the following is the most common side effect of antihyperlipidemic drug therapy? (　　)
   A. Elevated blood pressure　　B. Gastrointestinal disturbance
   C. Neurologic problems　　D. Heart palpitations
   E. Migraine headaches
7. Which drug can be used to prevent hypercholesterolemia by exerting antioxidant effects? (　　)
   A. Probucol　　B. Cholestyramine　　C. Pravastatin
   D. Ezetimibe　　E. Nicotinic acid
8. Which of the adverse reactions of fenofibrate is incorrect? (　　)
   A. Anorexia　　B. Fatigue　　C. Headache
   D. Rash　　E. Skin flushing
9. Which of the following drugs can significantly improve HDL? (　　)
   A. Ezetimibe　　B. Nicotinic acid　　C. Cholestyramine
   D. Polyenoic fatty acids　　E. Chondroitin sulfate
10. Which drug can significantly reduce plasma triglycerides? (　　)
    A. Bile acid binding resin　　B. Antioxidants
    C. Statins　　D. Polyenoic fatty acids
    E. Fibrates

第二十六章案例学习和选择题答案

第二十七章 抗心绞痛药

知识要点

一、心绞痛的病理生理基础与用药策略

1. 心肌需氧与供氧的平衡失调

心肌暂时性缺血缺氧，且静脉回流同时减少，代谢产物积聚后刺激心肌感觉神经末梢引起痛感。

2. 心绞痛分型及特点

劳累型心绞痛时心肌需氧增加而供氧不足；变异性（自发性）心绞痛主要因为冠状动脉痉挛性收缩导致供氧减少；混合型心绞痛时心肌需氧量可增加或不增加。

3. 用药策略

(1) 降低心肌耗氧量。

(2) 增加缺血区心肌供血供氧量。

(3) 抗血小板药及抗血栓药，另外保护血管内皮细胞。

二、常用抗心绞痛药物

1. 硝酸酯类

硝酸酯类主要有：硝酸甘油（nitroglycerin）、戊四硝酯、硝酸异山梨酯（消心痛）、单硝酸异山梨酯。

(1) 药理作用：通过作为外源性一氧化氮（NO）供体，释放出 NO 松弛血管平滑肌。①小剂量可以扩张静脉减少回心血量及心室容积，降低室壁肌张力及心肌耗氧量，迅速缓解心绞痛，还因为降低左心室充盈压增加心内膜下供血。②可选择性扩张较大冠状动脉及侧支血管，增加缺血区供血。③NO 可促进内源性 PGI_2 及 CGRP（降钙素基因相关肽）等物质合成和释放，对心肌细胞产生保护作用，减轻缺血性损伤。

(2) 临床应用：可用于各型心绞痛，也可用于急性心肌梗死及心衰治疗。口服时首过消除明显，一般采用舌下含服或静脉给药。

(3) 不良反应：①面颈部血管扩张引起皮肤潮红、颅内血管搏动性头痛；②剂量过大会明显降压导致反射性交感兴奋可能加重心绞痛；③超剂量会引起高铁血红蛋白血症。连续应用会有耐受现象。

2. β肾上腺素受体阻断药

常用于治疗心绞痛的β肾上腺素受体阻断药(β adrenoceptor antagonists)：如普萘洛尔(propranolol)、美托洛尔(metoprolol)、阿替洛尔(atenolol)。

(1)抗心绞痛作用。①降低心肌耗氧量：β肾上腺素受体阻断药通过减弱心肌收缩力、减慢心率、降低血压、从而降低心肌耗氧量。②阻断非缺血区冠脉血管的$β_2$受体使血管平滑肌收缩压力加大，促使血液向因缺血扩张的冠脉血管流动，增加缺血区侧支循环和血流量。心率减慢、舒张期延长也有利于血液更多流向心内膜区。③促进氧自血红蛋白解离增加心肌供氧。

(2)临床应用。适用于除变异性心绞痛之外的各种心绞痛，对伴有心律失常及高血压者尤为适用，用于心肌梗死可缩小梗死区范围。β受体阻断药与硝酸酯类合用可起到相互取长补短的协同效应。β受体阻断药能对抗硝酸酯类引起的反射性交感兴奋对心脏的影响，硝酸酯类可缩小β受体阻断药所致的心室前负荷增大和射血时间延长。合用时两药均可减量。

(3)不良反应。①突然停用β受体阻断药可能导致心绞痛加剧甚或诱发心肌梗死。②有严重心功能不全、支气管哮喘或有哮喘病史者慎用。③长期应用可能引起血脂异常。

3. 钙通道阻滞药

常用于治疗心绞痛的钙通道阻滞药有：硝苯地平(nifedipine)、维拉帕米(verapamil)、地尔硫䓬、哌克昔林及普尼拉明等。

(1)抗心绞痛作用及机制。阻滞细胞膜L型Ca^{++}通道，抑制Ca^{++}内流产生以下作用：①降低心肌收缩力，且舒张血管平滑肌后降低血压减轻心脏负荷，降低心肌耗氧量。②舒张冠状动脉，打开侧支血管，增加缺血区心肌供血供氧。③抑制缺血心肌细胞钙超载，保护缺血心肌细胞结构及功能。④降低血小板内Ca^{++}浓度，抑制血小板聚集，避免冠脉内形成血栓。

(2)临床应用。适用于各种心绞痛，是变异性心绞痛首选药。此外可用于以下三类：①并发支气管哮喘者。②并发外周血管痉挛性疾病者。③硝苯地平适合与β受体阻断药合用。

(3)不良反应。维拉帕米及地尔硫䓬抑制心肌收缩力及抑制窦房结和房室传导作用强，对伴有心衰或心动过缓者禁用。

案例学习

学习要点：

(1)心绞痛的病理生理机制、用药策略及药物分类。

(2)硝酸酯类的抗心绞痛作用特点和机制、临床应用及不良反应。

(3)β受体阻断药的抗心绞痛机制、临床应用及不良反应。

(4)钙通道阻滞药的抗心绞痛机制、临床应用特别是变异性心绞痛首选。

关键词：心绞痛；血氧供需平衡；硝酸甘油；β受体阻断药；钙通道阻滞药

案例

张先生今年50岁，有30年吸烟史和约5年高血压病史。近2年来偶尔在体力活动时出现心前区疼痛，休息后可自行好转。今晨因用力排便再次出现胸痛，并放射至左肩背部被送至急诊室。查体心率96次/min，血压160/100 mmHg，心电图显示ST段明显抬高，诊断为劳力型心绞痛。医生立即给予硝酸甘油片0.5 mg舌下含化，一会儿疼痛开始缓解并逐渐消失。医生询问他高血压病治疗的情况，他说一般在血压高到引起他不舒服的时候才用药。医生嘱咐他必须戒烟，避免进行剧烈体力活动，便秘时适当使用通便药物；随身携带硝酸甘油片；重要的是遵医嘱坚持规律应用降压药。

问答题

1. 为什么心绞痛发病后不首选止痛药治疗？
2. 试述硝酸酯类的抗心绞痛作用机制、临床应用及不良反应。
3. 吸烟、高血压病与心绞痛之间有什么关系？
4. 对于这位病人如何指导预防心绞痛发作？

选择题

1. 心绞痛患者宜随身携带的最重要的药是(　　)。
   A. 普萘洛尔　　B. 硝苯地平　　C. 肾上腺素　　D. 硝酸甘油　　E. 氢氯噻嗪
2. 变异性心绞痛宜首选用的药物是(　　)。
   A. 硝酸甘油　　B. 硝苯地平　　C. 普萘洛尔　　D. 阿司匹林　　E. 酚妥拉明
3. 硝酸甘油舌下含服能快速缓解心绞痛的机理是(　　)。
   A. 舌下含服硝酸甘油可被迅速吸收并代谢为NO，增加细胞内过氧亚硝基浓度，抑制鸟苷酸环化酶相关的心外膜动脉收缩，增加心肌供氧。
   B. 舌下含服硝酸甘油可被迅速吸收并在冠状动脉上皮细胞通过代谢被激活后抑制NO降解，增强NO相关的心外膜动脉舒张和心肌供氧。
   C. 舌下含服硝酸甘油可被迅速吸收并代谢为NO，扩张肺动脉后缓解肺动脉高压，增加心肌供氧。
   D. 舌下含服硝酸甘油可被迅速吸收并代谢为NO，扩张体循环静脉和心外膜动脉，降低心肌耗氧量并增加心肌供氧。
   E. 舌下含服硝酸甘油可被迅速吸收并代谢为NO，扩张体循环动脉降低血管阻力从而降低心肌耗氧量。
4. 普萘洛尔治疗心绞痛的缺点是(　　)。
   A. 无冠状动脉及外周血管扩张作用　　B. 抑制心肌收缩力，心室容积增加
   C. 延长心室射血时间　　　　　　　　D. 突然停药有"反跳"现象
   E. 以上都是
5. 硝酸甘油不具有下列哪种作用？(　　)
   A. 扩张容量血管　　B. 减少回心血量　　C. 降低心肌耗氧量
   D. 增加室壁肌张力　　E. 扩张冠状动脉

6. 硝酸甘油用药后常见的不良反应是(　　)。
   A. 短暂失明　　B. 头痛　　C. 肝功能异常　　D. 心动过缓　　E. 恶心
7. 普萘洛尔治疗心绞痛的主要作用机制是(　　)。
   A. 抑制心脏收缩功能,降低耗氧量　　B. 选择性阻断 $β_2$ 受体,舒张冠脉
   C. 延长心室射血时间　　D. 减慢心率,增加心室容积
   E. 降低氧合血红蛋白解离
8. 硝酸甘油通常采用舌下含服给药是因为(　　)。
   A. 起效比口服用药快速　　B. 不会刺激胃肠道产生恶心的副作用
   C. 这样用药不需喝水　　D. 较少出现头痛反应
   E. 可以避免首过消除
9. 不属于硝苯地平抗心绞痛机制的是(　　)。
   A. 降低平滑肌细胞内钙浓度,舒张冠状动脉　　B. 抑制心肌收缩力,降低氧耗量
   C. 降低血钙浓度　　D. 减慢心率　　E. 抗血小板功能
10. 通常不用于治疗心绞痛的药物是(　　)。
    A. 硝酸甘油　　B. 杜冷丁　　C. 普萘洛尔　　D. 阿司匹林　　E. 硝苯地平

Case study

Key points:

(1) The pathophysiological mechanism of angina pectoris, tactics for angina drug treatment and drug classification for angina.

(2) The antianginal characteristics and mechanisms, clinical uses and adverse reactions of nitrates.

(3) The antianginal mechanisms, clinical uses and adverse reactions of β blockers.

(4) The antianginal mechanisms and clinical uses of calcium channel blockers, especially for angina pectoris at rest.

Key words: angina pectoris; balance between oxygen supplication and requirement; nitroglycerin; β blocker; calcium channel blocker

Case

Mr. Zhang was 50-years old, with a history of smoking 30 years and hypertension about 5 years. He has been occasionally feeling transient precordial pain following force work or exercise for 2 years, generally recovered after rest, and he was sent to the emergency room because of severe chest pain which radiate to the left shoulder and back while he taking a shit forcibly this morning. Physical examination found his heart rate was 96/min, BP 160/100 mmHg, and ECG showed a significant ST segment elevation. He was diagnosed as exertional angina. Nitroglycerin tablet 0. 5 mg was administrated sublingually, his chest pain began to alleviate soon and gradually gone. The doctor asked him about the treatment of his hypertension, he said only took medicine when the BP was high enough to make him uncomfortable. The doctor told him that he must stop smoking; to avoid force activity; to administrate laxative while constipation; to carry nitroglycerin tablet with him in daily life; and another important thing was taking anti-hypertensives under directions of doctor regularly.

◎ **Essay questions**

1. Why are painkillers not preferred after the onset of angina pectoris?
2. Antianginal mechanism of action, clinical application and adverse effects of nitrates.
3. What is the relationship between smoking, hypertension and angina?
4. How can this patient be counseled to prevent an angina attack?

✎ **Multiple-choice questions**

1. The most important medicine an angina patient should take with is (　　).
   A. propranolol   B. nifedipine   C. adrenaline
   D. nitroglycerin   E. hydrochlorothiazide
2. The first choice for variant angina patient should be (　　).
   A. nitroglycerin   B. nifedipine   C. propranolol
   D. aspirin   E. phentolamine
3. What is the mechanism by which sublingual nitroglycerin acts so quickly to relieve chest pain? (　　)
   A. Sublingual nitroglycerin is rapidly absorbed and metabolized to NO, which increases intracellular concentrations of peroxynitrite and inhibit guanlate cyclase-associated vasoconstriction of epicardial arteries, and increases myocardial oxygen supply.
   B. Sublingual nitroglycerin is rapidly absorbed and activated by a first pass metabolism in the coronary artery epithelial cells to inhibit NO breakdown and increase NO-associated epicardial arterial dilation and myocardial oxygen supply.
   C. Sublingual nitroglycerin is rapidly absorbed and metabolized to NO, which dilates the pulmonary vasculature, relieving pulmonary hypertension and increasing myocardial oxygen supply.
   D. Sublingual nitroglycerin is rapidly absorbed and metabolized to NO, which dilate systemic veins and epicardial arteries, decreasing myocardial oxygen demand and increasing myocardial oxygen supply.
   E. Sublingual nitroglycerin is rapidly absorbed and metabolized to NO, which dilate systemic arterioles, decreasing systemic vascular resistance and reducing myocardial oxygen demand.
4. The disadvantage of propranolol in the treatment of angina is (　　).
   A. no coronary and peripheral vasodilating effect
   B. inhibits myocardial contractility and increases ventricular volume
   C. prolongation of ventricular ejection time

D. sudden discontinuation of the drug "rebound" phenomenon

E. all of the above

5. Nitroglycerin does not have which of the following effects? (   )

   A. Dilates volumetric vessels. B. Decrease return blood flow.

   C. Decrease myocardial oxygen consumption. D. Increase ventricular wall tone.

   E. Dilate coronary arteries.

6. The common adverse reaction after nitroglycerin administration is (   ).

   A. transient blindness   B. headache   C. abnormal liver function

   D. bradycardia   E. nausea

7. The main mechanism of action of propranolol in the treatment of angina pectoris is (   ).

   A. inhibit cardiac contractile function, reduce oxygen consumption

   B. selectively blocking β_2 receptors and dilating coronary arteries.

   C. prolonging ventricular ejection time

   D. slowing the heart rate and increasing ventricular volume

   E. decrease oxygenated hemoglobin dissociation

8. Nitroglycerin is usually given sublingually because (   ).

   A. it works faster than oral medication

   B. it does not irritate the gastrointestinal tract and cause nausea as a side effect

   C. it does not require water

   D. headache is less likely to occur

   E. first pass elimination can be avoided

9. What is not part of the antianginal mechanism of nifedipine (   ).

   A. lowering intracellular calcium concentration in smooth muscle cells and dilating coronary arteries

   B. inhibiting myocardial contractility and reducing oxygen consumption

   C. lowering blood calcium concentration

   D. slowing the heart rate

   E. antiplatelet function

10. The drug not usually used to treat angina is (   ).

    A. nitroglycerin   B. dolantin   C. propranolol   D. aspirin   E. nifedipine

第二十七章案例学习和选择题答案

第二十八章 作用于血液及造血系统的药物

知识要点

血液及造血系统的药物导图见图28-1：

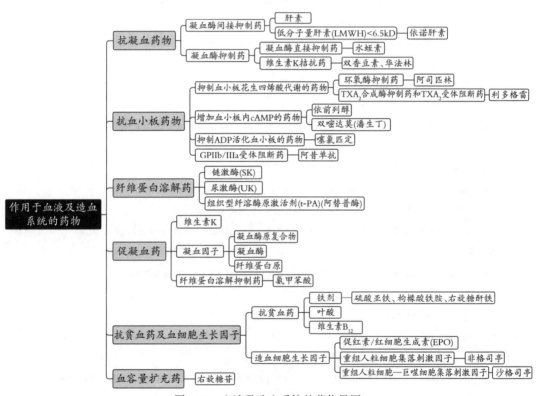

图28-1 血液及造血系统的药物导图

一、抗凝血药

(一) 凝血酶间接抑制药

1. 肝素

1) 药理作用

肝素在体内、体外均有强大的抗凝作用。静脉注射后，抗凝血作用立即发生，可使多种凝血因子灭活。该作用依赖于抗凝血酶Ⅲ(AT Ⅲ)。肝素还可使血管内皮释放脂蛋白脂酶，发挥降脂作用；抑制炎症介质活性和炎症细胞活动，有抗炎作用及抑制血管平滑肌增生；抑制血小板聚集。

2) 临床应用

(1) 血栓栓塞性疾病：防止血栓形成与扩大。

(2) 弥散性血管内凝血。

(3) 体外抗凝：心导管检查、血液透析。

3) 不良反应

(1) 出血：应用过量易引起自发性出血，注射带有阳电荷的强碱性鱼精蛋白解救。

(2) 血小板减少症：一般是肝素引起的一过性血小板聚集作用所致。

2. 低分子量肝素(low molecular weight heparin, LMWH)

1) 药理作用

从普通肝素中分离或由普通肝素降解后得到的短链制剂，分子量一般低于 7kDa。作用特点：①LMWH 的 $\frac{抗凝血因子\ Xa\ 活性}{抗凝血因子\ Ⅱa\ 活性}$ 比值(1.5~4.0)高于肝素(1.0)，使抗血栓作用与致出血作用分离，保持了抗血栓作用而降低了出血的危险；②LMWH 抗凝血因子 Xa 活性的 $t_{1/2}$ 长(图 28-2)。

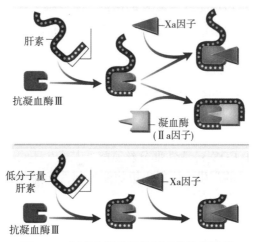

图 28-2 肝素和低分子量肝素的抗凝机制

2) 临床应用和不良反应

临床应用和不良反应与肝素相似。常用药物包括有依诺肝素、替地肝素、弗希肝素、洛吉肝素、洛莫肝素。

(二) 凝血酶抑制药

1. 凝血酶直接抑制药：水蛭素、阿加曲班

1) 药理作用

水蛭素直接与凝血酶的催化位点和阴离子外位点结合，抑制凝血酶活性。

2)临床应用

预防术后血栓形成,预防经皮冠状动脉成形术术后冠状动脉再阻塞,血液透析及体外循环。

2. 维生素K拮抗药:双香豆素、华法林和醋硝香豆素

1)药理作用

香豆素类为口服抗凝药,是维生素K拮抗剂,在肝脏抑制维生素K由环氧化型向氢醌型转化,从而阻止维生素K的反复利用,抑制凝血因子Ⅱ、Ⅶ、Ⅸ、Ⅹ的活化。

2)临床应用

一般采用先用肝素或者先与肝素合用,后用香豆素类维持治疗的序贯疗法。

防治血栓栓塞性疾病:风湿性心脏病、心脏瓣膜修复手术后防止静脉血栓发生。

3)不良反应

应用过量易致自发性出血,严重的出血需静脉注射大量维生素K或输新鲜血液解救。

4)药物相互作用

(1)有较高血浆蛋白结合率的药物阿司匹林、保泰松等可使血浆中游离香豆素类浓度升高,抗凝作用增强。

(2)降低维生素K生物利用度的药物或各种病理状态导致胆汁减少均可增强香豆素类的作用。

(3)广谱抗生素抑制肠道产生维生素K的菌群,减少维生素K的生成,增强香豆素类的作用。

二、抗血小板药

(一)抑制血小板花生四烯酸代谢的药物

1. 环氧酶抑制药:阿司匹林

1)药理作用

阿司匹林可与环氧酶(COX-1)活性部分丝氨酸残基发生不可逆的乙酰化反应,使酶失活,减少血栓素A_2(TXA_2)的产生,使血小板功能抑制;能部分拮抗纤维蛋白原溶解导致的血小板激活,还可抑制t-PA的释放。

2)临床应用

(1)临床应用最广泛的抗血小板药。

(2)血小板功能亢进而引起血栓栓塞性疾病:冠状动脉硬化性疾病、心肌梗死、脑梗死、深静脉血栓形成和肺梗死。

(3)对急性心肌梗死或不稳定型心绞痛患者,可降低再梗死率及死亡率。

(4)对一过性脑缺血也可减少发生率及死亡率。

2. TXA_2合成酶抑制药和TXA_2受体阻断药:利多格雷

1)药理作用

利多格雷为强大的TXA_2合成酶抑制药,并具有中度的TXA_2受体拮抗作用。对血小板血栓和冠状动脉血栓的作用较强。

2）临床应用

降低再栓塞、反复心绞痛和缺血性中风的发生率，但疗效不肯定。

（二）增加血小板内 cAMP 的药物

1. 依前列醇

1）药理作用

依前列醇为人工合成的 PGI_2，是活性最强的血小板聚集内源性抑制药。通过激活血小板中腺苷酸环化酶，升高细胞内 cAMP 水平，降低胞质内游离 Ca^{2+} 浓度，使血小板处于静止状态。

2）临床应用

体外循环、血栓性血小板减少性紫癜、微血栓形成、出血倾向。性质不稳定，作用短暂，临床应用受限。

2. 双嘧达莫

1）药理作用

(1) 抑制磷酸二酯酶（PDE）活性，减少 cAMP 降解，增加血小板内 cAMP 含量。

(2) 血管内皮细胞 PGI_2 的生成，增强 PGI_2 活性。

(3) 抑制腺苷再摄取，激活腺苷酸环化酶，cAMP 生成增多。

(4) 抑制血小板的环氧化酶，减少 TXA_2 合成。

2）临床应用

血栓栓塞性疾病、人工心脏瓣膜置换术后、缺血性心脏病、脑卒中和短暂性脑缺血发作。

（三）抑制 ADP 活化血小板的药物：噻氯匹定

1）药理作用

能选择性及特异性地干扰 ADP 介导的血小板活化，不可逆地抑制血小板聚集和黏附。

2）临床应用

预防脑卒中、心肌梗死及外周动脉血栓性疾病的复发。

（四）血小板膜糖蛋白 II_b/III_a 受体阻断药

1）药理作用

多种因素引起血小板聚集的最终共同通路都是暴露血小板膜表面的糖蛋白 II_b/III_a 受体（GP II_b/III_a 受体），GP II_b/III_a 受体拮抗药可抑制各种物质通过与血小板 GP II_b/III_a 受体结合诱发的血小板聚集。

2）临床应用

急性心肌梗死、溶栓治疗、不稳定型心绞痛和血管成形术后再梗死。常用药物包括阿昔单抗、拉米非班、夫雷非班等。

三、纤维蛋白溶解药

1）药理作用

通过降解纤维蛋白和纤维蛋白原而限制血栓增大和溶解血栓。

2）临床应用

血栓栓塞性疾病的溶栓治疗，如急性心肌梗死、肺栓塞、脑栓塞。常用药物包括链激酶、尿激酶、阿尼普酶、葡激酶、阿替普酶、瑞替普酶。

四、促凝血药

（一）维生素 K

1）药理作用

维生素 K 作为 γ-羧化酶的辅酶，参与凝血因子 Ⅱ、Ⅶ、Ⅸ、Ⅹ 的活化。

2）临床应用

维生素 K 缺乏引起的出血：梗阻性黄疸、胆瘘、慢性腹泻、早产儿、新生儿出血，香豆素类、水杨酸类药物所致出血；预防长期应用广谱抗菌药继发的维生素 K 缺乏症。

（二）凝血因子：凝血酶原复合物、抗血友病球蛋白、纤维蛋白原、凝血酶

凝血酶原复合物：由健康人静脉血分离而得的含有凝血因子 Ⅱ、Ⅶ、Ⅸ、Ⅹ 的混合制剂。

（三）纤维蛋白溶解抑制药：氨甲苯酸和氨甲环酸

1）药理作用

竞争性抑制纤溶酶原激活因子，阻止纤溶酶原转变为纤溶酶，抑制纤维蛋白的溶解，产生止血作用。

2）临床应用

纤维蛋白溶解症所致的出血：内脏器官手术所致的出血、产后出血、前列腺肥大出血、上消化道出血。

五、抗贫血药及造血细胞生长因子

（一）抗贫血药

1. 铁剂

1）体内过程

非血红素铁和无机铁必须还原为 Fe^{2+} 才能被吸收。胃酸、维生素 C、果糖、半胱氨酸等有助于铁的还原，可促进吸收。胃酸缺乏以及食物中高磷、高钙、鞣酸等物质使铁沉淀，妨碍吸收。四环素等与铁络合，也不利于铁吸收。

2）药理作用

吸收到骨髓的铁，吸附在有核红细胞膜上并进入细胞内的线粒体，与原卟啉结合形成血红素。后者再与珠蛋白结合，形成血红蛋白。

3）临床应用

口服铁剂包括硫酸亚铁、枸橼酸铁铵、右旋糖酐铁，主要用于缺铁性贫血治疗。

2. 叶酸

1）药理作用

叶酸为细胞生长分裂所必需的物质。叶酸在体内还原成四氢叶酸，以辅酶的形式参与一碳单位的传递过程，参与核酸及蛋白质的合成，并与维生素 B_{12} 共同促进红细胞的生长

和成熟。

2）临床应用

巨幼细胞贫血。

3. 维生素 B_{12}

1）体内过程

维生素 B_{12} 必须与胃壁细胞分泌的糖蛋白即"内因子"结合才能免受胃液消化而进入空肠吸收。胃黏膜萎缩所致"内因子"缺乏可影响维生素 B_{12} 吸收，引起"恶性贫血"。

2）药理作用

（1）维生素 B_{12} 参与 5-甲基四氢叶酸转变为四氢叶酸过程，提供一碳单位参与核酸及蛋白质的合成。

（2）促使脂肪酸中间代谢产物甲基丙二酸变成琥珀酸，维持神经髓鞘的完整性。

3）临床应用

恶性贫血和巨幼细胞贫血，以及神经炎、神经萎缩等神经系统疾病。常用药物包括氰钴胺、羟钴胺。

4）不良反应

可致过敏反应，甚至过敏性休克，不宜滥用。不可静脉给药。

(二)造血细胞生长因子

1. 促红素（细胞生成素）

促使红细胞生成，对多种原因引起的贫血有效。

2. 非格司亭（重组人粒细胞集落刺激因子）

促进中性粒细胞成熟、释放、趋化和吞噬功能。用于骨髓移植及肿瘤化疗后严重中性粒细胞缺乏症。

六、血容量扩充药：右旋糖酐

右旋糖酐 70：中分子右旋糖酐，平均分子量约为 70kDa；

右旋糖酐 40：低分子右旋糖酐，平均分子量约为 40kDa；

右旋糖酐 10：小分子右旋糖酐，平均分子量约为 10kDa。

1）药理作用

右旋糖酐分子量较大，能提高血浆胶体渗透压，从而扩充血容量，维持血压，其作用强度与维持时间随分子量减少而逐渐降低。

2）临床应用

低血容量性休克。

案例学习

学习要点：

（1）熟悉影响血液凝固过程的药物的类别。

（2）掌握抗血栓药物的作用机制、临床应用、不良反应。

关键词：肝素、抗血小板药、埃替非巴肽、氯吡格雷、阿司匹林

案例

周先生，60岁，有高血压和吸烟史。一天半夜，他从梦中惊醒，并感到胸骨下压榨性疼痛，并向左肩放射，伴有出汗和气短。他拨打了120电话，救护车把他送到了急救室。心电图检查结果发现，T波倒置，从V2变为V5。生化检查结果显示，肌酸激酶水平800 IU/L（正常值60~400 IU/L）其中MB片段为10%（心脏特异性亚型），提示已出现心肌梗死。经静脉注射了硝酸甘油、阿司匹林、依诺肝素、埃替非巴肽后，周先生的持续胸痛仍无缓解。经心导管检查，发现他有冠状动脉左前降支血栓，已占据90%管腔，所以导致其远端血流迟缓。医生成功地给他进行了血管成形术，并放置了支架。支架放置过程中，给他口服了负荷剂量的氯吡格雷。停用肝素，埃替非巴肽静脉注射持续了16个多小时，而后他被转移监护室。5个小时后，周先生的右腿动脉插管入口下方出现了扩张性血肿。埃替非巴肽被停用，对出血部位进行压迫止血，使血肿停止扩张。两天后，周先生出院，并遵医嘱回家服用氯吡格雷和阿司匹林以防止支架处的亚急性血栓的形成。

问答题

1. 周先生冠状动脉里的血栓是怎么形成的？
2. 阿司匹林、肝素、氯吡格雷、埃替非巴肽是如何解除血凝块阻滞，并阻止血栓再形成的？
3. 当观察到扩展性血肿时，除了停用埃替非巴肽外，是否还有其他措施可以减轻血肿的形成？
4. 如果使用低分子量肝素代替肝素，该如何监控患者的凝血状态？

选择题

1. 不可用于血栓栓塞性疾病的药物是以下哪种？（ ）
   A. 肝素　　　B. 阿司匹林　　　C. 氨甲苯酸　　　D. 双嘧达莫　　　E. 噻氯匹定
2. 肝素过量引起自发性出血选用什么药物解救？（ ）
   A. 维生素K　　　B. 氨甲苯酸　　　C. 鱼精蛋白　　　D. 垂体后叶素　　　E. 以上都不是
3. 体内、外均有抗凝血作用的药物是以下哪种？（ ）
   A. 双香豆素　　　B. 肝素　　　C. 尿激酶　　　D. 阿司匹林　　　E. 华法林
4. 治疗巨幼细胞贫血首选什么药物？（ ）
   A. 维生素 B_{12}　　　B. 叶酸+维生素 B_{12}　　　C. 甲酰四氢叶酸钙
   D. 维生素 B_6　　　E. 铁剂
5. 以下哪种药物可降低双香豆素抗凝血作用？（ ）
   A. 水杨酸类　　　B. 甲磺丁脲　　　C. 甲硝唑　　　D. 苯巴比妥　　　E. 西咪替丁
6. 阿司匹林是通过作用于以下哪种物质而抑制血小板代谢的？（ ）
   A. TXA_2　　　B. PGI_2　　　C. COX-1　　　D. PGE_2　　　E. PDE
7. 长期使用广谱抗菌药继发的出血宜选用以下哪种药物？（ ）
   A. 氨甲苯酸　　　B. 维生素C　　　C. 维生素K　　　D. 鱼精蛋白　　　E. 垂体后叶素

8. 以下描述中，哪项是氨甲苯酸(PAMBA)的药理作用？（　　）
   A. 抑制纤溶酶原　　　　B. 对抗纤溶酶原激活因子　C. 增加血小板聚集
   D. 促使毛细血管收缩　　E. 促进肝脏合成凝血酶原
9. 叶酸可用于治疗以下哪种疾病？（　　）
   A. 小细胞低色素性贫血　　B. 溶血性贫血　　　　C. 妊娠期巨幼细胞贫血
   D. 再生障碍性贫血　　　　E. 乙胺嘧啶所致巨幼细胞贫血
10. 过量链激酶引起出血时可选用的拮抗药是哪种？（　　）
    A. 维生素K　　B. 氨甲苯酸　　C. 鱼精蛋白　　D. 垂体后叶素　　E. 华法林

Case study

Key points：
(1) The classification of drugs affecting blood coagulation.
(2) The mechanism of actions, therapeutic uses, adverse effects, and adverse effects of antithrombotic medicines.

Key words： heparin; antiplatelet drugs; eptifibatide; clopidogrel; aspirin

Case

Mr. Zhou is a 60-year old man and has a 20-year history of hypertension and cigarette smoking. One night, he is awakened with a crushing pain behind the sternum radiated to his left shoulder. He also feels shortness of breath accompanied by sweating. He calls 120 and is taken to the emergency department. An electrocardiogram shows deep T-wave inversions in leads V2 to V5. A cardiac biomarker panel shows a creatine kinase level of 800 IU/L (normal, 60-400 IU/L) with 10% MB fraction (the heart-specific isoform), suggesting myocardial infarction. He is administered with intravenous nitroglycerin, aspirin, unfractionated heparin, and eptifibatide, but his chest pain is not alleviated. Therefore, the doctor decides to do cardiac catheterization to confirm the diagnosis and to locate the thrombus. Mr. Zhou is found to have a 90% mid-LAD (left anterior descending artery) thrombus with sluggish distal flow, so the doctor does an angioplasty and stent placement to dredge the artery. At the time of stent placement, an oral loading dose of clopidogrel is administered. The heparin is stopped, intravenous eptifibatide is continued for 16 more hours, and Mr. Zhou is transferred to ICU. Five hours later, Mr. Zhou is noted to have an expanding hematoma (an area of localized hemorrhage) in his right thigh below the arterial access site. The doctor stops eptifibatide and gives pressure to the access site to stop further bleeding, and the hematoma ceases to expand. Mr. Zhou is discharged 3 days later with prescriptions including clopidogrel and aspirin, which are administered to prevent subacute thrombosis of the stent.

◎ **Essay questions**
1. How did a blood clot arise in Mr. Zhou's coronary artery?

2. How do aspirin, heparin, clopidogrel, and eptifibatide act in the attempt to treat Mr. Zhou's blood clot and to prevent recurrent thrombus formation?
3. When the expanding hematoma was observed, could any measure other than stopping the eptifibatide have been used to reverse the effect of this agent?
4. If low-molecular-weight heparin had been used instead of unfractionated heparin, how would the monitoring of the patient's coagulation status during the procedure have been affected?

Multiple-choice questions

1. Which of the medicines can not be used for treatment of thromboembolic disease? (   )
   A. Heparin   B. Aspirin   C. Aminomethylbenzoic acid
   D. Dipyridamole   E. Ticlopidine
2. Which of the following should be used for heparin induced hematostaxis? (   )
   A. Vitamin K   B. Aminomethylbenzoic acid C. Protamine
   D. Hypophysin   E. None of above
3. Which of the following has anticoagulation effects in vitro and vivo? (   )
   A. Bishydroxycoumarin B. Heparin   C. Urokinase
   D. Aspirin   E. Warfarin
4. Which medication is recommended for the treatment of megaloblastic anemia? (   )
   A. Vitamin B_{12} B. Folic acid + vitamin B_{12} C. Calcium formyltetrahydrofolate
   D. Vitamin B_6 E. Iron supplements
5. Which of the following drugs reduces dicoumarol's anticoagulant effects? (   )
   A. Salicylates   B. Sulfonylurea   C. Metronidazole
   D. Phenobarbital   E. Cimetidine
6. Aspirin works on which of the following substances to inhibit platelet metabolism? (   )
   A. TXA_2 B. PGI_2 C. COX-1
   D. PGE_2 E. PDE
7. Which medication is recommended for bleeding caused by long-term use of broad-spectrum antimicrobials? (   )
   A. Aminomethylbenzoic acid B. Vitamin C   C. Vitamin K
   D. Protamine   E. Posterior pituitary hormone
8. Which of the following is the pharmacologic effect of PAMBA? (   )
   A. Inhibits fibrinogen   B. Inhibits fibrinogen-activating factor
   C. Increases platelet aggregation   D. Promotes capillary constriction
   E. Promotes hepatic synthesis of thrombinogen
9. Which of the following diseases is an indication of folic acid? (   )
   A. Hypochromic microcytic anemia   B. Hemolytic anemia
   C. Megaloblastic anemia in pregnancy   D. Aplastic anemia
   E. Ethambutol-induced Megaloblastic anemia

10. What is the antagonist for streptokinase-induced hemorrhage?(　　)
    A. Vitamin K
    B. Aminomethylbenzoic acid
    C. Protamine
    D. Posterior pituitary hormone
    E. Warfarin

第二十八章案例学习和选择题答案

第二十九章 作用于呼吸系统的药物

知识要点

呼吸系统的药物导图见图 29-1：

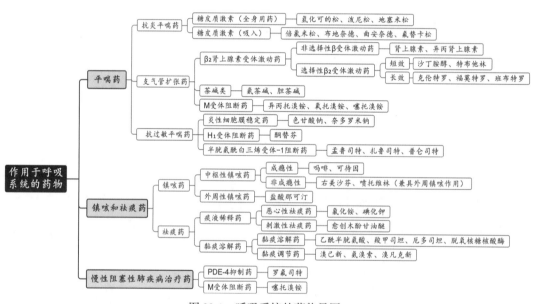

图 29-1 呼吸系统的药物导图

一、平喘药

（一）抗炎平喘药

糖皮质激素（glucocorticoids，GCs），如布地奈德（budesonide，BUD）、丙酸倍氯米松（beclomethasone dipropionate，BDP）。

1）药理作用

抗炎平喘药通过抑制气道炎症反应，可以达到长期防止哮喘发作的效果，已成为平喘药中的一线药物。

2）临床应用

用于支气管扩张药不能有效控制的慢性哮喘患者，但不能缓解急性症状。吸入糖皮质激素在气道内可获得较高的药物浓度，即可充分发挥局部抗炎作用，亦可避免或减少全身性的不良反应。因此，目前常用吸入剂型糖皮质激素；全身应用仅在吸入剂型糖皮质激素无效时使用。

3）不良反应

吸入糖皮质激素长期用药时，可沉积在咽部，引起声音嘶哑、声带萎缩变形、诱发口咽部念珠菌感染等；当吞咽到胃肠道吸收后，对下丘脑-垂体-肾上腺轴产生抑制作用，但远比口服制剂轻微。

(二) 支气管扩张药

1. 肾上腺素受体激动药(adrenoceptor agonists)

非选择性 β 受体激动药，如异丙肾上腺素(isoprenaline)、肾上腺素(adrenaline)；选择性 β_2 受体激动药，如沙丁胺醇(salbutamol)(短效)、克仑特罗(clenbuterol)(长效)。

1）药理作用

人气道中 β 肾上腺素受体主要是 β_2 受体，β 受体激动药可结合并激活气道平滑肌细胞膜上的 β_2 受体，使支气管平滑肌松弛。非选择性 β 受体激动剂平喘作用强大，但可引起严重的心脏不良反应。选择性 β_2 受体激动药对 β_2 受体有强大的兴奋性，对 β_1 受体的亲和力低，常规剂量口服或吸入给药时很少产生心血管反应，是平喘药中的一线药物。

2）临床应用

主要用于支气管哮喘、喘息性支气管炎及伴有支气管痉挛的呼吸道疾病。吸入给药最为常用，而在哮喘急性发作时，由于气道痉挛，吸入给药效果不佳，静脉给药仍是首选。

3）不良反应

(1) 心脏反应：β_2 受体激动药对心脏的作用较轻，但在大剂量或注射给药时，仍可引起心脏反应。

(2) 肌肉震颤：激动骨骼肌慢收缩纤维的 β_2 受体，引起肌肉震颤，好发于四肢与面颈部。

(3) 代谢紊乱：增加肌糖原分解，引起血乳酸、丙酮酸升高，产生酮体。糖尿病患者应用时应注意引起酮中毒或乳酸性酸中毒；兴奋骨骼肌细胞膜上的 Na^+-K^+-ATP 酶，使 K^+ 进入细胞内而引起血钾降低，过量应用或与糖皮质激素合用时，可能引起低钾血症。

2. 茶碱类(theophylline)：氨茶碱、胆茶碱

3. 抗胆碱药(M 胆碱受体阻断药)：异丙托溴铵

(三) 抗过敏平喘药

1. 炎症细胞膜稳定药：色甘酸钠、奈多罗米钠
2. H_1 受体阻断药：酮替芬
3. 半胱氨酰白三烯受体-1 阻断药：扎鲁司特(zafirlukast)、孟鲁司特(montelukast)

二、镇咳药

1. 中枢性镇咳药：直接抑制延髓咳嗽中枢而发挥镇咳作用

(1) 成瘾性中枢性镇咳药：主要指阿片类生物碱，如吗啡。

(2) 非成瘾性中枢性镇咳药：氢溴酸右美沙芬、枸橼酸喷托维林。

2. 外周性镇咳药

通过抑制咳嗽反射弧中的感受器、传入神经、传出神经或效应器中任何环节而发挥镇咳作用，如盐酸那可汀。

三、祛痰药

1. 痰液稀释药

口服后增加痰液中水分含量，稀释痰液。

(1) 恶心性祛痰药：氯化铵(ammonium chloride)。

(2) 刺激性祛痰药：愈创甘油醚(guaifenesin)。

2. 黏痰溶解药

使痰液黏稠度降低或调节黏液成分，使痰液容易排出。

(1) 黏痰溶解药：乙酰半胱氨酸、脱氧核糖核酸酶。

(2) 黏痰调节药：溴己新。

案例学习

学习要点：

1. 吸入型糖皮质激素和全身应用糖皮质激素的药理作用特点和各自的适应证。
2. 糖皮质激素停药反应发生的机制及相应的处理措施。
3. 长期大剂量应用糖皮质激素引起的不良反应及相关机制。

关键词：糖皮质激素；哮喘；给药途径；停药反应

案例

龙龙今年7岁，两年前开始不时感到呼吸困难，在运动时尤其明显。他被诊断患有支气管哮喘。由于龙龙的支气管哮喘病情反复发作，症状始终得不到完全缓解。尽管担心会干扰龙龙的生长发育，医生最终还是给他开了口服泼尼松(一种糖皮质激素类似物)治疗，并嘱咐龙龙的父母一定要确保龙龙每天遵医嘱服药。几周后，龙龙的哮喘病情有所缓解，终于能够像正常孩子那样踢足球和游泳了。在此期间，医生仍密切监视龙龙的生长情况。三年后，医生认为吸入型的糖皮质激素对龙龙的治疗更为安全，于是医生给龙龙停用了口服泼尼松，改为吸入型糖皮质激素治疗。四天后，龙龙因高热(40℃)到急诊室就诊，伴有低血压，诊断为呼吸道感染。鉴于龙龙有既往口服泼尼松的治疗史，医生立即对龙龙进行氢化可的松(皮质醇)和生理盐水静脉注射。随后，龙龙的病情开始好转，之后的12个月内，龙龙在继续吸入糖皮质激素治疗的同时逐步减少口服泼尼松的剂量。最后，单独应用吸入型糖皮质即可有效治疗龙龙的哮喘。

问答题

1. 为什么像泼尼松这样的皮质醇类似物可用于治疗哮喘？

2. 为什么口服泼尼松突然停用会导致龙龙的病情突发变化，表现出在急诊室出现的症状？

3. 为什么在支气管哮喘的长期治疗中吸入型糖皮质激素比口服糖皮质激素更为安全？
4. 为什么医生要监测龙龙的生长情况？

选择题

1. 针对服用大剂量糖皮质激素持续6个月的病人，以下哪种策略是最好的撤药方法（　　）。
   A. 维持量的糖皮质激素加上美替拉酮　　B. 维持量的糖皮质激素加上安体舒通
   C. 开始隔日给予糖皮质激素　　　　　　D. 每日给予维持量的糖皮质激素
   E. 在1~2周内缓慢减少糖皮质激素的用量

2. 某病人由于炎症而出现严重的肩痛，该病人经萘普生治疗后症状无改善，后改用口服地塞米松治疗。作为一种更有效的抗炎药物，糖皮质激素的作用机制是什么？（　　）
   A. 糖皮质激素抑制前列腺素的合成和炎症细胞的功能
   B. 糖皮质激素抑制环氧酶的作用比萘普生更强
   C. 糖皮质激素抑制环氧酶 COX-1 和 COX-2 的生物合成
   D. 糖皮质激素缓解炎症部位的水肿
   E. 在1~2周内缓慢减少糖皮质激素的用量

3. 一位32岁的女性因脸部和手臂的毛发过度生长而服用药物。服药后，她晚上如厕的次数明显增多。以下哪种表述能更好地解释病人出现夜尿症的原因（　　）。
   A. 药物的糖尿病尿崩症效应　　　　B. 药物转运系统对肾脏的渗透性负荷
   C. 药物对末端肾小管的作用　　　　D. 药物的促血糖增高效应
   E. 药物对近曲小管的作用

4. 沙丁胺醇的突出优点是（　　）。
   A. 兴奋心脏的作用与肾上腺素相似　　B. 对 β_2 受体的作用明显大于 β_1 受体
   C. 气雾吸入作用比异丙肾上腺素快　　D. 适于口服给药
   E. 作用强而持久

5. 预防支气管哮喘发作的首选治疗药物是（　　）。
   A. 可待因　　　　B. 麻黄碱　　　　C. 异丙肾上腺素
   D. 喷托维林　　　E. 苯丙哌林

6. 氨茶碱的平喘机制是（　　）。
   A. 促使儿茶酚胺释放及阻断腺苷受体　　B. 抑制腺苷酸环化酶
   C. 激活磷酸二酯酶　　　　　　　　　　D. 抑制磷酸二酯酶
   E. 激活鸟苷酸环化酶

7. 色甘酸钠的作用机制是（　　）。
   A. 选择性阻断 β_2 受体　　B. 抗炎、抗免疫作用　　C. 抑制炎症介质释放
   D. 稳定肥大细胞膜　　　　　E. 选择性激动 β_2 受体

8. N-乙酰半胱氨酸的祛痰作用机制是（　　）。
   A. 恶心性祛痰作用
   B. 使痰量逐渐减少，产生化痰作用

C. 增强呼吸道纤毛运动，促使痰液排出

D. 使蛋白多肽链中的二硫链断裂，降低痰的黏滞性，易于咳出

E. 使呼吸道分泌的总蛋白量降低，使痰液易咳出

9. 有较强局麻作用的止咳药是（　　）。

　　A. 可待因　　　B. 喷托维林　　　C. 苯丙哌林　　　D. 苯佐那酯　　　E. N-乙酰半胱氨酸

10. 非成瘾性中枢性镇咳药是（　　）。

　　A. 可待因　　　B. 麻黄碱　　　C. 肾上腺素　　　D. 喷托维林　　　E. 氢化可的松

 Case study

Key points：

（1）The characteristics and indications of inhaled and systemic glucocorticoids.

（2）The mechanisms underlying glucocorticoids withdrawal syndrome.

（3）The mechanisms of the adverse effects caused by continued use of supraphysiological glucocorticoid doses.

Key words：glucocorticoid；asthma；administration route；withdrawal syndrome

Case

A 7-year-old boy, Longlong, has been frequently feeling difficult to catch his breath for 2 years, especially when he is exercising, and he is diagnosed with asthma. His asthma comes and goes, and the symptoms are never completely alleviated. Although his doctor is concerned that it could retard Longlong's growth, he eventually decides to prescribe oral prednisone (a glucocorticoid analogue), and urges Longlong's parents to make sure he takes the medication every day. After a month, Longlong's asthma attacks subside, and he is able to play football and swim as a normal boy. During this time, the doctor pays close attention to Longlong's linear growth. Three years later, Longlong's doctor decides that a new inhaled glucocorticoid couldbe a safer medication for him. Therefore, his doctor switches Longlong's oral prednisone to an inhaled glucocorticoid, and stops oral prednisone completely. Four days later, Longlong is brought to the emergency department with a temperature of 40℃ and low blood pressure, and diagnosed with respiratory infection. Based on his history of oral prednisone use, Longlong is immediately administered intravenous hydrocortisone (Cortisol), as well as a saline infusion. Longlong finally recovers from the respiratory infection, and for the next 12 months his doctor slowly tapers his oral prednisone dose with continued use of the inhaled glucocorticoid. Eventually, he is able to take the inhaled glucocorticoid alone as an effective therapy for his asthma.

◎ **Essay questions**

1. Why are Cortisol analogues such as prednisone used for treating asthma?

2. Why did abrupt cessation of oral prednisone precipitate Longlong's clinical presentation in the emergency department?

3. Why are inhaled glucocorticoids safer than oral glucocorticoids for long-term treatment of asthma?
4. Why did the doctor monitor Longlong's linear growth?

Multiple-choice questions

1. Which of the following best describes appropriate protocols for the withdrawal of glucocorticoids from a patient who has been taking large doses for 6 months? (　　)
   A. Maintain the dose of glucocorticoids and addmetyrapone
   B. Maintain the dose of glucocorticoids and add spironolactone
   C. an alternate-day dosage regimen of glucocorticoids should begin
   D. Slow reduction of the glucocorticoid dose over 1-2 weeks
   E. Stop the medication immediately
2. A patient with severe shoulder pain resulting from inflammation is not responding to treatment with naproxen. You elect to begin a course of treatment with oral dexamethasone. What is the basis that the glucocorticoid will be more effective as an anti-inflammatory agent? (　　)
   A. Glucocorticoids inhibit both prostaglandin production and inflammatory cells
   B. Glucocorticoids are more potent inhibitors of cyclooxygenase than naproxen
   C. Glucocorticoids inhibit the biosynthesis of both COX-1 and COX-2.
   D. Glucocorticoids will reduce the edema in the inflamed area
   E. Slowly reduce glucocorticoid dosage over 1-2 weeks
3. A 32-year-old woman is prescribed a pill for excessive hair on her face and arms. She notes that she has been going to the bathroom at night more often. What is the most likely explanation for the nocturia? (　　)
   A. Diabetes insipidus effect of the medication
   B. Osmotic load to the kidney from the medication delivery system
   C. Distal renal tubule effect of the medication
   D. Hyperglycemic effect from the medication
   E. Effects on the proximal tubule of the medication
4. The significant advantage of salbutamol is (　　).
   A. the excitatory effect on the heart is similar to that of adrenaline
   B. its effect on β_2 receptors is significantly greater than its effects on β_1 receptors
   C. salbutamol aerosol inhalation has a faster effect than isoprenaline
   D. oral administration
   E. strong and long-lasting effects
5. The preferred medication for preventing bronchial asthma attacks is (　　).
   A. codeine　　　　　　B. ephedrine　　　　　　C. isoprenaline
   D. pentoxyverine　　　E. benproperine
6. The anti-asthmatic mechanism of aminophylline is (　　).

A. inducing catecholamine release and blocking adenosine receptors

B. adenylyl cyclase inhibition

C. phosphodiesterase activation

D. phosphodikinase inhibition

E. guanylate cyclase activation

7. Sodium cromoglycate's mechanism of action is (   ).

   A. selective blockade of β_2 receptors
   B. anti-inflammatory and anti-immune effects
   C. inhibition of inflammatory mediator release
   D. mast cell membrane stabilization
   E. selective agonism of β_2 receptors

8. The mechanism of expectorant action of N-acetylcysteine is (   ).

   A. nauseating expectorant effect

   B. producing an expectorant effect to reduce the amount of sputum gradually

   C. breaking the disulfide chain in the protein polypeptide chain to lower the viscosity of mucous sputum to make it easy to cough up

   D. increasing respiratory ciliary movement to promote the sputum expulsion

   E. reducing the amount of protein secreted by the respiratory tract to make sputum easy to cough up

9. The cough medicine with local anesthetic effects is (   ).

   A. codeine   B. pentoxyverine   C. benproperine
   D. benzonatate   E. n-acetylcysteine

10. The non-addictive central cough suppressant is (   ).

    A. codeine   B. ephedrine   C. epinephrine
    D. pentoxyverine   E. hydrocortisone

第二十九章案例学习和选择题答案

第三十章 作用于消化系统的药物

知识要点

消化系统的药物导图见图 30-1：

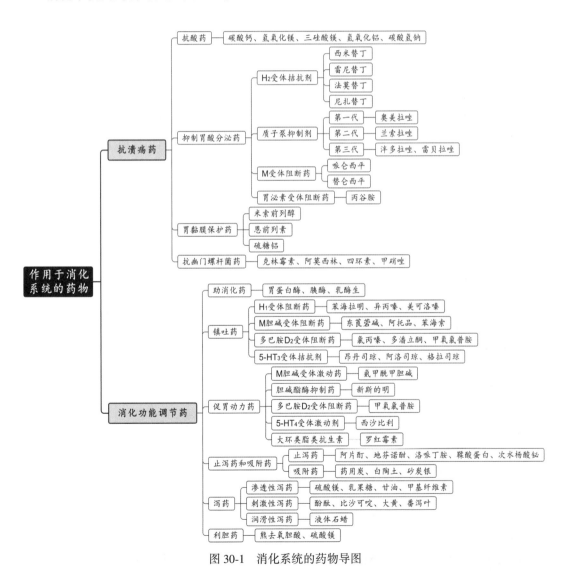

图 30-1 消化系统的药物导图

一、抗消化性溃疡药

消化性溃疡主要发生于胃和十二指肠暴露于胃酸和胃蛋白酶的黏膜部位。在黏膜防御机制不全时，黏膜上皮不能对抗胃酸和胃蛋白酶的消化作用，就可能形成溃疡。

(一) 抗酸药

1) 药理作用

抗酸药(antacids)为弱碱性物质，作用主要有两方面：①口服后在胃内直接中和胃酸，升高胃内容物 pH；②降低胃蛋白酶活性，从而解除胃酸和胃蛋白酶对胃、十二指肠黏膜的侵蚀和对溃疡面的刺激。

2) 临床应用

常用的抗酸药有氢氧化镁、三硅酸镁、氢氧化铝、碳酸钙、碳酸氢钠等。该类药物常用于治疗消化性溃疡和反流性食管炎。

(二) 抑制胃酸分泌药

1. H_2 受体阻断药

1) 药理作用

竞争性阻断胃壁细胞基底膜 H_2 受体，减少胃酸分泌。

2) 临床应用

常用药物有包括西咪替丁、雷尼替丁、法莫替丁等，为治疗消化性溃疡的常用药，亦可用于无并发症的胃食管反流综合征和预防应激性溃疡的发生。

3) 不良反应

长期大剂量使用西咪替丁，因西咪替丁结合并拮抗雄激素受体，偶见男性性功能减退和乳腺发育、女性溢乳等内分泌系统症状。西咪替丁是肝药酶抑制剂，可抑制其他药物的体内转化。

2. H^+-K^+-ATP 酶抑制药

1) 药理作用

H^+-K^+-ATP 酶抑制药属于弱酸性的苯并咪唑类化合物，在酸性的壁细胞分泌小管内，转化为次磺酸和亚磺酰胺。后者与 H^+-K^+-ATP 酶 α 亚单位的巯基不可逆的共价结合使酶失活，而发挥强大、持久的抑酸作用，还具有抑制幽门螺杆菌的作用。

2) 临床应用

常用药物有奥美拉唑、兰索拉唑、潘多拉唑等，可用于胃、十二指肠溃疡、反流性食道炎、卓-艾综合征、非甾体类抗炎药所致的胃溃疡的治疗。

3. M 胆碱受体阻断药

1) 药理作用

M 胆碱受体阻断药抑制胃酸分泌的机制：①阻断壁细胞上的 M 受体，抑制胃酸分泌；②阻断胃黏膜中嗜铬细胞上的 M 受体，减少组胺的释放；③阻断胃窦 G 细胞上的 M 受体抑制胃泌素的分泌，而间接减少胃酸的分泌。此外，M 受体阻断药还有解痉作用。

2) 临床应用

常用药物有哌仑西平、替仑西平。由于其抑制胃酸分泌的作用较弱，不良反应较多，目前已较少用于溃疡病的治疗。

4. 胃泌素受体阻断药

1）药理作用

（1）与胃泌素竞争胃泌素受体，抑制胃酸分泌。

（2）促进胃黏膜黏液合成，增强胃黏膜的黏液-HCO_3^-保护屏障。

2）临床应用

常用药物丙谷胺可用于消化性溃疡的治疗。

（三）增强胃黏膜屏障功能的药物

本类药物通过增强胃黏膜的细胞屏障、黏液-HCO_3^-盐屏障而发挥抗溃疡作用。

1. 米索前列醇

1）药理作用

（1）抑制壁细胞的胃酸分泌。

（2）促进浅表细胞分泌黏液和HCO_3^-。

（3）抑制胃蛋白酶分泌。

（4）增加胃黏膜血流，促进胃黏膜上皮细胞增殖重建。

2）临床应用

对长期应用非甾体抗炎药引起的消化性溃疡、胃出血，作为胃黏膜细胞保护药有特效。

3）不良反应

发生率较高，孕妇及前列腺素类过敏者禁用。

2. 硫糖铝

1）药理作用

聚合成不溶性的带负电荷的胶体黏稠多聚体，黏附于胃、十二指肠黏膜溃疡面，形成保护屏障，阻止胃酸和消化酶的侵蚀，可抑制幽门螺杆菌。

2）临床应用

消化性溃疡、反流性食管炎、慢性糜烂性胃炎及幽门螺杆菌感染。

3）不良反应

最常见的不良反应为便秘。

3. 胶体次枸橼酸铋

1）药理作用

在溃疡表面或溃疡基底肉芽组织形成一种坚固的氧化铋胶体沉淀，成为保护性薄膜，减少胃内容物对溃疡部位的侵蚀作用，对幽门螺杆菌有一定抑制作用。

2）临床应用

临床应用主要为消化性溃疡。

（四）抗幽门螺杆菌药

临床常用的抗幽门螺杆菌的抗菌药包括阿莫西林、四环素、红霉素、甲硝唑等，非抗生素药包括H^+-K^+-ATP酶抑制药、硫糖铝、枸橼酸铋钾等。

二、消化功能调节药

(一) 助消化药
助消化药多为消化液中的成分或促进消化液分泌的药物,如胃蛋白酶、胰酶、乳酶生,主要用于治疗消化不良、消化道功能减弱。

(二) 止吐药
1. H_1 受体阻断药:如苯海拉明、异丙嗪、美可洛嗪

1) 药理作用

中枢镇静作用和止吐。

2) 临床应用

预防和治疗晕动病、内耳性眩晕病。

2. M 胆碱受体阻断药:如东莨菪碱、苯海索

1) 药理作用

阻断呕吐中枢的和外周反射途径中的 M 受体,降低迷路感受器的敏感性,抑制前庭小脑通路的传导。

2) 临床应用

抗晕动病和防治胃肠刺激所致的恶心、呕吐。

3. 多巴胺(D_2)受体阻断药

1) 氯丙嗪

(1) 药理作用:阻断中枢催吐化学感受区 CTZ 的多巴胺 D_2 受体,发挥中枢止吐作用。

(2) 临床应用:减轻化疗引起的轻度恶心、呕吐,但不能控制化疗药物(如顺铂、多柔比星、氮芥等)引起的严重恶心、呕吐。

2) 甲氧氯普胺

(1) 药理作用:①中枢作用:阻断中枢 CTZ 多巴胺 D_2 受体发挥止吐作用,产生止吐作用;②外周作用:阻断胃肠多巴胺受体,增加胃肠运动,加速胃的正向排空。

(2) 临床应用:慢性功能性消化不良引起的胃肠运动障碍,如恶心、呕吐等症状。

(3) 不良反应:大剂量时可引起明显的锥体外系症状、男性乳房发育等。

3) 多潘立酮

(1) 药理作用:不易通过血脑屏障,阻断胃肠 D_2 受体,具有促进胃肠蠕动、加速胃肠排空、协调胃肠运动、防止食物反流和止吐的作用。

(2) 临床应用:①胃肠运动障碍性疾病(慢性食后消化不良和胃潴留);②放射治疗及肿瘤化疗药、偏头痛、颅外伤、手术、胃镜检查等引起的恶心、呕吐;③抗帕金森病药左旋多巴、溴隐亭、苯海索等引起的恶心、呕吐。

(3) 不良反应:头痛、溢乳、男性乳房发育。

4. 5-羟色胺受体阻断药:如昂丹司琼、阿洛司琼、格拉司琼

1) 药理作用

选择性地抑制外周神经系统突触前和呕吐中枢的 5-HT_3 受体,阻断呕吐反射。

2)临床应用

对肿瘤放疗和化疗导致的呕吐有良效,对晕动病及多巴胺受体激动药如阿扑吗啡引起的呕吐无效。

(三)增强胃肠动力药

增强胃肠动力药主要用于胃运动减弱和各种胃轻瘫、胃肠反流性疾病、反流性食管炎、慢性自发性便秘和结肠运动减弱(表30-1)。

表 30-1　　　　　　　　　　　　　增强胃肠动力药

药物种类	代表性药物	作用机制
M 胆碱受体激动药	氨甲酰甲胆碱	激动 M 胆碱受体
胆碱酯酶抑制药	新斯的明	抑制乙酰胆碱降解
多巴胺受体拮抗药	甲氧氯普胺	阻断突触前多巴胺 D_2 受体
5-HT 受体激动药	西沙必利	激动兴奋性神经元的 $5-HT_4$ 受体
大环内酯类抗生素	罗红霉素	增强促胃动素受体作用

(四)止泻药与吸附药

由胃肠道感染造成的腹泻应对因使用抗感染药物治疗,但对腹泻剧烈而持久的患者,可适当给予止泻药对症处理以缓解腹泻症状。

(1)阿片酊、复方樟脑酊、地芬诺酯、洛哌丁胺:通过激动肠道 μ 阿片受体,减少胃肠推进性蠕动发挥其止泻作用。

(2)鞣酸蛋白、次水杨酸铋、碱式碳酸铋:抑制肠道炎性渗出,发挥收敛、止泻作用。

(3)药用炭、白陶土、矽炭银:通过吸附肠道内液体、毒物,发挥止泻和阻止毒物吸收作用。

(五)泻药

泻药是刺激肠蠕动、软化粪便、润滑肠道促进排便的药物,主要用于治疗功能性便秘。

(1)渗透性泻药:口服后肠道吸收很少,增加肠容积而促进肠道推进性蠕动,产生泻下作用。常用药物有硫酸镁、乳果糖、甘油、山梨醇、植物纤维素和甲基纤维素。

(2)刺激性泻药:刺激结肠推进性蠕动,产生泻下作用。常用药物有酚酞、比沙可啶、大黄、番泻叶。

(3)润滑性泻药:通过局部润滑并软化粪便导泻作用,如液体石蜡、甘油等。

(六)利胆药

利胆药是具有促进胆汁分泌或胆囊排空的药物,如去氢胆酸、熊去氧胆酸、硫酸镁等,主要用于治疗胆囊炎、胆石症的治疗。

案例学习

学习要点:

(1)掌握常用抗酸药的名称、作用机制、临床应用和不良反应。

(2) 掌握 H_2 受体阻断剂和质子泵抑制剂常用药物名称、作用机制、临床应用和不良反应。

(3) 掌握加强胃黏膜保护作用的药物名称、作用机制、临床应用和不良反应。

关键词：消化性溃疡；质子泵抑制剂；H_2 受体阻断剂；抗酸药；硫糖铝；胶体铋；米索前列醇；幽门螺杆菌；抗菌药

案例

张振是一位 27 岁的白领。尽管他喜欢抽烟喝酒，他的身体状况仍然良好。居高不下的房价影响了他和女朋友的结婚计划，他感到非常焦虑。因为在一次篮球比赛中扭伤了手肘，在过去的 2 个月里，他每天都服用两片阿司匹林。

最近两周以来，张振经常在进食后 1~2 小时感到上腹灼痛，而且频繁地在凌晨 3 点被痛醒，吃些食物和服用抗酸药能使他的疼痛得到缓解。当疼痛不断加剧后，张振去看了医生。医生给他做了腹部检查，结果显示除了上腹压痛外其他都正常。在医生的建议下，张振做了内镜检查。在检查过程中，医生在张振十二指肠近端部分的后壁发现了溃疡，溃疡直径 0.5 cm，医生还取了胃窦部的黏膜组织用于检测幽门螺杆菌的感染。张振被诊断为十二指肠溃疡，医生给他开了一种质子泵抑制剂奥美拉唑。第二天，病检结果显示张振感染了幽门螺杆菌，于是医生又给他开了铋剂、克拉霉素和羟氨苄青霉素。医生建议张振停止抽烟和饮酒，而且最重要的是停止服用阿司匹林。

34 岁时，张振患上了肩周炎，并开始每天服用阿司匹林。两个月后，张振感到上腹灼痛。在吐出咖啡渣样呕吐物和发现自己排黑便后，他去看了医生。经过胃镜检查，医生发现张振患上了胃溃疡，而且有并发出血。这意味着消化性溃疡病复发了。张振的呼吸试验结果显示其幽门螺杆菌感染为阴性，因此服用阿司匹林最有可能是他溃疡复发的原因。医生给他开了抗酸药和雷尼替丁（H_2 受体阻断剂），并要求他停止服用阿司匹林。医生也给张振讲解了哪些止痛药物属于非甾体类抗炎药（NSAIDs）。

两周后，张振告诉医生，他肩膀的疼痛加剧，已无法忍受，他必须继续服用阿司匹林才能静心工作。医生告诉他，如果他把 H_2 受体拮抗剂换成质子泵抑制剂，他就可以服用阿司匹林。

◎ 问答题

1. 哪些危险因素促使张振患上消化性溃疡？幽门螺杆菌和非甾体类抗炎药在消化性溃疡病中的地位如何？

2. 为什么张振第一次就诊时医生给他开了质子泵抑制剂？而第二次就诊医生先让他使用 H_2 受体拮抗剂，而后又换成质子泵抑制剂？

3. 为什么医生要让张振使用克拉霉素而不是甲硝唑来治疗幽门螺杆菌感染？

选择题

1. 以下哪项是奥美拉唑最常见的不良反应？（　　）
   A. 黑便　　　B. 便秘　　　C. 头痛　　　D. 呕吐　　　E. 性功能减退

2. 雷尼替丁抑制下列哪项作用或哪个分子？（　　）
   A. 胃泌素与壁细胞结合　　B. 组胺与壁细胞结合　　C. H^+-K^+-ATP 酶

D. 壁细胞前列腺素受体　　E. 乙酰胆碱与 M 受体结合
3. 下列哪项是对西咪替丁的正确描述？（　　）
   A. 它是前列腺素 E_1 的同源物　　B. 它是前体药物
   C. 它与老年患者的精神错乱和幻觉有关　D. 它减少了其他药物的作用时间
   E. 抑制幽门螺杆菌
4. 奥美拉唑属于以下哪类药物？（　　）
   A. H^+-K^+-ATP 酶抑制药　　B. H_2 受体阻断药　　C. M 胆碱受体阻断药
   D. 胃泌素受体阻断药　　E. H_1 受体阻断药
5. 以下哪种药物在酸性环境中保护胃十二指肠黏膜，且不宜与碱性药合用？（　　）
   A. 氧化镁　　B. 氢氧化铝　　C. 西咪替丁　　D. 枸橼酸铋钾　　E. 奥美拉唑
6. 以下哪种药物主要通过增强胃黏膜屏障功能而治疗消化性溃疡？（　　）
   A. 雷尼替丁　　B. 哌仑西平　　C. 奥美拉唑　　D. 米索前列醇　　E. 比沙可啶
7. 以下哪种药物可抑制幽门螺杆菌繁殖、减少黏膜中幽门螺杆菌密度？（　　）
   A. 米索前列醇　　B. 恩前列素　　C. 硫糖铝　　D. 替普瑞酮　　E. 麦滋林
8. 以下哪种药物可选择性阻断 5-HT_3 受体，发挥止吐作用？（　　）
   A. 昂丹司琼　　B. 苯海拉明　　C. 多潘立酮　　D. 硫乙拉嗪　　E. 西沙必利
9. 哪种药物通过阻断 CTZ 的 D_2 受体发挥止吐作用？（　　）
   A. 苯海拉明　　B. 东莨菪碱　　C. 甲氧氯普胺　　D. 地芬诺酯　　E. 昂丹司琼
10. 服用某些驱肠虫药后的导泻，应选用以下哪种药物（　　）。
    A. 氢氧化镁　　B. 甘油　　C. 氯丙嗪　　D. 地芬诺酯　　E. 硫酸镁

Case study

Key points：

（1）List the antacid agents and describe their mechanisms of action, therapeutic uses, and adverse effects.

（2）List the histamine H_2-receptor antagonists and PPIs that inhibit gastric acid production and describe their mechanisms of action, therapeutic uses, and adverse effects.

（3）List the drugs used therapeutically to promote the defense of the GI tract from the effects of acid, and describe their mechanisms of action, therapeutic uses, and adverse effects.

Key words： peptic ulcer; proton pump inhibitor (ppi); h2-receptor antagonist; antacid; sucralfate; colloidal bismuth; misoprostol; *H. pylori*; antibiotics

Case

Zhang Zhen is a white-collar worker. He is 27 years old. Although helikes to smoke cigarettes and drink alcohol, He is still in good health. He is very anxious about the high housing cost, because it affects his marriage plan with his girlfriend. He has been taking two aspirin daily for the past 2 months because of an elbow injury in a basketball competition.

During the past 2 weeks, Zhang Zhen has suffered a burning pain in his upper abdomen after eating which may last 1-2 hours. It is more often to awake him at approximately 3:00 AM. Eating some food or taking antacids can always make him feel better.

Zhang Zhen visits a doctor when the pain increases in intensity. His abdominal examination is normal except for epigastric tenderness. Zhang Zhen undergoes the endoscopic examination with the doctor's advice. During the examination, an ulcer is identified in the proximal portion of the duodenum on the posterior wall. The ulcer is 0.5 cm in diameter. A mucosal biopsy of the gastric antrum is performed for detection of *Helicobacter pylori*. Zhang Zhen is diagnosed with a duodenal ulcer. The doctor prescribes omeprazole, a proton pump inhibitor. The following day, when the pathology report indicates the presence of an H. pylori infection, the doctor prescribes bismuth, clarithromycin, and amoxicillin in addition to the proton pump inhibitor. The doctor also advises Zhang Zhen to stop smoking and drinking alcohol and, importantly, to avoid taking aspirin.

At age 37, Zhang Zhen develops scapulohumeral periarthritis and begins to take several aspirin daily for the pain. Two months later, Zhang Zhen develops a burning pain in his upper abdomen. After vomiting "coffee grounds" material and noticing the black stool, he visits the doctor. With the gastroscopic examination, the doctor discovers that Zhang Zhen has a gastric ulcer and that the ulcer has recently bled. It means that he has a recurrence of peptic ulcer disease. His breath test is negative for H. pylori, so aspirin is the most likely cause of this recurrence. Zhang Zhen is treated with antacids and ranitidine, an H_2 receptor antagonist, and is told to stop taking aspirin. The doctor goes over with Zhang Zhen which pain-relieving medications are considered nonsteroidal anti-inflammatory drugs (NSAIDs).

Two weeks later, Zhang Zhen informs the doctor that the pain in his shoulder has become unbearable and that he must continue taking aspirin to be able to concentrate at work. The doctor tells him that he can take aspirin as long as he switches his antiulcer medication from an H_2 antagonist to a proton pump inhibitor.

◎ **Essay questions**

1. What risk factors did Zhang Zhen have for the development of peptic ulcer disease? What are the roles of H. pylori and NSAIDs in this disease?
2. Why was Zhang Zhen given a proton pump inhibitor when he went to see the doctor for the first time? Why was an H_2 antagonist prescribed for him while he saw the doctor the second time, and then a proton pump?
3. Why was Zhang Zhen given clarithromycin rather than metronidazole for treatment of his H. pylori infection?

Multiple-choice questions

1. Which of the following is the most common adverse effect of omeprazole? (   )
   A. Black stools   B. Constipation   C. Headache   D. Vomiting   E. Hypogonadism
2. Ranitidine inhibits which of the following? (   )

A. Gastrin binding to parietal cells B. Histamine binding to parietal cells
C. H^+-K^+-ATPase D. Parietal cell prostaglandin receptors
E. Acetylcholine binding to M receptor

3. Which of the following is true of cimetidine? (   )
   A. It is a prostaglandin analog of PGE1
   B. It is a prodrug
   C. It is associated with confusion and hallucinations in elderly patients
   D. It reduces the duration of action of other drugs
   E. It inhibits Helicobacter pylori

4. Which of the following drug classes does omeprazole belong to? (   )
   A. H^+-K^+-ATPase inhibitors B. H_2 receptor blockers
   C. M receptor blockers D. Gastrin receptor blockers
   E. H_1 receptor blockers

5. Which drugs protect the gastroduodenal mucosa in an acidic environment and should not be combined with alkaline drugs? (   )
   A. Magnesium oxide B. Aluminum hydroxide C. Cimetidine
   D. Bismuth potassium citrate E. Omeprazole

6. Which of the following drugs treats peptic ulcers primarily by enhancing gastric mucosal barrier function? (   )
   A. Ranitidine B. Pirenzepine C. Omeprazole D. Misoprostol E. Bisacodyl

7. Which of the following drugs inhibits *H. pylori* colonization and decreases H. pylori density in the mucosa? (   )
   A. Misoprostol B. Enprostil C. Sucralfate D. Teprenone E. Marzulene

8. Which medications selectively inhibit 5-HT_3 receptors to provide antiemetic effects? (   )
   A. Ondansetron B. Diphenhydramine C. Domperidone
   D. Thiethylperazine E. Cisapride

9. Which drug acts as an antiemetic by blocking the D_2 receptor in the CTZ? (   )
   A. Diphenhydramine B. Scopolamine C. Metoclopramide
   D. Diphenoxylate E. Ondansetron

10. Which drugs should be used to induce diarrhea after taking anthelmintics? (   )
    A. Magnesium hydroxide B. Glycerin C. Chlorpromazine
    D. Diphenoxylate E. Magnesium sulfate

第三十章案例学习和选择题答案

第三十一章 肾上腺皮质激素类药物

知识要点

一、糖皮质激素

糖皮质激素包括可的松、氢化可的松等。

(一)药理作用

1. 对代谢的影响

(1) 糖代谢：促进糖原异生；减少葡萄糖氧化分解；减少组织对葡萄糖的利用。增加肝糖原和肌糖原含量，升高血糖。

(2) 蛋白质代谢：加速胸腺、肌肉、骨组织蛋白质分解，造成负氮平衡；长期用药会出现骨质形成障碍、影响生长发育、伤口愈合。

(3) 脂质代谢：长期大剂量使用促进皮下脂肪分解和重新向心性分布。

(4) 水和电解质代谢：具有保钠排钾(作用较弱)、利尿作用，并促进骨质脱钙。

(5) 核酸代谢：影响 DNA/RNA 代谢关键酶活性，诱导敏感组织 DNA 降解，以致细胞核酸合成代谢受到抑制，而分解代谢增强。

2. 抗炎作用

抗炎作用强大，可抑制各种原因所致炎症和炎症不同阶段。

3. 免疫抑制和抗过敏作用

小剂量可抑制细胞免疫，大剂量抑制体液免疫，用于治疗移植排斥反应、皮肤迟发性过敏反应、自身免疫性疾病。抑制肥大细胞脱颗粒，抑制过敏介质释放，起抗过敏作用。

4. 抗休克

糖皮质激素用于严重休克，特别是感染中毒性休克的治疗。

5. 允许作用

糖皮质激素对有些组织细胞虽无直接活性，但可给其他激素发挥作用创造有利条件。

6. 其他作用

(1) 退热作用：抑制体温中枢对致热原的反应，减少内源性致热原的释放，具有迅速、良好的退热作用。

(2) 血液与造血系统：刺激骨髓造血功能，导致红细胞、血红蛋白增加，血小板增多，提高纤维蛋白原浓度，缩短凝血酶原时间；提高中性白细胞数量，但其功能下降，减少淋巴细胞数量。

(3) 中枢神经系统：导致 CNS 兴奋性增强，欣快感、激动，可诱发精神病和癫痫。
(4) 骨骼：导致骨质脱钙，骨质疏松，特别是绝经期妇女。
(5) 消化系统：增加胃酸、胃蛋白酶分泌，大剂量诱发或加重溃疡。
(6) 心血管系统：增强血管对其他活性物质的反应性，可以增加血管壁肾上腺素受体的表达，可引起高血压。

(二) 临床应用

1. 严重感染和炎症

(1) 严重急性感染。适用于：中毒性感染或同时伴休克；结核病的急性期，特别是渗出为主的结核病，早期、短程、小剂量应用可迅速退热，减少炎症渗出。带状疱疹、水痘患者禁用。

(2) 抗炎治疗及防止某些炎症的后遗症。

2. 自身免疫性疾病、器官移植排斥反应及过敏性疾病

(1) 自身免疫性疾病：一般采用综合疗法，不宜单用。

(2) 器官移植排斥反应：用于预防与治疗，常与环孢素 A 合用。

(3) 过敏性疾病：对严重病例或其他药物无效时，可应用糖皮质激素辅助治疗。

3. 抗休克治疗

抗休克治疗时，宜及早、短时间、大量突击应用，作为辅助用药。

4. 血液病

多用于治疗儿童急性淋巴细胞性白血病，与抗肿瘤药合用；也可用于治疗再生障碍性贫血、粒细胞减少症、血小板减少症，过敏性紫癜等。

5. 局部应用

皮肤病：皮炎、湿疹、肛门瘙痒、银屑病等，眼部疾病：结膜炎、角膜炎、虹膜炎，肌肉韧带或关节劳损。

6. 替代治疗

用于急慢性肾上腺皮质功能不全(肾上腺危象)、脑垂体前叶功能减退、肾上腺次全切除术后韧带或关节损伤。

(三) 不良反应和注意事项

1. 长期大量应用引起的不良反应

(1) 医源性肾上腺皮质功能亢进综合征。表现为满月脸、水牛背、皮肤变薄、多毛、水肿、低钾血症、高血压、糖尿病等，停药后症状可自行消失。必要时可加用抗高血压药、抗糖尿病药治疗，并采用低盐、低糖、高蛋白饮食及加用氯化钾等措施。

(2) 诱发或加重感染。对于无有效药物可控制的感染(如病毒感染)，应慎用或禁用。

(3) 消化道溃疡、出血、穿孔。

(4) 心血管系统并发症，如高血压、动脉粥样硬化等。

(5) 骨质疏松、肌肉萎缩、伤口愈合延迟、影响生长发育等。骨质疏松多见于儿童、绝经妇女和老人，还可引起自发性骨折、股骨头无菌性缺血坏死。孕妇应用偶引起胎儿畸形。

(6) 糖尿病：这类糖尿病对降糖药物敏感性较差，所以应在控制原发病的基础上尽量

减少糖皮质激素的用量,最好停药。

(7) 糖皮质激素性青光眼:用药期间要定期检查眼内压、眼底、视野。

(8) 对妊娠的影响:胎盘功能不全、新生儿体重减少或死胎的发生率。

(9) 其他:癫痫或精神病史者禁用或慎用。

2. 停药反应

(1) 医源性肾上腺皮质功能不全或萎缩。表现为恶心、呕吐、乏力、低血压和休克等,须及时抢救。因此不可骤然停药,须缓慢减量,停用糖皮质激素后连续应用 ACTH 7 天左右;在停药 1 年内如遇应激情况(如感染或手术等),应及时给予足量的糖皮质激素。

(2) 反跳现象。常需加大剂量再行治疗,待症状缓解后再缓慢减量、停药。

(3) 糖皮质激素抵抗:此时对患者盲目加大剂量和延长疗程不但无效,而且会引起严重的后果。目前临床还未见解决糖皮质激素抵抗的有效措施。

(四) 禁忌证

严重精神病和癫痫、活动性消化性溃疡、骨折、创伤修复期、肾上腺皮质功能亢进、严重高血压、糖尿病、孕妇、抗菌药不能控制的感染。

案例学习

学习要点:

(1) 掌握糖皮质激素的药理作用、临床应用和不良反应。

(2) 熟悉常用的糖皮质激素制剂及用法。

关键词:糖皮质激素;强的松;布地奈德;停药反应

案例

小明,9 岁,因患哮喘经常感觉呼吸困难,尤其是运动后。因他的哮喘一直时好时坏,没有得到有效控制,医生予以口服强的松治疗,每天用药一次。用药几周后,小明的哮喘发作得到控制,生活和运动恢复正常。用药期间,医生高度关注小明身高和体重的增长情况。两年后,医生停用强的松,换用新型的吸入性糖皮质激素药物布地奈德进行治疗。几天后,小明因呼吸道感染出现低血压、高热,被紧急送往 ICU。了解到小明有强的松应用史,他被立即给予静脉点滴氢化可的松治疗,其症状逐渐恢复。其后 6 个月内,在应用吸入性布地奈德的同时,小明强的松的口服剂量逐渐减量至最后停用,单用吸入性布地奈德来控制哮喘。

问答题

1. 强的松为什么可以用来治疗哮喘?

2. 为什么口服强的松期间医生要监测小明的身高和体重的增长情况?

3. 突然停用强的松为什么会导致小明被紧急送往 ICU?给予静脉点滴氢化可的松治疗的原因?

4. 为什么吸入性糖皮质激素长期应用治疗哮喘比口服糖皮质激素更安全?

选择题

1. 水钠潴留作用最弱的糖皮质激素是（　　）。
   A. 泼尼松　　B. 泼尼松龙　　C. 甲泼尼松龙　　D. 地塞米松　　E. 氢化可的松
2. 糖皮质激素对血液系统的影响是（　　）。
   A. 中性粒细胞的数量增加　　B. 中性粒细胞的数量减少　　C. 红细胞数量减少
   D. 血小板数量减少　　E. 红细胞数和血红蛋白均减少
3. 糖皮质激素隔日疗法的给药时间最好是（　　）。
   A. 早上5点　　B. 上午8点　　C. 中午12点　　D. 下午5点　　E. 晚上8点
4. 糖皮质激素类药物对代谢的影响不包括（　　）。
   A. 升高血糖　　B. 增加肝、肌糖原含量　　C. 促进全身脂肪分解
   D. 促进蛋白质分解　　E. 抑制蛋白质合成
5. 下列药物中，抗炎作用最强的是（　　）。
   A. 可的松　　B. 泼尼松　　C. 曲安西龙　　D. 倍他米松　　E. 氢化可的松
6. 下列不良反应中，哪种不是糖皮质激素产生的？（　　）
   A. 高血压、高血糖　　B. 高血钙、高血钾　　C. 加重感染
   D. 诱发癫痫　　E. 肌肉萎缩
7. 糖皮质激素可用于下列哪种疾病的治疗？（　　）
   A. 活动性消化性溃疡　　B. 角膜溃疡　　C. 再生障碍性贫血
   D. 肾上腺皮质功能亢进　　E. 霉菌感染
8. 男，24岁，咽炎，注射青霉素后1分钟，呼吸急促、面部发绀、心率130次/分，血压60/40 mmHg。抢救药物是（　　）。
   A. 地塞米松+去甲肾上腺素　　B. 地塞米松+多巴胺　　C. 曲安西龙+异丙肾上腺素
   D. 地塞米松+肾上腺素　　E. 地塞米松+山莨菪碱
9. 男，60岁，风湿性关节炎，口服泼尼松和多种非甾体抗炎药5个月，今日突发自发性胫骨骨折，原因可能与哪种药物有关？（　　）
   A. 阿司匹林　　B. 吲哚美辛　　C. 布洛芬　　D. 泼尼松　　E. 保泰松
10. 男，50岁，大叶性肺炎，并发感染性休克。药物治疗方案是（　　）。
    A. 头孢拉定+口服泼尼松　　B. 头孢拉定+口服可的松　　C. 头孢拉定+口服泼尼松龙
    D. 头孢拉定+肌内注射泼尼松　　E. 头孢拉定+静脉点滴氢化可的松

Case study

Key points:

(1) Master the pharmacological action, clinical application and adverse reactions of glucocorticoids.

(2) Familiar with commonly used glucocorticoid preparations and their usage.

Key words: glucocorticoid; prednisone; budesonide; withdrawal reaction

Case

Xiao Ming, 9 years old, finds that he can barely catch his breathe because of asthma, especially while exercising. His asthma comes and goes, but no therapy seems to stop the asthma attacks completely. His doctor prescribed oral prednisone, and tells his parents to make sure he takes the medication once daily. After a few weeks, Xiao Ming's asthma attack subside, and he is able to have a fairly normal childhood. During the medication, the doctor pays close attention to Xiao Ming's growth in height and weight. Two years later, the doctor decides that a new inhaled glucocorticoid budesonide could be a safer medication for him. Xiao Ming switches to the inhaled budesonide and discontinues oral prednisone. A few days later, Xiao Ming developed a respiratory infection and is brought to ICU with low blood pressure and high fever. Based on his history of prednisone use, he is immediately given intravenous hydrocortisone treatment, and his symptoms gradually recovers. And for the next 6 months slowly tapers his oral prednisone dose with continued use of the inhaled budesonide. Eventually, he is able to take the inhaled budesonide alone as an effective therapy for his asthma.

◎ **Essay questions**

1. Why are prednisone used to treat asthma?
2. Why does the doctor monitor Xiao Ming's height and weight growth during the use of oral prednisone?
3. Why does abrupt cessation of oral prednisone precipitate Xiao Ming's clinical presentation in ICU? Why is the intravenous hydrocortisone therapy given?
4. Why are inhaled glucocorticoids safer for long-term treatment of asthma than oral glucocorticoids?

Multiple-choice questions

1. Which of the glucocorticoids has the weakest water-sodium retention effect? (   )
    A. Prednisone   B. Prednisolone   C. Methylprednisolone
    D. Dexamethasone   E. Hydrocortisone
2. The effect of glucocorticoids on blood cells is (   ).
    A. increasing the number of neutrophils   B. reducing the number of neutrophils
    C. reducing the number of red cells   D. reducing the number of platelets
    E. reducing the number of red cells and hemoglobins
3. The administration time of glucocorticoids in the alternate-day treatment therapy is at (   ).
    A. 5 AM   B. 8 AM   C. 12 at noon   D. 5 PM   E. 8 PM
4. The effects of glucocorticoids on metabolism do not include (   ).
    A. increasing the blood glucose level
    B. increasing the glycogen level in the liver and the muscles
    C. promoting lipolysis of the whole body

D. causing protein breakdown

E. inhibiting protein synthesis

5. Which of the glucocorticoids has the strongest anti-inflammatory effects? (   )

   A. Cortisone　　　　　B. Prednisone　　　　　C. Triamcinolone

   D. Betamethasone　　　E. Hydrocortisone

6. Which of the following is not the side effects of glucocorticoids? (   )

   A. Hypertension and hyperglycemia　　　B. Hypercalcemia and hyperkalemia

   C. Aggravate infection　　　　　　　　D. Induce epilepsy

   E. Amyotrophy

7. Glucocorticoids can be used to treat (   ).

   A. active peptic ulcer　　B. keratohelcosis　　C. aplastic anemia

   D. hypercorticism　　　　E. fungal infection

8. A 24-year male had pharyngitis. One minute after the injection of penicillin G, he suffered shortness of breath and facial cyanosis, his heart rate was 130 bpm, blood pressure was 60/40mmHg. The emergency treatment should include (   ).

   A. dexamethasone + noradrenaline　　　B. dexamethasone + dopamine

   C. triamcinolone + isoprenaline　　　　D. dexamethasone + epinephrine

   E. dexamethasone + anisodamine

9. A 60-year male of rheumatic arthritis has taken prednisone and NSAIDs orally for 5 months. He suffered spontaneous tibial fracture suddenly today. Which medicine might cause his fracture? (   )

   A. Aspirin　　　　　　B. Indomethacin　　　　C. Ibuprofen

   D. Prednisone　　　　　E. Butazodine

10. A 50-year male had lobar pneumonia and septic shock. The medicine therapy should be (   ).

    A. cefradine + oral prednisone　　　　B. cefradine + oral cortisone

    C. cefradine + oral prednisolone　　　D. cefradine + intramuscular prednisone

    E. cefradine + intravenous hydrocortisone

第三十一章案例学习和选择题答案

第三十二章 甲状腺激素及抗甲状腺药

知识要点

一、甲状腺激素

(一) 合成、分泌和调节

甲状腺腺泡细胞主动摄取碘,在过氧化物酶作用下进行碘的活化和酪氨酸碘化。碘化酪氨酸偶联生成 T_4 和 T_3。在蛋白水解酶作用下甲状腺球蛋白分解并释放出 T_4 和 T_3 进入血液。甲状腺激素的合成和分泌受垂体分泌的促甲状腺激素(TSH)和下丘脑分泌的促甲状腺激素释放激素(TRH)的调节。血中的 T_3 和 T_4 可反馈性调节 TSH 和 TRH 的释放。

(二) 药理作用和不良反应

T_3 作用快而强,T_4 作用弱而慢。甲状腺激素在细胞核内与其受体结合,诱导靶基因转录而发挥效应。其药理作用有维持正常生长发育、促进代谢和增加产热、提高交感-肾上腺系统的反应性等。主要用于甲状腺功能低下(呆小症或粘液性水肿)的替代疗法;也用于治疗单纯性甲状腺肿,减轻甲亢患者服用抗甲亢药后的突眼、甲状腺肿大及防止甲状腺功能低下、甲状腺癌术后减少复发、T_3 抑制试验等。过量可引起甲亢症状、腹泻、呕吐、发热、脉搏快而不规则,甚至心绞痛、心衰、肌肉震颤等。

二、抗甲状腺药

(一) 硫脲类

硫脲类包括硫氧嘧啶类(甲硫氧嘧啶、丙硫氧嘧啶)和咪唑类(甲巯咪唑、卡比马唑)。

1. 药理作用

(1) 作为过氧化物酶的底物被氧化,影响酪氨酸的碘代和偶联,从而抑制甲状腺激素合成。起效慢,需 2~3 周。

(2) 丙硫氧嘧啶还能抑制外周组织的 T_4 转化为 T_3。

(3) 减慢 β 受体介导的糖代谢。

(4) 轻度抑制免疫球蛋白生成,减少甲状腺刺激性免疫球蛋白水平,具有免疫抑制作用。

2. 临床应用

(1) 甲亢内科保守治疗,适用于轻症、不宜手术及放射性碘治疗者。

(2) 甲状腺手术前准备,使甲状腺功能控制正常,以便手术;但会使甲状腺增生、变脆、充血,需在术前 2 周加服碘剂。

(3)甲状腺危象的辅助治疗,除消除病因、对症治疗外,给予大剂量碘剂抑制甲状腺激素释放,并立即应用大剂量丙基硫氧嘧啶,阻止甲状腺素合成。

3. 不良反应

(1)胃肠道反应,如厌食、呕吐、腹痛腹泻等。

(2)过敏反应,如皮肤瘙痒、药疹、发热等。

(3)粒细胞缺乏症,为最严重的不良反应。需定期查血象,并注意与甲亢本身引起的白细胞数偏低相区别。

(4)甲状腺肿和甲状腺功能减退。甲状腺癌、结节性甲状腺肿并甲亢等患者禁用。孕妇慎用或不用,服用本类药物的妇女应避免哺乳。

(二)碘和碘化物

常用复方碘溶液(卢戈液)。小剂量碘剂促进甲状腺激素合成,用于预防单纯性甲状腺肿。大剂量碘剂有抗甲状腺作用,作用机制为:抑制谷胱甘肽还原酶,抑制甲状腺激素释放;抑制过氧化酶,抑制甲状腺激素合成;拮抗 TSH,使腺体缩小、血管减少。其作用特点为快而强、短暂,用药 2~7 天起效,10~15 天达最大效应,其后失去抑制激素合成的效应,不能单独用于甲亢内科治疗。临床应用于:①甲亢的术前准备,术前 2 周应用,使腺体缩小变韧,血管减少,利于手术。②甲状腺危象的治疗。2 周内逐渐停服,同时配合服用硫脲类药物。不良反应包括:①一般反应,如喉头不适、口内金属味、呼吸道刺激等;②过敏反应,如发热、皮疹、血管神经性水肿、上呼吸道水肿、喉头水肿等;③诱发甲状腺功能紊乱,长期服用碘化物可诱发甲亢、甲减、甲状腺肿。可进入乳汁并通过胎盘引起新生儿甲状腺肿,孕妇及乳母慎用。

(三)β 受体阻断药

普萘洛尔等是甲亢及甲状腺危象的辅助治疗药。通过阻断 β 受体改善甲亢所致的交感神经激活症状;普萘洛尔与氧烯洛尔还能减少 T_3 生成。适用于不宜用其他抗甲状腺治疗者,并能改善甲状腺危象的症状,与硫脲类合用作术前准备,甲亢患者因故需紧急手术,也可用 β 受体阻断药保护患者。

(四)放射性碘

^{131}I 的 β 射线在组织中射程仅为 2 mm,损伤甲状腺,起到类似手术切除部分甲状腺的作用。少量 γ 射线可在体外测得,用于测定甲状腺摄碘功能。^{131}I 适用于不宜手术、术后复发、硫脲类无效或过敏的甲亢患者,作用缓慢,1 月起效,3~4 月甲状腺功能恢复正常。剂量过大可导致甲状腺功能低下。^{131}I 不宜用于妊娠和哺乳期妇女、20 岁以下患者、肾功能不良者。禁用于甲状腺危象、重症浸润性突眼症及甲状腺不能摄碘者。

案例学习

学习要点:
掌握硫脲类药物的作用机制、作用特点、不良反应和干预措施。

关键词:硫脲类;作用机制;不良反应

案例

22岁女性被诊断为初发 Graves 病，甲状腺中度弥漫性肿。服用卡比马唑片 5 mg，3 次/天治疗。2 周后症状开始好转，3 个月后完全得到控制，甲状腺肿消退。其后按 5 mg，2 次/天继续服用卡比马唑。一年以后她发现脖子粗的现象再次出现，体重也增长了 3 kg，但没有出现之前的症状。相反，她总是觉得嗜睡、反应迟钝、沮丧。血浆 TSH 为 15 μU/mL，血浆游离 T_4 水平为 8 pmol/L。

问答题

1. 为什么服用卡比马唑 2 周后才出现症状的改善？可以用什么药物让她能更快速地改善症状吗？
2. 1 年后她再次出现脖子粗的原因是什么？这次可以用什么药物进行治疗？

选择题

1. 以下药物可用于妊娠期甲亢的是（　　）。
   A. 甲硫氧嘧啶　　B. 丙硫氧嘧啶　　C. ^{131}I　　D. 大剂量碘剂　　E. 卡比马唑
2. 甲硫氧嘧啶最严重的不良反应是（　　）。
   A. 过敏反应　　B. 胃肠道反应　　C. 粒细胞减少　　D. 甲状腺肿　　E. 甲状腺功能减退
3. 关于碘和碘化物的描述不正确的是（　　）。
   A. 小剂量碘可预防单纯性甲状腺肿　　B. 大剂量碘可抑制甲状腺激素释放
   C. 大剂量碘的抗甲状腺作用快而强　　D. 大剂量碘可单独用于甲亢的内科治疗
   E. 大剂量碘可抑制谷胱甘肽还原酶
4. 甲状腺素的适应证是（　　）。
   A. 甲状腺危象　　B. 轻中度甲状腺功能亢进
   C. 甲亢的手术前准备　　D. 交感神经活性增强引起的病变
   E. 单纯性甲状腺肿
5. 治疗甲状腺危象无效的药物是（　　）。
   A. 大剂量碘剂　　B. 丙硫氧嘧啶　　C. 普萘洛尔　　D. 甲苯磺丁脲　　E. 糖皮质激素
6. 甲亢的内科治疗患者服用一段时间甲巯咪唑后突眼症加重，适宜加用什么药物治疗？（　　）
   A. 复方碘溶液　　B. T_3　　C. T_4　　D. 卡比马唑　　E. 放射性碘
7. ^{131}I 不适用于（　　）。
   A. 对硫脲类过敏者　　B. 不宜行甲亢手术者　　C. 甲亢手术后复发者
   D. 儿童甲亢者　　E. 对硫脲类无效者
8. 女性患者，38 岁，因多汗、多食、消瘦、心悸 3 个月就诊，查体有甲状腺肿大。根据同位素扫描和血 T_3、T_4 检查，诊断为 Graves 病。该病人应选用以下哪项治疗？（　　）
   A. 甲状腺素片　　B. 丙硫氧嘧啶+普萘洛尔　　C. 碘剂+卡比马唑
   D. 放射性碘　　E. 肾上腺皮质激素+普萘洛尔
9. 女性患者，44 岁，甲亢 5 年，不规则治疗。因乏力、腹泻 4 天，昏迷 1 天入院，诊断为甲亢危象。该病人应选用以下哪项治疗？（　　）

A. 肾上腺皮质激素+丙硫氧嘧啶+大剂量碘剂　　B. 甲状腺素片+普萘洛尔+卡比马唑
C. 大剂量碘剂+普萘洛尔　　D. 肾上腺皮质激素+丙硫氧嘧啶
E. 肾上腺皮质激素+大剂量碘剂

10. 硫脲类抗甲状腺药的药理作用不包括（　　）。
    A. 抑制甲状腺素的合成　　B. 抑制甲状腺素的释放
    C. 抑制外周组织的 T_4 转化为 T_3　　D. 抑制免疫球蛋白的生成
    E. 减弱糖代谢

Case study

Key points:

Master the mechanism of action, action characteristics, adverse reactions and intervention measures of thiourea drugs.

Key words: thiourea; mechanism of action; adverse effects

Case

A 22-year girl was diagnosed as a case of recent onset Graves' disease with mild diffuse pulsatile thyroid enlargement. She was treated with tab. Carbimazole 5 mg 3 times a day. Her symptoms started subsiding after 2 weeks and were fully controlled after 3 months. The thyroid swelling also subsided and she was maintained on a dose of carbimazole 5 mg twice daily. After one year she noticed that the neck swelling was reappearing and her body weight increased by 3 kg in the last one month, but without recurrence of her earlier symptoms. She rather felt dull, sleepy and depressed. The serum TSH was 15 μU/mL and free thyroxine (FT_4) was 8 pmol/L.

◎ **Essay questions**

1. Why was the initial response to carbimazole delayed? Could any additional medicine be given to her initially to afford more rapid symptomatic relief?
2. What was the cause of reappearance of the neck swelling and her condition after 1 year? What measures need to be taken at this stage?

Multiple-choice questions

1. Which medicine is used to treat Grave's disease in pregnancy? (　　)
   A. Methylthiouracil　　B. Propylthiouracil　　C. ^{131}I
   D. High dose of iodine　　E. Carbimazole
2. The most serious adverse effect of methylthiouracil is (　　).
   A. anaphylaxis　　B. gastrointestinal reaction　　C. agranulocytosis
   D. thyroid goiter　　E. hypothyroidism
3. Which of the following is incorrect? (　　)
   A. Low dose of iodine is used to treat simple thyroid goiter
   B. High dose of iodine inhibits the release of thyroid hormone

C. High dose of iodine has strong and quick anti-thyroid effects

D. High dose of iodine can be used to treat thyrotoxicosis alone

E. High dose of iodine inhibits glutathione reductase

4. Thyroid hormone is used to (   ).

    A. thyroid storm
    B. mild or moderate hyperthyroidism
    C. preparation for surgery in thyrotoxic patients
    D. increased sympathetic nerve activity
    E. simple thyroid goiter

5. Which is useless to thyroid storm? (   )

    A. High dose of iodine
    B. Propylthiouracil
    C. Propranolol
    D. Tolbutamide
    E. Glucocorticoid

6. The exophthalmia of the Grave's disease patient is aggravated after a period use of methimazole. What drug treatment is appropriate? (   )

    A. Compound iodine solution
    B. T_3
    C. T_4
    D. Carbimazole
    E. Radioactive iodine

7. ^{131}I is contraindicated to (   ).

    A. the patients allergic to thioureas
    B. the patients not suitable for surgery
    C. recurrence after surgery
    D. child hyperthyroidism
    E. the patients who have no effect to thioureas

8. Female, 38 years old, has symptoms of hyperhidrosis, hyperphagia, weight loss and palpitation for 3 months. The physical examination showed goiter. According to the isotope scanner and blood T_3, T_4 level, she was diagnosed as Graves' disease. This patient should be treated with (   ).

    A. thyroxine tablet
    B. propylthiouracil+ propranolol
    C. iodine+ carbimazole
    D. radioactive iodine
    E. adrenocortical hormone + propranolol

9. Female, 44 years old, has been treated unregularly for hyperthyroidism for 5 years. She came to hospital due to fatigue, diarrhea for 4 days, and coma for 1 day. She was diagnosed as thyroid storm. The patient should be treated with (   ).

    A. adrenocortical hormone + propylthiouracil + high dose of iodine
    B. thyroxine tablet + propranolol + carbimazole
    C. high dose of iodine + propranolol
    D. adrenocortical hormone + propylthiouracil
    E. adrenocortical hormone + high dose of iodine

10. The pharmacological effects of thioamides do not include (   ).

    A. inhibiting the synthesis of thyroid hormone
    B. inhibiting the release of thyroid hormone
    C. inhibiting the conversion of T_4 to T_3
    D. inhibiting the synthesis of immunoglobulin
    E. inhibiting glucose metabolism

第三十三章 胰岛素及其他降血糖药

知识要点

一、胰岛素

1. 药理作用

(1) 促进脂肪合成，抑制脂肪分解，减少游离脂肪酸和酮体生成，增加脂肪酸的转运。

(2) 促进糖原的合成和贮存，增加葡萄糖的转运，加速葡萄糖的氧化和酵解，抑制糖原分解和异生。

(3) 增加氨基酸的转运和核酸、蛋白质的合成，抑制蛋白质的分解。

(4) 加快心率，加强心肌收缩力，减少肾血流。

(5) 促进钾离子进入细胞，降低血钾浓度。

2. 临床应用

(1) 1 型糖尿病(T1DM)。

(2) 新诊断的 2 型糖尿病(T2DM)有明显的高血糖症状和(或)血糖及糖化血红蛋白水平升高。

(3) T2DM 经饮食控制或用口服降糖药未能控制者。

(4) 发生急性或严重并发症的糖尿病，如酮症酸中毒或非酮症高渗性昏迷。

(5) 合并严重感染、消耗性疾病、高热、妊娠、创伤及手术的各型糖尿病。

(6) 细胞内缺钾，与葡萄糖同用促进钾内流。

3. 不良反应

(1) 低血糖症：最重要、最常见的不良反应。轻者饮用糖水或摄食，重者立即静注 50% 葡萄糖。低血糖昏迷要与酮症酸中毒昏迷和非酮症糖尿病昏迷相鉴别。

(2) 过敏反应：用 H_1 受体阻断药、糖皮质激素治疗，换用高纯度制剂或人胰岛素。

(3) 胰岛素抵抗

①急性型：多因合并感染、创伤、手术等应激状态所致。需要正确处理诱因，调节酸碱、电解质平衡，加大胰岛素剂量。

②慢性型：指胰岛素用量超过 200 U/天，且无并发症者。形成原因可能与受体前、受体水平、受体后因素有关。

(4) 脂肪萎缩：见于注射部位。

二、其他降糖药

其他降糖药有：双胍类、促胰岛素分泌药磺酰脲类和格列奈类、胰高血糖素样肽-1 (GLP-1)受体激动药、二肽基肽酶-4(DPP-4)抑制药、钠-葡萄糖共转运体 2(SGLT-2)抑制药、胰岛素增敏药、α-葡萄糖苷酶抑制药等。

(一) 双胍类

双胍类常用的有二甲双胍和苯乙双胍。

1. 药理作用和机制

(1)激活 AMP 活化的蛋白激酶(AMPK)，减少肝脏葡萄糖、脂肪酸和胆固醇的生成。

(2)增加外周肌肉组织对葡萄糖的摄取。

(3)增强胰岛素信号转导，降低肥胖或胰岛素抵抗的 T2DM 患者的血糖。

2. 临床应用

治疗 T2DM 的首选药物和联合用药中的基础用药，尤适用于肥胖及单用饮食控制无效者；对 T1DM，与胰岛素联合应用可减少胰岛素用量和血糖波动。

3. 不良反应

食欲下降、恶心、腹部不适、腹泻、乳酸性酸血症、酮血症。肝肾功能不全、慢性心肺功能不全、酗酒者等禁用。

(二) 磺酰脲类

磺酰脲类的代表药有格列齐特、格列美脲等。

1. 药理作用和机制

(1)降血糖：降低正常人血糖，对胰岛功能尚存的患者有效。其降血糖的主要机制是刺激胰岛 β 细胞释放胰岛素。

(2)对水排泄的影响：氯磺丙脲促进 ADH 分泌和增强其作用，有抗利尿作用，可用于尿崩症。

(3)对凝血功能的作用：格列齐特使血小板黏附力减弱，刺激纤溶酶原的合成。

2. 临床应用

(1)用于胰岛功能尚存的 2 型糖尿病且单用饮食控制无效者。

(2)氯磺丙脲可用于尿崩症治疗。

3. 不良反应

低血糖、过敏反应、胃肠不适、黄疸和肝损害、嗜睡、眩晕、白细胞、血小板减少及溶血性贫血等。需定期检查肝功能和血象，老人及肝、肾功能不良的糖尿病患者慎用。

(三) 瑞格列奈

"第一个餐时血糖调节药"上市，是一种短效的促胰岛素分泌药。主要用于 T2DM 患者，老年糖尿病患者也可服用，且适用于糖尿病肾病患者。因其结构中不含硫，对磺酰脲类药物过敏者仍可使用。常见不良反应为低血糖，较磺酰脲类药物少见。

(四) 胰高血糖素样肽-1(GLP-1)受体激动药

GLP-1 的生理作用为：

(1)以葡萄糖依赖的方式作用于 β 细胞，促进胰岛素基因的转录，使胰岛素的合成和分泌增加。

(2) 刺激 β 细胞的增殖和分化，抑制凋亡，增加 β 细胞数量。

(3) 抑制 α 细胞的胰高血糖素分泌。

(4) 促进胰岛 δ 细胞生长抑素分泌，进而抑制胰高血糖素的分泌。

(5) 抑制食欲与摄食。

(6) 延缓胃内容物排空。

GLP-1 受体激动药的短效制剂有艾塞那肽、利司那肽、利拉鲁肽和贝那鲁肽等；长效制剂有司美格鲁肽、杜拉鲁肽、阿必鲁肽等。除司美格鲁肽可口服外，其他均需皮下注射给药。

本类药物的作用机制为与 GLP-1 受体结合后，产生与 GLP-1 相似的作用：促进胰岛素合成和分泌、抑制胰高血糖素分泌、抑制食欲与摄食、增加能量消耗、延迟胃排空等。GLP-1 受体激动药可降低血糖、糖化血红蛋白和体重，由于其降血糖作用是葡萄糖依赖性的，单独应用一般不会引起低血糖。此外，还可降低心血管疾病高危人群发生心血管事件的风险，可能有肾脏保护作用。常见的不良反应为胃肠道反应。艾塞那肽的禁忌证包括严重的胃肠道疾病和肾功能不全。司美格鲁肽还有荨麻疹等过敏反应，可增加胰腺炎风险。对本品过敏者、甲状腺髓样瘤个人既往病史或家族病史、多发性内分泌肿瘤综合征患者禁用。

(五) 二肽基肽酶-4 (DPP-4) 抑制药

二肽基肽酶-4 (DPP-4) 抑制药包括西格列汀、沙格列汀、维格列汀、利格列汀、阿格列汀等。作用机制为抑制 DPP-4 水解 GLP-1，降低空腹和餐后血糖，一般不会引起低血糖和体重增加。可单独或与其他降血糖药物合用治疗 T2DM。不良反应偶见过敏、血管性水肿、皮疹等皮肤损害等。

(六) 钠-葡萄糖共转运体 2 (SGLT-2) 抑制药

钠-葡萄糖共转运体 2 抑制药包括卡格列净、达格列净、依帕列净等。SGLT-2 抑制药主要通过抑制肾脏近曲小管的 SGLT-2，减少肾脏葡萄糖重吸收，降低肾糖阈，促进尿中葡萄糖排泄，从而降低血糖水平。其降糖作用不依赖于胰岛素的分泌或胰岛素的作用，可降低糖化血红蛋白水平，还可减轻体重、降低血压、保护肾脏等。SGLT-2 抑制药单独或与其他口服降血糖药物及胰岛素合用治疗 T2DM。达格列净用于降低有症状的慢性心力衰竭成人的心血管死亡、心力衰竭住院或紧急心力衰竭就诊的风险；还可用于治疗合并或不合并 T2DM 的慢性肾脏病成人患者。SGLT-2 抑制药的主要不良反应为尿道感染、生殖器感染，与胰岛素和磺酰脲类合用易引起低血糖；酮症酸中毒是不常见但严重的不良反应，不建议用于 T1DM 或糖尿病酮症酸中毒的患者。

(七) 胰岛素增敏药

噻唑烷二酮类，包括罗格列酮、吡格列酮、曲格列酮等。

1. 作用机制

竞争性激活 PPARγ，调节胰岛素反应性基因的转录。

2. 药理作用

(1) 改善胰岛素抵抗、降低高血糖。

(2) 改善脂肪代谢紊乱。
(3) 防治 2 型糖尿病血管并发症。
(4) 改善胰岛 β 细胞功能。
3. 临床应用
临床应用于治疗胰岛素抵抗和 T2DM。
4. 不良反应
不良反应主要有水肿、体重增加、嗜睡、肌肉和骨骼痛、头痛、消化道症状等。

(八) α 葡萄糖苷酶抑制药

阿卡波糖和伏格列波糖，竞争性抑制小肠上皮刷状缘 α-葡萄糖苷酶，抑制寡糖分解为单糖，减少小肠中淀粉、糊精和双糖的吸收，降低餐后血糖和糖化血红蛋白，不增加体重。单用或与其他降糖药合用降低患者的餐后血糖。主要副作用为胃肠道反应，与胰岛素或磺酰脲类合用易发生低血糖。胃肠功能紊乱、妊娠、哺乳期妇女和儿童不宜使用。

案例学习

学习要点：
(1) 掌握胰岛素的作用机制、临床应用和不良反应。
(2) 掌握口服降糖药的分类、作用机制、临床应用和不良反应。
(3) 熟悉不同类型糖尿病的选择用药。

关键词： 胰岛素；口服降糖药；磺酰脲类；双胍类

案例

王女士，59 岁，15 年前因多饮多尿乏力，查空腹血糖 12.0 mmol/L，诊断为 2 型糖尿病，口服二甲双胍治疗。因血糖控制不理想，加用格列本脲。后因数次出现低血糖现象，患者不能耐受，因此，将格列本脲换成格列吡嗪。近两年来出现血糖控制欠佳，且常有波动。目前空腹血糖 18.0 mmol/L，餐后 2 小时血糖>20.0 mmol/L，糖化血红蛋白 14.1%。患者体胖，体温、血压均正常，尿糖 3+，尿酮体阴性，胰岛素抗体、胰岛细胞抗体阴性，肝肾功能正常。入院后控制饮食，适当运动，予胰岛素泵强化降糖治疗，血糖逐渐下降，后改为口服二甲双胍、格列美脲、阿卡波糖联合控制血糖；血糖控制平稳后，予以出院。

问答题

1. 二甲双胍的作用机制、适应证和不良反应？
2. 格列本脲、格列吡嗪、格列美脲属于哪一类口服降糖药？作用有何异同点？
3. 阿卡波糖的作用机制和适应证？
4. 胰岛素的作用机制？为什么本案例中给予患者胰岛素泵强化降糖治疗？

选择题

1. 胰岛素与磺酰脲类药的共同不良反应是（   ）。

A. 过敏反应　　B. 粒细胞缺乏　　C. 低血糖　　D. 胃肠反应　　E. 黄疸
2. 噻唑烷二酮类治疗2型糖尿病的机制为(　　)。
　　A. 抑制胰岛素降解　　　　B. 促进胰岛素分泌　　　　C. 降低血清糖原水平
　　D. 促进外周组织对葡萄糖的摄取和利用　　E. 抑制碳水化合物在小肠的吸收
3. 主要降低餐时血糖的口服降糖药是(　　)。
　　A. 阿卡波糖　　B. 格列吡嗪　　C. 二甲双胍　　D. 罗格列酮　　E. 瑞格列奈
4. 长期使用二甲双胍的患者应重视潜在(　　)缺乏的早期筛查。
　　A. Vit D　　B. Vit B_{12}　　C. Vit B_2　　D. Vit C　　E. Vit B_6
5. 对糖尿病昏迷患者，应立即采取的措施是(　　)。
　　A. 静脉注射普通胰岛素　　　　　　B. 皮下注射普通胰岛素
　　C. 皮下注射低精蛋白锌胰岛素　　　D. 皮下注射珠蛋白锌胰岛素
　　E. 皮下注射精蛋白锌胰岛素
6. 餐时血糖调节药的作用机制是(　　)。
　　A. 关闭钾离子通道　　B. 抑制α-葡萄糖苷酶　　C. 抑制钠-葡萄糖联合转运体
　　D. 抑制二肽基肽酶-4　　E. 激动PPARγ
7. 胰岛素增敏药的药理作用不包括(　　)。
　　A. 增强胰岛素信号传递　　　　B. 激活胰高血糖素样肽-1受体
　　C. 降低TNFα的表达　　　　　 D. 改善胰岛β细胞功能
　　E. 增加葡萄糖的摄取和转运，激活糖酵解
8. 在降糖药中，对于胰岛功能完全丧失的患者，无效的是(　　)。
　　A. 氯磺丙脲　　B. 胰岛素　　C. 二甲双胍　　D. 罗格列酮　　E. 阿卡波糖
9. 患者，女，55岁，患糖尿病多年，现在饮食控制并服用格列本脲治疗中，糖尿病控制良好。近日受凉后出现高热、咳嗽，X光证实为肺炎，尿糖+++，住院治疗。除了按肺炎常规治疗外，对糖尿病的治疗方案应调整为(　　)。
　　A. 加强饮食控制，继续服用格列本脲　　B. 加大格列本脲用量
　　C. 改用二甲双胍　　D. 加用二甲双胍　　E. 改用胰岛素
10. 胰岛素耐受的形成原因错误的是(　　)。
　　A. 严重创伤　　　　B. 产生胰岛素抗体　　　　C. 感染
　　D. 酮症酸中毒　　　E. 合并手术

Case study

Key points:

(1) Master the mechanism of action, clinical application and adverse reactions of insulin.

(2) Master the classification, mechanism of action, clinical application and adverse reactions of oral hypoglycemic drugs.

(3) Be familiar with the choice of medication for different types of diabetes.

Key words: insulin; oral hypoglycemic agents; sulfonylureas; biguanides

Case

Ms. Wang, 59 years old, was diagnosed as type 2 diabetes mellitus 15 years ago due to excessive drinking and urine and fatigue, and her fasting blood glucose was 12.0 mmol/L. She was treated with metformin orally and glabenluide was added due to unsatisfactory blood glucose control. Later, due to several episodes of hypoglycemia, the patient could not tolerate it, so glibenzide was replaced by glipizide. In the past two years, the blood sugar control was poor and often fluctuated. At present, the fasting blood glucose was 18.0 mmol/L, the blood glucose was > 20.0 mmol/L 2 hours after meals, and the glycosylated hemoglobin was 14.1%. The patient is obese, body temperature and blood pressure was normal, urine sugar 3+, urine ketone body was negative, insulin antibody and islet cell antibody were negative, liver and kidney function was normal. After admission, diet and proper exercise were controlled, and intensive hypoglycemic treatment with insulin pump was given. Blood glucose was gradually decreased, and then metformin, glimepiride and acarbose were taken orally to control blood glucose. After the blood sugar was control stably, he was discharged.

◎ **Essay questions**

1. What are the mechanism of action, indications and adverse reactions of metformin?
2. What kind of oral hypoglycemic drugs do glibenclamide, glipizide and glimepiride belong to? What are the differences and similarities between the functions of these drugs?
3. What are the mechanism and indications of acarbose?
4. What is the mechanism of insulin? Why was the patient given intensive hypoglycemic therapy with insulin pump in this case?

Multiple-choice questions

1. The common adverse reaction of insulin and sulfonylureas is (   ).
   A. anaphylaxis   B. agranulocytosis   C. low blood sugar
   D. gastrointestinal reactions   E. jaundice
2. The mechanism of thiazolidinones in the treatment of type 2 diabetes is (   ).
   A. inhibiting insulin degradation
   B. promoting insulin secretion
   C. decreasing serum glycogen levels
   D. promoting glucose uptake and utilization in peripheral tissues
   E. inhibiting the absorption of carbohydrates in the small intestine
3. The main oral hypoglycemic agent that lower blood sugar during meals is (   ).
   A. acarbose   B. glipizide   C. metformin
   D. rosiglitazone   E. repaglinide
4. Patients with long-term use of metformin should pay attention to early screening for potential (   ) deficiencies.

A. Vit D B. Vit B$_{12}$ C. Vit B$_2$
D. Vit C E. Vit B$_6$

5. For diabetic coma patients, which immediate measure should be taken (　　).
    A. intravenous injection of regular insulin
    B. subcutaneous injection of regular insulin
    C. subcutaneous injection of hypoprotamine zinc insulin
    D. subcutaneous injection of globin zinc insulin
    E. subcutaneous injection of zinc protamine insulin

6. The mechanism of mealtime blood glucose regulators is (　　).
    A. close potassium ion channels
    B. inhibition of alpha-glucosidase
    C. inhibition of sodium-glucose co-transporters
    D. inhibition of dipeptidyl peptidase-4
    E. activation of PPARγ

7. Pharmacological effects of insulin sensitizers do not include (　　).
    A. enhancing insulin signaling
    B. activation of glucagon-like peptide-1 receptors
    C. decreased the expression of TNF-α
    D. improving the function of islet beta cells
    E. increase glucose uptake and metonymy you to activate glycolysis

8. Among hypoglycemic drugs, which is ineffective to the patients with complete loss of islet function (　　).
    A. chlorpropamide B. insulin C. metformin
    D. rosiglitazone E. acarbose

9. Patient, female, 56 years old, has been suffering from diabetes for many years. Now, with diet control and glibenclamide therapy, the diabetes was well controlled. Recently, she had high fever and cough after cold, X ray confirmed pneumonia, urine sugar +++, hospitalized. In addition to the usual treatment of pneumonia, the treatment of diabetes should be adjusted to (　　).
    A. strengthen diet control and continue to take glibenclamide
    B. increase the dosage of glibenclamide
    C. switch to use meformin
    D. add use meformin
    E. switch to use of insulin

10. The cause of insulin tolerance is wrong (　　).
    A. severe trauma B. insulin resistance
    C. infection D. ketoacidosis
    E. combined surgery

第三十三章案例学习和选择题答案

第三十四章 抗菌药物概论

知识要点

一、基本概念

(1)化学治疗：针对致病原(包括细菌、真菌、病毒等其他微生物和寄生虫)和癌细胞所致疾病的药物治疗。治疗目的在于选择性消灭或抑制致病原或肿瘤，同时尽可能小地对宿主机体造成损伤。

(2)抗菌药：能杀灭病原菌或抑制其生长繁殖的药物，用于防治细菌感染性疾病。

(3)抑菌药：仅抑制病原菌生长繁殖，不能杀灭病原菌的药物。

(4)杀菌药：不但抑制病原菌生长繁殖，还能杀灭病原菌的药物。

(5)抗菌谱：药物抗菌活性所覆盖的病原菌范围。

(6)窄谱抗菌药：药物抗菌范围窄，仅针对某一种或某一类的细菌具有抗菌活性。

(7)广谱抗菌药：药物抗菌范围广，对不同种类的多种病原菌具有抗菌活性。

(8)化疗指数：导致半数实验动物死亡的剂量(LD_{50})与在半数实验动物中产生抗感染疗效的剂量(ED_{50})的比值或 LD_5(5%致死剂量)与 ED_{95}(95%有效剂量)的比值。一般地，化疗指数越大，药物安全性越高、毒性越小。但不能以化疗指数作为评判药物安全性的唯一指标。

(9)最小抑菌浓度：抑制培养基中细菌生长所需的最低药物浓度，反映药物的体外抑菌活性。

(10)最小杀菌浓度：杀死培养基中99.9%的细菌所需的最低药物浓度，反应药物的体外杀菌能力。

(11)耐药性：包括固有耐药性和获得性耐药。固有耐药性是指病原体对药物天然不敏感。获得性耐药是指致病原在与药物多次接触后，对药物的敏感性下降乃至消失，导致药物的抗感染疗效降低甚至失效。提高药物剂量不能克服耐药性。

(12)抗生素后效应：体内药物浓度虽然降至最小抑菌浓度以下，但细菌的生长在一段时间内仍持续受到抑制的现象。这是设计抗菌药临床给药方案的重要参考依据。

(13)交叉耐药性：病原菌对某一种抗菌药产生耐药性后，对其他作用机制相似的药物也产生耐药性。

(14)多重耐药性：病原菌对化学结构和抗菌机制不同的多种药物产生耐药。

(15)二重感染：正常人的口、咽喉部和下消化道中存在完整的微生态系统，即正常菌群。长期口服或注射使用广谱抗菌药时，正常菌群被抑制，使得对药物不敏感的微生物得以乘机大量繁殖，由原来的劣势菌群变为优势菌群造成新的感染，称作二重感染或菌群交替症。

二、抗菌药物的分类

1. 根据来源

(1) 天然来源：即抗生素，多为真菌分泌的细菌毒素，如青霉素、头孢菌素、红霉素、林可霉素、氯霉素等。

(2) 人工合成：如磺胺类和喹诺酮类药物。

2. 根据化学结构

(1) β-内酰胺类：如青霉素、头孢菌素。

(2) 大环内酯类：如红霉素、阿奇霉素和克拉霉素等。

(3) 林可酰胺类：林可霉素、克林霉素等。

(4) 多肽类：万古霉素、多黏菌素等。

(5) 氨基苷类：链霉素、庆大霉素、妥布霉素、卡那霉素、新霉素和阿米卡星等。

(6) 四环素类：四环素、多西环素和米诺环素等。

(7) 氯霉素、喹诺酮类、磺胺类、甲硝唑和替硝唑等。

3. 根据作用结果

(1) 繁殖期杀菌药：如β-内酰胺类、万古霉素。

(2) 静止期杀菌药：如氨基苷类、喹诺酮类、多黏菌素等。

(3) 快速抑菌药：如大环内酯类、林可酰胺类、四环素、氯霉素等。

(4) 慢速抑菌药：磺胺类。

三、药物的抗菌作用机制

1. 抑制细胞壁合成

(1) β-内酰胺类药物抑制细胞壁黏肽合成酶，使繁殖期的细胞壁合成受阻，细胞壁发生缺损，大量水分进入菌体，导致菌体溶胀、变形，最终裂解。

(2) 万古霉素与细胞壁肽聚糖的前体D-丙氨酰-D-丙氨酸结合，抑制细胞壁肽聚糖的合成，导致细菌溶解。

(3) 环丝氨酸抑制D-丙氨酰-D-丙氨酸连接酶，阻断细胞壁中丝氨酸二肽的形成，从而干扰结核菌细胞壁的合成。

2. 破坏细胞膜完整性

(1) 多黏菌素与革兰氏阴性杆菌细胞膜上的磷酸基团结合，引起细胞膜通透性增加，菌体内的重要物质外漏，同时细菌膨胀溶解。

(2) 两性霉素与真菌细胞膜上的麦角甾醇结合，在细胞膜上形成孔道，细胞膜通透性增加，细胞内重要物质外漏。

3. 抑制蛋白质合成

(1) 大环内酯类药物不可逆地与细菌核糖体50S亚基结合，阻断转位作用，也可使肽酰 tRNA 在肽链延长阶段过早地脱离核糖体。

(2)氨基苷类药物抑制蛋白质合成的全过程：①与核糖体 70S 始动复合物结合，抑制肽链合成的起始；②与核糖体 30S 亚基的 16S rRNA 结合，使 mRNA 密码发生误读错译，从而产生错误的蛋白质；③阻止终止密码与核糖体结合。

(3)氯霉素与细菌 70S 核糖体的 50S 亚基结合，抑制肽酰基转移酶，阻断肽链延长。

(4)四环素特异性地与细菌核糖体 30S 亚基的 A 位置结合，阻断氨酰基-tRNA 与核糖体 A 位的结合，从而阻止肽链延长。

4. 抑制核酸代谢

(1)喹诺酮类药物抑制细菌的 DNA 回旋酶和拓扑异构酶Ⅳ，干扰细菌 DNA 复制和 RNA 转录，同时细菌 DNA 也无法形成正常的超螺旋结构，使得染色体易受损，最终导致细菌死亡。

(2)利福平与细菌的DNA依赖性RNA多聚酶的β亚基结合，抑制结核杆菌RNA的合成。

5. 抑制叶酸代谢

(1)对氨基苯甲酸(PABA)是细菌从头合成叶酸所必需的中间产物。磺胺类药物是 PABA 类似物，可竞争性抑制二氢叶酸合成酶，干扰二氢叶酸的合成。

(2)甲氧苄啶选择性抑制细菌的二氢叶酸还原酶，使二氢叶酸不能还原为四氢叶酸。

四、细菌耐药的类型及机制

1. 类型

细菌耐药可分为固有耐药性和获得性耐药。

(1)固有耐药性又称天然耐药性，是细菌与生俱来的结构特点或生化机制使其对药物作用不敏感，如链球菌对氨基苷类抗生素天然耐药。

(2)获得性耐药，是指细菌在药物作用后发生基因突变或获得外源性耐药基因(多由质粒介导)，从而获得新的性状或机制使其能避免或抵抗药物的作用。如金黄色葡萄球菌通过产生 β-内酰胺酶对 β-内酰胺类抗生素耐药。获得性耐药可因脱离药物接触而消失，也可由质粒将耐药基因转入染色体而成为可遗传的固有耐药性。

2. 机制

(1)产生药物灭活酶：通过产生的酶将药物灭活，这是细菌耐药性的重要机制。某些细菌可产生 β-内酰胺酶，该酶可破坏青霉素类和头孢霉素类药物分子中结构的 β-内酰胺环。一些细菌可产生酯酶灭活大环内酯类抗生素。另一些细菌则可产生钝化酶，包括乙酰化酶、腺苷化酶和磷酸化酶等。这些酶可将乙酰基、腺苷酰基和磷酰基连接到氨基苷类药物的氨基或羟基上，使药物分子结构发生改变因而失去抗菌活性。还有些细菌可产生乙酰转移酶来灭活氯霉素或产生核苷转移酶来灭活林可霉素。

(2)改变药物作用靶点：①改变靶蛋白结构(即产生同工酶)，使抗菌药对其亲和力降低甚至不能与其结合。肺炎链球菌可通过此机制对青霉素耐药。②增加靶蛋白数量，当部分靶蛋白被药物抑制时，其余的靶蛋白仍足以维持细菌的形态和机能。如肠球菌可通过增加青霉素结合蛋白的数量对 β-内酰胺类药物产生耐药。

(3)改变细菌外膜通透性：革兰阴性菌细胞壁的外膜能抵抗很多抗菌药的穿透，因而对这些药物具有天然耐药性。某些抗菌药(如 β-内酰胺类、喹诺酮类)需要经由外膜上的孔道蛋白进入菌体,而细菌也会通过改变这些孔道蛋白的结构和数量来减少药物的进入从而产生耐药。

(4)表达外排机制:某些细菌可表达转运机制(又称为外排泵),通过消耗能量将进入菌体的药物逆浓度差转运至菌体外。该转运机制的底物可包含分子结构和抗菌机制不同的多种药物,是引起细菌多重耐药的重要机制。金黄色葡萄球菌、表皮葡萄球菌和铜绿假单胞菌等可通过此机制对 β-内酰胺类、大环内酯类、氟喹诺酮类、四环素和氯霉素等药物产生多重耐药。

(5)形成生物膜:生物膜是指细菌在无机物体或有机体表面形成菌落,并分泌大量多糖、蛋白质等大分子将细菌包裹组织起来而形成的膜状物。生物膜中的大量多糖形成分子屏障和电荷屏障,可阻碍药物的穿透。生物膜中还含有大量细菌分泌的水解酶,可灭活抗菌药。此外,生物膜深部含氧量低、营养匮乏,此处的细菌代谢低下、生长缓慢,对绝大多数抗生素不敏感。因此,抗菌药仅能杀死生物膜表层的细菌,不但无法清除生物膜,还会诱导耐药细菌的产生。

(6)改变代谢途径:比如某些细菌可通过摄取利用哺乳动物细胞合成好的叶酸来对磺胺类药物产生耐药。

3. 避免细菌耐药性的产生

原则:合理用药、剂量和疗程足够、必要时联合用药、开发新药。

五、抗菌药物的合理应用的基本原则[①]

(1)用药须有指征(细菌性感染)。
(2)尽早确定病原,根据病原种类及药敏试验结果选用药物。
(3)根据药物的抗菌作用及其药动学特点选用药物。
(4)结合患者病情、病原种类及抗菌药物特点制订治疗方案。

六、抗菌药物的联合应用[②]

1. 目的

发挥协同作用以提高疗效,对混合感染或病原不明的感染扩大抗菌范围,降低单一药物的毒副作用,延缓或减少细菌耐药的产生。

2. 原则

(1)原菌未明的严重感染,包括免疫缺陷者的严重感染。
(2)单一抗菌药物不能控制的需氧菌及厌氧菌混合感染,2 种或 2 种以上病原菌感染。
(3)单一抗菌药物不能有效控制的感染性心内膜炎或败血症等重症感染。
(4)需长程治疗,但病原菌易对某些抗菌药物产生耐药性的感染,如结核病、深部真菌病。

---

① 参见中国药学会医院药学专业委员会:抗菌药物临床应用指导原则。
② 中国药学会医院药学专业委员会:抗菌药物临床应用指导原则。

(5) 由于药物协同抗菌作用，联合用药时应将毒性大的抗菌药物剂量减少。

(6) 宜联合使用具有协同或相加抗菌作用的药物。

(7) 通常采用 2 种药物联合，3 种及 3 种以上药物联用仅适用于个别情况，如结核病的治疗。

3. 联合用药的可能效果

(1) 协同：联合用药的疗效强于各药单用的疗效之和。如繁殖期杀菌药和静止期杀菌药合用可产生协同作用。又如青霉素与氨基苷类抗生素合用时，前者破坏细菌细胞壁，有利于后者进入细菌内部。

(2) 相加：联合用药的疗效等于各药单用的疗效之和。如静止期杀菌药和速效抑菌药合用可产生相加作用，因为后者迅速抑制细菌蛋白质合成后，不影响甚至有利于前者充分发挥作用。繁殖期杀菌药也可与慢性抑菌药合用产生相加作用。

(3) 无关：联合用药的疗效等于作用较强的药物单用之疗效。

(4) 拮抗：联合用药的疗效弱于单一用药之疗效。繁殖期杀菌药与速效抑菌药可发生拮抗。如青霉素与氯霉素或四环素合用时，后两药迅速抑制蛋白质合成使细菌处于静止状态，致使繁殖期杀菌的青霉素不能充分发挥抑制细胞壁合成的作用。

案例学习

学习要点：
选择合适的抗菌药物需要考虑的因素：病原菌的类型、药物敏感性、抗菌药的抗菌机制、药动学特点、抗菌谱、适应证、患者自身状态等。

关键词： 抗菌机制；抗菌谱；药敏试验

案例一

一名 30 岁男子就诊诉尿道分泌物。查体发现尿道分泌物为脓性，阴茎无溃疡、水泡，腹股沟淋巴结未见异常。革兰氏染色显示分泌物的白细胞内有革兰氏阴性双球菌。

◎ 问答题

男子诊断为淋病奈瑟氏球菌引起的无并发症性尿道炎，治疗时应考虑使用何种作用机制的抗生素？

案例二

一女怀孕，来院进行第一次产前检查。查体显示正常妊娠 12 周，但非螺旋体和荧光螺旋体抗体测试均为阳性。患者不记得此前一年有过梅毒的表现，并否认接受过梅毒治疗。亦无此前的梅毒血清学资料可资比较。患者经治疗痊愈，后终产一子。男孩现 3 岁半，因面部皮疹就诊。经询问得知，小患者的托儿所今天还有其他几个孩子也出现类似的皮疹。查体发现患儿一般情况良好，但在双颊上有离散性红斑丘疹，无小水疱或大泡。皮疹表面有蜜样硬壳，提示脓疱病。

◎ 问答题

1. 该孕妇诊断为处于梅毒潜伏期，宜选用何种治疗药物为最佳？如患者为非孕妇，可考虑选用哪些治疗药物？

2. 经诊断男孩患小儿脓疱疮，在氨苯砜、酮康唑、强力霉素、双氯西林和喷昔洛韦这些药物中，哪一种适用于男孩的治疗？

选择题

1. 关于微生物对抗生素产生耐药性，下列表述中准确的是（　　）。
   A. 需要同时使用多种抗生素　　　　B. 是对牲畜使用抗生素引起的
   C. 万古霉素可以克服这一问题　　　D. 主要原因是人类对抗生素的滥用
   E. 可以通过提高药物剂量来克服
2. 以下哪种药物属于窄谱抗生素？（　　）
   A. 头孢曲松　　B. 环丙沙星　　C. 异烟肼　　D. 亚胺培南　　E. 米诺环素
3. 以下哪种抗生素具有浓度依赖性的杀菌作用？（　　）
   A. 克林霉素　　B. 利奈唑胺　　C. 万古霉素　　D. 红霉素　　E. 达托霉素
4. 以下哪种抗生素具有较长的抗生素后效应，可以每天用药一次？（　　）
   A. 庆大霉素　　B. 青霉素G　　C. 万古霉素　　D. 氨曲南　　E. 头孢克洛
5. 丙型肝炎合并肝硬化患者使用以下哪种抗生素时需要密切监测并调整剂量？（　　）
   A. 青霉素G　　B. 妥布霉素　　C. 红霉素　　D. 万古霉素　　E. 亚胺培南
6. 红霉素和林可霉素合用可导致下列哪种结果？（　　）
   A. 扩大抗菌谱　　　　　B. 降低毒性　　　　　C. 相互拮抗
   D. 降低细菌耐药性　　　E. 增强抗菌活性
7. 一名20岁女性患者，因身体不适来就诊。发现患有淋病，因其有青霉素过敏史，那么她应该使用（　　）进行治疗。
   A. 磺胺类　　　　　　　B. 第三代喹诺酮类　　C. 第一代头孢菌素
   D. 第二代头孢菌素　　　E. 第三代头孢菌素
8. 药物抑制或杀灭病原菌的能力称为（　　）。
   A. 抗菌谱　　　　　　　B. 抗菌活性　　　　　C. 最低抑菌浓度
   D. 最低杀菌浓度　　　　E. 化学治疗学
9. 下列何种药物为繁殖期杀菌药？（　　）
   A. 氨基苷类　　　　　　B. 头孢菌素类　　　　C. 四环素类
   D. 氯霉素类　　　　　　E. 磺胺类
10. 化疗指数可用下面哪个比例关系来衡量？（　　）
    A. ED_{95}/LD_5　　B. ED_5/LD_{95}　　C. ED_{50}/LD_{50}　　D. LD_{50}/ED_{50}　　E. LD_1/ED_{99}

Case study

Key points：

Aspects to be considered in deciding appropriate antimicrobial drugs: types of pathogenic bacteria, drug susceptibility, antimicrobial mechanism, pharmacokinetic characteristics, antimicrobial spectrum, indications, patient condiction, and etc.

Key words: antimicrobial mechanism; antimicrobial spectrum; drug sensitivity test

Case 1

A thirty-year-old man presented with a complaint of urethral discharge. On examination, the urethral discharge was found to be purulent. There were no ulcers or blisters on the penis, and the inguinal lymph nodes appeared normal. Gram staining showed Gram-negative diplococci in the leucocytes of the discharge.

◎ **Essay question**

The man is diagnosed with uncomplicated urethritis caused by Neisseria gonorrhoeae. Antibiotics with what mechanisms of action should be considered for the treatment of the patient's infection?

Case 2

A woman became pregnant and came to the hospital for her first prenatal examination. The examination showed 12 weeks of normal gestation. However, both the non-treponemal syphilis serological test and fluorescent treponemal antibody-absorption test came back positive. The patient did not recall any manifestation of syphilis in the previous year and denied having received any treatment for syphilis. There was no previous syphilis serological results for comparison, either. The woman eventually gave birth to a boy after treatment. The boy, now 3.5 years old, was brought to doctor for a facial rash. It was learnt that several other children from the young patient's nursery were presenting with similar rashes the same day. Examination revealed that the boy was in a generally good condition but had discrete erythematous papules on both cheeks, but no small blisters or large vacuoles. The rash had a honey-like crust on the surface, suggesting impetigo.

◎ **Essay questions**

1. The woman is diagnosed with latent syphilis. What is the best drug treatment for this pregnant woman? If the patient is non-pregnant, what therapeutic agents might be considered?
2. The boy is diagnosed with pediatric impetigo. Which drug among ampicillin, ketoconazole, doxycycline, dicloxacillin and penciclovir would be appropriate for the boy's treatment?

Multiple-choice questions

1. Which of the following statements regarding microbial resistance to antibiotics is accurate? (　　)
    A. Multiple antibiotics should be used at the same time to overcome the problem.
    B. The problem is caused by the use of antibiotics on livestock.
    C. Vancomycin can overcome this problem.
    D. The main cause of the problem is antibiotics abuse by humans.

E. The resistance can be overcome by increasing the dose of the antibiotics.

2. Which of the following is a narrow spectrum antimicrobial agent? (   )

    A. Ceftriaxone   B. Ciprofloxacin   C. Isoniazid   D. Imipenem   E. Minocycline

3. Which of the following agents has a concentration-dependent bactericidal effect? (   )

    A. Clindamycin   B. Linezolid   C. Vancomycin   D. Clindamycin   E. Daptomycin

4. Which of the following agents has a long post-antibiotic effect and can be administered once daily? (   )

    A. Gentamicin   B. Penicillin G   C. Vancomycin   D. Aztreonam   E. Cefaclor

5. Which of the following agents requires close monitoring and dosage adjustment when administered to a patient with hepatitis C and liver cirrhosis? (   )

    A. Penicillin G   B. Tobramycin   C. Erythromycin   D. Vancomycin   E. Imipenem

6. The combination of erythromycin and lincomycin leads to which of the following outcomes? (   )

    A. Expansion of the antimicrobial spectrum   B. Reduced toxicity
    C. Mutual antagonism   D. Reduction of bacterial resistance
    E. Enhancement of antibacterial activity

7. A 20-year-old female patient comes to the clinic because she is not feeling well. She is diagnosed with gonorrhea. Because of her history of allergy to penicillin, she should be treated with (   ).

    A. sulfonamides   B. third-generation quinolones
    C. first-generation cephalosporins   D. second-generation cephalosporins
    E. third-generation cephalosporins

8. The ability of a drug to inhibit or kill pathogenic bacteria is termed as (   ).

    A. antimicrobial spectrum   B. antimicrobial activity
    C. minimum bacteriostatic concentration   D. minimum bactericidal concentration
    E. chemotherapeutics

9. Which of the following drugs is a bactericidal agent to bacteria in the proliferating phase? (   )

    A. Aminoglycosides   B. Cephalosporins   C. Tetracyclines
    D. Chloramphenicol   E. Sulfonamides

10. The chemotherapeutic index is calculated as which of the following ratios? (   )

    A. ED_{95}/LD_5 B. ED_5/LD_{95} C. ED_{50}/LD_{50} D. LD_{50}/ED_{50} E. LD_1/ED_{99}

第三十四章案例学习和选择题答案

第三十五章 β-内酰胺类抗生素

知识要点

一、β-内酰胺类抗生素的概念、分类、抗菌机制和细菌耐药机制

1. 概念

β-内酰胺类抗生素是指化学结构中含有 β-内酰胺环的一类抗生素。

2. 分类

（1）青霉素类：窄谱青霉素，如青霉素 G 和青霉素 V；耐酶青霉素，如甲氧西林、氯唑西林和氟氯西林；广谱青霉素，如氨苄西林和阿莫西林；抗铜绿假单胞菌广谱青霉素，如羧苄西林、拉西林；抗革兰阴性菌青霉素，如美西林和匹美西林。

（2）头孢菌素类：按抗菌谱、耐药性和肾毒性分为一、二、三、四、五代。第一代，如头孢拉定和头孢氨苄；第二代，如头孢呋辛和头孢克洛；第三代，如头孢哌酮、头孢噻肟和头孢克肟；第四代，如头孢匹罗；第五代，如头孢洛林、头孢吡普。

（3）其他 β-内酰胺类，如碳青霉烯、头霉素、氧头孢烯、单环 β-内酰胺类等。

（4）β-内酰胺酶抑制剂，如棒酸和舒巴坦。

（5）β-内酰胺类抗生素的复方制剂。

3. 抗菌机制

与细菌菌体内的青霉素结合蛋白（PBPs）结合，抑制细菌细胞壁合成，使菌体失去渗透屏障而发生膨胀、裂解；同时还能促进细菌自溶。

4. 耐药机制

（1）产生水解酶。如 β-内酰胺酶，水解药物分子中的 β-内酰胺环，破坏药物分子结构，从而使药物失活。

（2）产生与药物结合的酶。如 β-内酰胺酶可与某些耐酶 β-内酰胺类抗生素结合，使药物停留在胞浆膜外间隙中，不能到达作用靶点。

（3）改变药物作用靶点。如细菌可改变 PBPs 的结构，降低其与 β-内酰胺类抗生素的亲和力；细菌也可通过增加 PBPs 的产量来稀释药物作用。

（4）降低菌膜对药物的通透性。比如革兰氏阴性菌可改变跨膜通道孔蛋白的结构或减少跨膜通道蛋白的表达，从而产生耐药。

（5）增加药物外排。细菌可以增加菌膜上的主动外排蛋白的表达，从而促进菌体内药物的排出。

(6)减少自溶酶的表达。

二、青霉素类药物

1. 青霉素 G

1)抗菌作用

青霉素 G 属于繁殖期杀菌剂,机制为抑制细菌细胞壁四肽侧链和五肽交连桥的连接而抑制细胞壁合成。对敏感病菌有良好的抗菌活性,对宿主无明显毒性。抗菌谱为:①多数革兰氏阳性球菌(如溶血性链球菌、肺炎链球菌、草绿色链球菌等);②革兰氏阳性杆菌(如白喉杆菌、炭疽杆菌及革兰氏阳性厌氧杆菌);③革兰氏阴性球菌(如脑膜炎球菌和淋球菌);④少数革兰氏阴性杆菌(如流感嗜血杆菌和百日咳鲍特氏菌);⑤梅毒螺旋体、钩端螺旋体、回归热螺旋体、鼠咬热螺菌、放线杆菌等高度敏感。青霉素 G 对多数革兰氏阴性杆菌和肠球菌活性较弱,对真菌、立克次体、病毒和原虫无活性。金黄色葡萄球菌、肺炎球菌、脑膜炎球菌和淋球菌对本药易产生耐药。

2)临床应用

首选青霉素 G 静脉滴注或肌肉注射来治疗敏感的革兰氏阳性球菌和杆菌、革兰氏阴性球菌以及螺旋体所致的感染,如溶血性链球菌所致蜂窝织炎、扁桃体炎、心内膜炎、猩红热、咽炎和丹毒等。以下感染也可优先考虑青霉素 G:肺炎球菌所致大叶性肺炎、支气管炎、脓胸,肺炎链球菌感染所致肺炎、中耳炎、脑膜炎和菌血症等,不产青霉素酶葡萄球菌感染、破伤风、气性坏疽等,梭状芽孢杆菌感染、炭疽、梅毒、钩端螺旋体、白喉、回归热等。对于草绿色链球菌所致心内膜炎,由于药物不易分布到病灶,需要超大剂量静脉滴注并联用氨基苷类药物。

3)不良反应

(1)过敏反应:是青霉素类最常见的不良反应。可出现各种类型的变态反应,常见 II 型(哮喘、药疹、溶血性贫血、接触性皮炎、间质性肾炎)和 III 型(血清病)变态反应,多数不严重,停药后消失。I 型变态反应即过敏性休克最为严重,发生率低但死亡率高。引发变态反应的不是青霉素本身而是其降解产物如青霉噻唑蛋白、青霉烯酸、6-APA 高分子聚合物等。机体首次接触后约在一周内产生抗体,再次接触时即引发变态反应,可立即发生也可延迟数日发生。过敏性休克的临床表现主要表现是呼吸、循环衰竭和中枢抑制。防治措施:①仔细询问是否有青霉素过敏史,对青霉素过敏者禁用;②避免局部用药;③必须在有抢救药物和设施的条件下用药;④初次用药、间隔 3 日以上用药或使用不同批次药物之前必须做皮试,阳性反应者禁用;⑤药液现用现配,不可久置后使用;⑥患者用药后留观 30 分钟,无反应方可离去;⑦一旦发生过敏反应,应立即皮下注射 1 mL 0.1%盐酸肾上腺素(抢救过敏性休克首选),严重者可静脉滴注,必要时可静脉注射糖皮质激素(地塞米松)。对呼吸抑制者应立即进行人工呼吸,并肌肉注射呼吸兴奋剂(如尼可刹米)。喉头水肿导致窒息时,应尽快行气管切开术。

(2)赫氏反应:在使用青霉素治疗螺旋体感染(梅毒、钩体、雅司病)或炭疽等感染时,病原体崩解释放大量毒素和异体蛋白刺激机体产生的不良反应,表现为急起畏寒、高热、寒战、头痛、全身酸痛、皮疹、肌痛甚至休克。

(3) 其他：青霉素 G 肌注可引起给药局部疼痛、红肿或硬结。鞘内注射可产生脑膜刺激征或诱发惊厥和癫痫。

2. 氨苄西林

1) 抗菌作用

为半合成广谱青霉素，耐酸且可口服，可杀灭革兰氏阳性菌和革兰氏阴性菌，活性与青霉素 G 相当，但不耐 β-内酰胺酶，故对耐药金黄色葡萄球菌感染无效。对革兰氏阴性杆菌有较强的活性，如大肠埃希菌、痢疾志贺菌、流感杆菌、百日咳杆菌、伤寒与副伤寒杆菌、痢疾杆菌、奇异变形杆菌、布氏杆菌等。革兰氏阴性的淋球菌、脑膜炎球菌也对本药敏感。本药对草绿色链球菌和肠链球菌的活性优于青霉素 G。本药对铜绿假单胞菌、肺炎杆菌和吲哚阳性变形杆菌无效，对革兰氏阳性杆菌和螺旋体的作用不及青霉素 G。

2) 临床应用

用于治疗敏感菌所致的泌尿系统、呼吸系统、胆道、肠道感染以及脑膜炎、心内膜炎、软组织感染和败血症等。重症感染者应将本药与氨基苷类抗生素合用。本品与氯唑西林按 1:1 组成合剂（氨唑西林）可提高疗效，采用肌内或静脉给药。

3) 不良反应

与青霉素 G 相似，与青霉素 G 有交叉过敏。可引起二重感染。

3. 阿莫西林

1) 抗菌作用

广谱半合成青霉素，耐酸且可口服，可杀灭革兰氏阳性菌和革兰氏阴性菌，活性与青霉素 G 相似。不耐酶，对耐药金黄色葡萄球菌无效。抗菌谱和抗菌活性与氨苄西林相似，但对肺炎球菌、肠球菌、沙门氏菌、幽门螺杆菌的活性强于氨苄西林。本品与氟氯西林按 1:1 组成复方制剂"新灭菌"可提高疗效，肌内或静脉给药。

2) 临床应用

作为口服 β-内酰胺类抗生素的首选，可用于治疗多种敏感菌所致的感染，包括急性中耳炎、链球菌性咽炎、肺炎、皮肤感染、胆道感染、尿路感染、沙门氏菌感染、莱姆病和衣原体感染，也可用于治疗幽门螺杆菌相关的慢性活动性胃炎和消化性溃疡。

3) 不良反应

恶心、呕吐、腹泻等消化道反应和皮疹多见。可有血清转氨酶升高，偶见嗜酸性粒细胞增多、白细胞减少和二重感染。对青霉素 G 过敏者禁用。

三、头孢菌素类药物的抗菌作用、分类与临床应用

头孢菌素类药物为杀菌药，机制与青霉素相同。细菌对头孢菌素可产生耐药性，并与青霉素类药物有部分交叉耐药。

第一代头孢菌素对革兰氏阳性菌的活性强于第二、三代药物，主要用于治疗敏感菌所致的呼吸道、尿路、皮肤及软组织感染。但第一代头孢菌素不能耐受革兰氏阴性菌的 β-内酰胺酶，故革兰氏阴性菌（如吲哚阳性变形杆菌、产气杆菌、假单胞菌、沙雷杆菌、拟杆菌和肠链球菌）对第一代头孢菌素易于耐药。

第二代头孢菌素对革兰氏阳性菌的活性弱于第一代药物，对革兰氏阴性菌（大肠杆

菌、奇异变形杆菌等)有显著作用,对厌氧菌也有一定活性,但对铜绿假单胞菌无效。第二代头孢菌素对多种 β-内酰胺酶比较稳定,其抗菌谱也大于第一代药物。可用于治疗敏感菌所致的肺炎、菌血症、胆道、尿路和其他组织器官感染。

第三代头孢菌素对革兰氏阳性菌的活性弱于第一、二代药物,但对革兰氏阴性菌(如肠杆菌、铜绿假单胞菌、沙雷杆菌、不动杆菌等)以及厌氧菌有较强的活性。第三代头孢菌素对 β-内酰胺酶较为稳定,抗菌谱也进一步扩大。可用于治疗危及生命的败血症、脑膜炎、肺炎、骨髓炎及尿路严重感染,也能有效控制严重的铜绿假单胞菌感染。

第四代头孢菌素对 β-内酰胺酶高度稳定,对革兰氏阴性菌具有强大的活性,其对革兰氏阳性球菌(如金黄色葡萄球菌)的活性也强于第三代药物,可用于治疗对第三代头孢菌素耐药的细菌感染。

第五代头孢菌素对革兰氏阴性菌的作用与第四代药物相似,但对革兰氏阳性菌的作用更强、抗菌谱也更宽,尤其对耐甲氧西林金黄色葡萄球菌、耐万古霉素金黄色葡萄球菌、耐甲氧西林表皮葡萄球菌和耐青霉素的链球菌有效,对一些厌氧菌也有很好的抗菌活性。第五代头孢菌素对大部分 β-内酰胺酶高度稳定,但对金属 β-内酰胺酶和超广谱 β-内酰胺酶耐受性不高,主要用于复杂性皮肤或软组织感染、革兰氏阴性菌所致的糖尿病足感染、社区或医院获得性肺炎等。

四、万古霉素类

1. 抗菌作用及机制

对革兰氏阳性菌具有强大杀菌作用,尤其是对甲氧西林耐药的金黄色葡萄球菌、表皮葡萄球菌。抗菌作用机制是与细胞壁前体肽聚糖结合,阻断细胞壁合成,造成细胞壁缺陷而发挥杀菌作用,对分裂增殖期的细菌呈现快速杀菌作用。

2. 耐药性

耐药菌株可产生一种能修饰细胞壁前体肽聚糖的酶,阻止药物与前体肽聚糖结合从而产生耐药。

3. 临床应用

仅用于严重革兰氏阳性菌感染,特别是对甲氧西林耐药的金黄色葡萄球菌和表皮葡萄球菌和肠球菌属所致感染,如败血症、心内膜炎、骨髓炎、呼吸道感染等。可用于对 β-内酰胺类过敏的患者。口服给药用于治疗假膜性结肠炎和消化道感染。

4. 不良反应

(1)耳毒性。血药浓度超过 800 mg/L 且持续数天即可引起耳鸣、听力减退,甚至耳聋。及早停药可恢复正常,少数患者停药后仍有致聋危险。应避免同时使用耳毒性和肾毒性的药物。

(2)肾毒性。主要损伤肾小管,表现为蛋白尿和管型尿、少尿、血尿、氮质血症甚至肾功能衰竭。

(3)过敏反应。可引起斑块皮疹和过敏性休克。万古霉素快速静注时可出现极度皮肤潮红、红斑、荨麻疹、心动过速和低血压等表现,称为"红人综合征"。

(4)静注时偶发疼痛和血栓性静脉炎。

案例学习

学习要点：
(1) 青霉素和头孢菌素的作用机制和耐药机制。
(2) 抗生素的经验性使用。

关键词： β-内酰胺；脑膜炎；耐药性

案例

急诊科收治一名神志不清的中年男子。患者入院时已发热超过 24 小时，期间患者曾诉剧烈头痛，并伴有恶心和呕吐。腰椎穿刺显示开口压升高，脑脊液检查结果为蛋白水平升高、葡萄糖水平降低和中性粒细胞增多。脑脊液涂片显示革兰氏阳性双球菌，初步诊断为化脓性脑膜炎。从本地分离的肺炎双球菌株约有 25% 对青霉素 G 的最小抑制浓度为 20 μg/mL。

问答题

1. 需立即对该患者进行治疗。现有如下药物：阿莫西林、头孢菌素、头孢曲松加万古霉素、萘夫西林、哌拉西林。应使用其中哪种静脉注射为宜？

2. 如果该患者为 80 岁的老年人，脑脊液涂片显示白喉样革兰氏阳性杆菌，则应考虑经验性地给予何种抗生素治疗？

选择题

1. 青霉素类的主要抗菌作用机制是抑制(　　)。
   A. β-内酰胺酶　　　B. 细胞膜合成　　　C. N-乙酰氨基酸的合成
   D. 肽聚糖交联　　　E. 转糖基化

2. 关于 β-内酰胺类抗生素，以下说法中错误的是(　　)。
   A. 头孢唑啉和其他第一代头孢菌素不能通过血脑屏障
   B. 头孢曲松和萘夫西林都主要通过胆汁分泌排出体外
   C. 青霉素类药物对胃酸不稳定因此限制其口服吸收
   D. 丙磺舒抑制肾小管对阿莫西林的重吸收
   E. 替卡西林对几种革兰氏阴性杆菌有活性

3. 肺炎球菌对青霉素 G 产生耐药性的原因是(　　)。
   A. 孔蛋白结构改变
   B. 产生 β-内酰胺酶
   C. 改变靶标青霉素结合蛋白的化学结构
   D. 肽聚糖前体的 d-Ala-d-Ala 结构单元发生改变
   E. 青霉素 G 在细胞内的富集减少

4. 原发梅毒的最佳治疗方案是(　　)。
   A. 单次口服磷霉素　　　B. 单剂头孢曲松　　　C. 肌肉注射苄星青霉素 G

D. 口服四环素7天　　　E. 使用万古霉素治疗
5. 以下哪项不是青霉素的常见适应证？（　　）
   A. 脑膜炎　　　　B. 肺炎或慢性支气管炎　　C. 尿路感染
   D. 耐甲氧西林金黄色葡萄球菌感染　　E. 淋病或梅毒
6. 以下哪一种属于超广谱抗生素，可用于假性杆菌、肠杆菌属、变形杆菌、脆弱杆菌和克雷伯杆菌感染？（　　）
   A. 奥西西林　　B. 氨苄青霉素　　C. 阿莫西林　　D. 青霉素　　E. 哌拉西林
7. 以下哪一种头孢菌素容易被β-内酰胺酶破坏？（　　）
   A. 头孢噻吩　　B. 头孢孟多　　C. 头孢噻肟　　D. 头孢吡肟　　E. 头孢洛林
8. 以下哪种药物不会引起酒精不耐受？（　　）
   A. 头孢呋辛　　B. 拉氧头孢　　C. 头孢哌酮　　D. 头孢曲松　　E. 头孢他啶
9. 下列关于第三代头孢菌素的叙述中，错误的是（　　）。
   A. 体内分布较广，一般从肾脏排泄
   B. 对各种β-内酰胺酶高度稳定
   C. 对革兰氏阴性菌作用不如第一、二代药物
   D. 对铜绿假单胞菌作用很强
   E. 基本无肾毒性
10. 关于万古霉素，以下说法中准确的是（　　）。
    A. 对耐甲氧西林葡萄球菌有活性　　　B. 为抑菌药
    C. 与青霉素结合蛋白（PBPs）结合　　D. 经肝脏代谢
    E. 口服生物利用度高

Case study

Key points：
（1）Mechanisms of action and resistance of penicillins and cephalosporins.
（2）Empirical use of antibiotics.
Key words：β-lactam；meningitis；drug resistance

Case

A middle-aged man in a state of confusion and delirium was admitted to the emergency department. The patient had been febrile for more than 24 hours on admission, during which time he had complained of severe headache with nausea and vomiting. A lumbar puncture revealed an elevated opening pressure, and cerebrospinal fluid examination revealed increased protein, decreased glucose, and an increased neutrophil count. Cerebrospinal fluid smear showed Gram-positive diplococci and a preliminary diagnosis of purulent meningitis was made. About 25 per cent of the locally isolated S. pneumoniae strains had a minimum inhibitory concentration of 20 μg/mL of penicillin G.

◎ **Essay questions**

1. The patient requires immediate treatment. The following drugs are available, amoxicillin, cephalosporin, ceftriaxone plus vancomycin, nafcillin and piperacillin. Which of these should be administered intravenously to the patient?

2. If this patient is 80 years old and a cerebrospinal fluid smear shows diphtheria-like gram-positive bacilli, empiric treatment of what antibiotics can be considered?

📝 **Multiple-choice questions**

1. The main mechanism of antimicrobial action of penicillins is inhibition of (   ).
    A. β-lactamases
    B. Cell membrane synthesis
    C. Synthesis of N-acetylamino acids
    D. Peptidoglycan cross-linking
    E. Transglycosylation

2. Which of the following statements regarding β-lactam antibiotics is incorrect? (   )
    A. Cefazolin and other first-generation cephalosporins do not cross the bloodbrain barrier
    B. Both ceftriaxone and nafcillin are excreted mainly through bile secretion.
    C. The instability of penicillins in gastric acid limits their oral absorption
    D. Probenecid inhibits tubular reabsorption of amoxicillin
    E. Ticarcillin is active against several Gram-negative bacilli

3. Resistance of pneumococci to penicillin G is due to (   ).
    A. structural changes in pore proteins
    B. production of beta-lactamase
    C. alteration of the chemical structure of the target penicillin-binding proteins
    D. changes in the d-Ala-d-Ala structural block of peptidoglycan precursors
    E. decreased intracellular enrichment of penicillin G

4. The best treatment for primary syphilis is (   ).
    A. single oral dose of phosphomycin
    B. single-dose ceftriaxone
    C. intramuscular injection of benzylpenicillin G
    D. oral tetracycline for 7 days
    E. treatment with vancomycin

5. Which of the following is not a common indication for penicillin? (   )
    A. Meningitis
    B. Pneumonia or chronic bronchitis
    C. Urinary tract infection
    D. Methicillin-resistant Staphylococcus aureus infections
    E. Gonorrhoea or syphilis

6. Which of the following is an ultra-broad-spectrum antibiotic that can be used for infections of pseudomonas aeruginosa, enterobacteriaceae, aspergillus, bacteroides fragilis and klebsiella? (   )

A. Oxacillin B. Ampicillin C. Amoxicillin
D. Penicillin E. Piperacillin

7. Which of the following cephalosporins is readily destroyed by β-lactamase? (   )

    A. Cephalothin B. Cefamandole C. Cefotaxime
    D. Cefepime E. Ceftarolin

8. Which of the following drugs does not cause alcohol intolerance? (   )

    A. Cefuroxime B. Latamoxef C. Cefoperazone
    D. Ceftriaxone E. Ceftazidime

9. Which of the following statements of the third-generation cephalosporins is incorrect? (   )

    A. Widely distributed in the body, generally excreted from the kidneys
    B. Highly stable to various β-lactamases
    C. Not as effective as the first and second generation against G-bacteria
    D. It has strong effect on Pseudomonas aeruginosa.
    E. Insignificant nephrotoxicity

10. Which of the following statements regarding vancomycin is accurate? (   )

    A. Active against methicillin-resistant staphylococci   B. Bacteriostatic drug
    C. Binding to PBPs   D. Via liver metabolism
    E. Good after oral administration bioavailability

第三十五章案例学习和选择题答案

第三十六章 大环内酯类抗菌药和林可霉素

知识要点

一、大环内酯类抗生素所包括的药物

大环内酯类(macrolides)是一类含有14、15和16元大环内酯环的抗生素。常首选用于需氧革兰氏阳性菌、革兰氏阴性球菌和厌氧球菌等感染的治疗，以及对β-内酰胺类抗生素过敏的患者。红霉素是第一代药物，抗菌谱窄、不良反应重、易发生细菌耐药。阿奇霉素、罗红霉素和克拉霉素属于第二代半合成大环内酯类抗生素，具有较强的抗生素后效应，广泛用于呼吸道感染的治疗。泰利霉素和喹红霉素属于第三代大环内酯类抗生素。

按化学结构分为：14元大环内酯类，包括红霉素、竹桃霉素、克拉霉素、罗红霉素、地红霉素、泰利霉素和喹红霉素等；15元大环内酯类，包括阿奇霉素；16元大环内酯类，包括麦迪霉素、乙酰麦迪霉素、吉他霉素、乙酰吉他霉素、交沙霉素螺旋霉素、乙酰螺旋霉素罗他霉素等。

二、大环内酯类抗生素的主要作用及特点

大环内酯类抗菌谱较窄，第一代药物的抗菌谱涵盖大多数革兰氏阳性菌、厌氧球菌和包括奈瑟菌、嗜血杆菌及白喉棒状杆菌在内的部分革兰氏阴性菌，有强大抗菌活性。对军团菌、弯曲菌、支原体、衣原体、弓形虫、非典型分枝杆菌等也有良好抗菌活性。对产β-内酰胺酶的葡萄球菌和耐甲氧西林金黄色葡萄球菌有一定抗菌活性。第二代药物的抗菌范围扩大，对革兰氏阴性菌的抗菌活性也得到提高。大环内酯类通常为抑菌药，高浓度时也有杀菌作用。

大环内酯类药物的主要抗菌机制为不可逆地结合到细菌核糖体50S亚基的靶位上，14元大环内酯类可阻断肽酰基t-RNA移位，而16元大环内酯类则抑制肽酰基的转移反应，由此选择性抑制细菌蛋白质合成。有的大环内酯类也能与50S亚基上的L27和L22蛋白结合，促使肽酰基t-RNA从核糖体上解离，从而抑制蛋白质合成。林可霉素、克林霉素和氯霉素在细菌核糖体50S亚基上的结合位点与大环内酯类相同或相近，故合用时可能发生相互拮抗，也易使细菌产生耐药。由于细菌核糖体为70S，由50S和30S亚基构成，而哺乳动物核糖体为80S，由60S和40S亚基构成，因此大环内酯类药物对哺乳动物核糖体几无影响。

三、红霉素

1. 抗菌作用

红霉素是第一代(14元)大环内酯类药物,与细菌核糖体 50S 亚基的靶位不可逆地结合,阻断肽酰基 t-RNA 移位,抑制细菌蛋白质合成。低浓度时有抑菌作用,高浓度时有杀菌作用。抗菌谱较窄,主要对大多数革兰氏阳性菌,如金黄色葡萄球菌、表皮葡萄球菌、厌氧球菌和部分革兰氏阴性菌,如脑膜炎/淋病耐瑟菌、流感嗜血杆菌及白喉棒状杆菌在内的有强大抗菌活性。对嗜肺军团菌,弯曲菌,支原体,衣原体,弓形虫,非典型分枝杆菌等也有良好活性。对产 β-内酰胺酶的葡萄球菌和耐甲氧西林金黄色葡萄球菌有一定活性。对某些螺旋体,肺炎支原体,立克次体和螺杆菌也有抗菌作用。

2. 临床应用

红霉素常用于治疗耐青霉素的金黄色葡萄球菌感染和对青霉素过敏者,还用于上述敏感菌所致的各种感染,也能用于厌氧菌引起的口腔感染和肺炎支原体、肺炎衣原体、解脲支原体等非典型病原体所致的呼吸、泌尿生殖系统感染。对于军团菌肺炎和支原体肺炎,红霉素可作为首选治疗药物。红霉素的不良反应主要为胃肠道反应。

四、阿奇霉素

1. 抗菌作用

阿奇霉素、为半合成的 15 元大环内酯类抗生素,抗菌谱较红霉素广。在对红霉素敏感的细菌,阿奇霉素的抗菌活性与红霉素相当,但阿奇霉素对革兰氏阴性菌的活性显著强于红霉素,甚至对某些细菌表现为快速杀菌作用。口服吸收快,组织分布广,细胞内游离浓度较同期血药浓度高 10~100 倍,半衰期长达 35~48 小时,为大环内酯类中最长者,每日仅需给药一次。

2. 临床应用

阿奇霉素用于治疗敏感细菌所致的上呼吸道感染(鼻窦炎、咽炎、扁桃体炎等)、下呼吸道感染(支气管炎、肺炎等)、急性中耳炎、皮肤和软组织感染等,也可用于沙眼衣原体和非多重耐药淋球菌所致的单纯性生殖器感染和杜克嗜血杆菌引起的软下疳。

五、林可霉素和克林霉素

1. 抗菌作用

克林霉素是林可霉素的半合成品,两药具有相同的抗菌机制:与核糖体 50S 亚基结合,抑制转肽反应,阻止肽链延长,从而抑制细菌的蛋白质合成。它们的抗菌谱与红霉素相近,但不属于大环内酯类药物。两药属于快速抑菌剂,但克林霉素的抗菌活性比林可霉素强 4~8 倍,药动学特点更佳且毒性更低。两药对各类厌氧菌有强大抗菌活性,对需氧革兰氏阳性菌有显著活性,对部分需氧革兰氏阴性球菌、人型支原体和沙眼衣原体也有抑制作用,但对肠球菌、革兰氏阴性杆菌、耐甲氧西林金黄色葡萄球菌、肺炎支原体作用微弱。

2. 临床应用

林可霉素和克林霉素主要用于厌氧菌（脆弱拟杆菌、产气荚膜梭菌、放线杆菌等）引起的口腔、腹腔和妇科感染，需氧革兰氏阳性球菌引起的呼吸道、骨及软组织、胆道感染以及败血症和心内膜炎等，可作为首选药物治疗金黄色葡萄球菌引起的骨髓炎。

案例学习

学习要点：
(1) 社区获得性肺炎及其治疗。
(2) 非典型病原体的种类。
关键词： 获得性肺炎；非典型病原体；药物联用

案例

一名 30 岁女性患者就诊，主诉干咳、头痛、发热和不适 4 天。患者有呼吸困难表现，胸部可闻及啰音，但无其他明显肺部体征。X 光胸片显示肺部广泛片状浸润样改变。痰液经革兰氏染色未检出病原菌。患者提到一位同事也出现了类似症状。初步诊断为社区获得性肺炎。患者无既往严重病史，喜晒日光浴，每日摄取 5 杯咖啡，日常补充铁剂，并于就诊前服用抗过敏药物氯雷他定。

◎ **问答题**

1. 现有氨苄西林、克林霉素、红霉素、多西环素、利奈唑胺和万古霉素，其中哪种药物最适合用于该患者的治疗？
2. 如使用红霉素进行治疗，患者应采取何种措施避免不良反应？
3. 拟给予抗菌药治疗 5 天。现有阿奇霉素、红霉素、克林霉素、多西环素和万古霉素，考虑疗效和药物相互作用，宜选用哪种药物？

选择题

1. 基于同一作用部位的拮抗作用，以下哪例抗生素联用是不恰当的？（　　）
   A. 克林霉素和红霉素　　B. 强力霉素和阿莫西林　　C. 替加环素和阿奇霉素
   D. 环丙沙星和阿莫西林　　E. 阿奇霉素和头孢克洛
2. 克拉霉素的抗菌活性与红霉素相似，但克拉霉素的优点在于（　　）。
   A. 不抑制肝脏药物代谢酶　　　　　　B. 一次用药即可根除支原体感染
   C. 对幽门螺杆菌具有更强的活性　　　D. 对耐甲氧西林的葡萄球菌有效
   E. 对耐红霉素的链球菌有效
3. 革兰氏阳性菌对大环内酯类抗生素产生耐药的主要机制是（　　）。
   A. 改变 30S 核糖体亚基　　　　　　B. 降低细胞膜对药物的通透性
   C. 产生乙酰转移酶使药物失活　　　　D. 产生水解内酯环的酯酶
   E. 50S 核糖体亚基上的药物结合位点发生甲基化
4. 患者在接受克林霉素治疗 3 周后出现腹泻，应考虑下列哪种不良反应？（　　）

A. 高胆红素血症　　B. 肾毒性　　C. 艰难梭菌感染　　D. 假性脑瘤　　E. 肝功能损害

5. 红霉素在下列哪种组织中浓度最高？（　　）
   A. 骨髓　　　　B. 肺　　　　C. 肠道　　　　D. 肾脏　　　　E. 胆汁

6. 治疗支原体肺炎和军团菌感染应首选（　　）。
   A. 青霉素　　　B. 氨苄青霉素　　C. 妥布霉素　　D. 红霉素　　　E. 链霉素

7. 急、慢性金黄色葡萄球菌性骨髓炎的首选用药是（　　）。
   A. 罗红霉素　　B. 万古霉素　　C. 林可霉素　　D. 庆大霉素　　E. 克拉维酸

8. 下列关于大环内酯类抗生素的叙述中，错误的是（　　）。
   A. 细菌对本类各药有不完全交叉耐药性
   B. 在酸性环境中抗菌活性较强
   C. 不易透过血脑屏障
   D. 血药浓度低，但组织中浓度相对较高
   E. 主要作用是抑制细菌蛋白质的合成

9. 红霉素对下述哪类病原体无效？（　　）
   A. 金黄色葡萄球菌　　　B. 肺炎支原体　　　C. 白喉棒状杆菌
   D. 淋球菌　　　　　　　E. 大肠杆菌

10. 红霉素的抗菌作用特点是（　　）。
    A. 抑制细菌蛋白质合成而抑菌　　　B. 抑制细菌蛋白质合成而杀菌
    C. 抑制细菌细胞膜合成而抑菌　　　D. 抑制细菌细胞膜合成而杀菌
    E. 抑制细菌蛋白质合成既可杀菌又可抑菌

Case study

Key points：
(1) Community-acquired pneumonia and its treatment.
(2) Types of atypical pathogens.

Key words：β-lactam；meningitis；drug resistance

Case

A 30-year-old female patient presented with complaints of dry cough, headache, fever and malaise for the last 4 days. The patient had some respiratory difficulty and there were no other significant pulmonary signs than rales in the chest. Chest X-ray film showed extensive patchy infiltrative changes in the lungs. Gram stain of expectorated sputum did not reveal any bacterial pathogen. The patient mentioned a colleague with similar symptoms. The patient denied any serious medical conditions in the past. She took the anti-allergic drug loratadine and daily iron supplements prior to the visit, and drank 5 cups of coffee every day. The initial diagnosis was community-acquired pneumonia.

◎ **Essay questions**

1. Available antibiotics include ampicillin clindamycin doxycycline linezolid and vancomycin. Which of the medications would be the most appropriate for the treatment of this patient?
2. If treated with erythromycin, what precautions should the patient take to ward off adverse effects of the drug?
3. The doctor planned to give the patient antimicrobial therapy for 5 days. Taking into account efficacy and drug interactions, which drug among azithromycin, clindamycin, doxycycline, erythromycin and vancomycin would be the appropriate choice?

Multiple-choice questions

1. Which of the following antibiotic combinations is inappropriate considering possible antagonism at the same site of action? (   )
    A. Clindamycin and erythromycin B. Doxycycline and amoxicillin
    C. Tigecycline and azithromycin D. Ciprofloxacin and amoxicillin
    E. Azithromycin and cefaclor
2. The antibacterial activity of clarithromycin is similar to that of erythromycin, but the advantages of clarithromycin is (   ).
    A. clarithromycin does not inhibit liver drug-metabolising enzymes
    B. mycoplasma infections can be eradicated with a single dose of medication
    C. clarithromycin is more active against H. pylori
    D. clarithromycin is effective against methicillin-resistant staphylococci
    E. clarithromycin is effective against erythromycin-resistant streptococci
3. The main mechanism whereby Gram-positive bacteria develop resistance to macrolide antibiotics is (   ).
    A. alteration of the 30S ribosomal subunit
    B. reducing the permeability of cell membranes to drugs
    C. production of drug-inactivating acetyltransferases
    D. production of esterases that hydrolyze the lactone ring
    E. methylation of the drug binding site on the 50S ribosomal subunit
4. Which of the following adverse reactions should be considered for a patient who develops diarrhoea after 3 weeks of clindamycin treatment? (   )
    A. Hyperbilirubinaemia   B. Nephrotoxicity   C. Clostridium difficile infection
    D. Pseudotumour cerebri   E. Hepatic impairment
5. Erythromycin has the highest concentration in which of the following tissues? (   )
    A. Bone marrow   B. Lungs   C. Intestine
    D. Kidney   E. Bile
6. The drug of choice for treatment of mycoplasma pneumonia and Legionella infections is (   ).

A. penicillin B. ampicillin C. tobramycin
D. erythromycin E. streptomycin

7. The drug of choice for acute and chronic aureus osteomyelitis is (   ).
   A. roxithromycin B. vancomycin C. lincomycin chronic osteomyelitis
   D. gentamicin E. clavulanic acid

8. Which of the the following statements about macrolide antibiotics is incorrect? (   )
   A. Bacteria are incompletely cross-resistant to the drugs in this class.
   B. Antibacterial activity is stronger in acidic environments
   C. They do not easily cross the blood-brain barrier
   D. Low blood concentration, but relatively high concentration in tissues
   E. The main function is to inhibit the synthesis of bacterial proteins

9. Erythromycin is ineffective against which of the following groups of pathogens? (   )
   A. Staphylococcus aureus B. Mycoplasma pneumoniae
   C. Corynebacterium diphtheriae D. Gonococci
   E. Escherichia coli

10. The antibacterial action of erythromycin is characterized by (   ).
    A. inhibition of bacterial protein synthesis and being bacteriostatic
    B. inhibition of bacterial protein synthesis and being bactericidal
    C. being bacteriostatic by inhibiting bacterial cell membrane synthesis.
    D. inhibition of bacterial cell membrane synthesis and being bactericidal
    E. inhibition of bacterial protein synthesis and being both bactericidal and bacteriostatic.

第三十六章案例学习和选择题答案

第三十七章 氨基苷类抗菌药

知识要点

一、氨基苷类抗生素的概念

氨基苷类是一类由氨基醇环与氨基糖分子以苷键相结合的碱性抗生素，包括天然和半合成产品两大类。天然来源的氨基苷类由链霉菌和小单胞菌产生，包括链霉素、卡那霉素、妥布霉素、大观霉素、新霉素、庆大霉素、小诺米星、西索米星、阿司米星等。半合成品包括奈替米星、依替米星、异帕米星、卡那霉素 B、阿米卡星、地贝卡星、阿贝卡星等。氨基苷类药物属于有机碱，对需氧革兰氏阴性杆菌尤其有效。该类药物不能与 β-内酰胺类混合，否则易失活。

二、氨基苷类抗生素的抗菌机制和特点

1. 作用及作用机制

氨基苷类药物属于静止期杀菌药，主要作用是抑制细菌蛋白质合成的全过程，机制包括：①抑制 70S 核糖体始动复合物的形成；②选择性地与核糖体 30S 亚基结合，造成 mRNA 上的三联密码发生误读，导致翻译错误，从而产生错误的蛋白；③阻止肽链释放因子的结合，导致合成好的肽链不能释放；④抑制 70S 复合物的解离，使核糖体无法循环利用去合成新的蛋白。氨基苷类药物还能破坏胞质膜的完整性，使其发生渗漏，导致胞内物质大量外泄。

本类药物的抗菌作用具有如下特点：①杀菌作用呈浓度依赖性；②仅对需氧菌有效，对需氧革兰氏阴性杆菌的活性最强；③抗生素后效应明显，且呈浓度依赖性；④具有首次暴露效应，即抗菌药在首次接触细菌时表现出强大活性，但短时间内再次或多次使用同种抗菌药时，其作用并不增强甚至减弱，待一段时间后才能恢复；⑤碱性环境可增强其抗菌活性。氨基苷类药物对各种需氧革兰氏阴性杆菌(大肠埃希菌、铜绿假单胞菌、变形杆菌、克雷伯菌、肠杆菌、志贺菌和枸橼酸杆菌等)具有强大抗菌活性，对沙雷菌、沙门菌、产碱杆菌、不动杆菌和嗜血杆菌有一定活性，对革兰氏阴性球菌(淋病奈瑟菌、脑膜炎奈瑟菌等)作用较弱，对多数革兰氏阳性菌(如肠球菌)效差。但庆大霉素、阿米卡星等对产酶和不产酶的金黄色葡萄球菌及耐甲氧西林金黄色葡萄球菌具有较强活性。链霉素和卡那霉素还对结核分枝杆菌有效。本类药物的抗菌作用依赖于氧，故对厌氧菌无效。

2. 不良反应

氨基苷类药物最主要的不良反应是耳毒性和肾毒性，尤其多见于儿童和老年人。药物毒性的产生因药而异，与用药剂量和疗程有关，停药后也可发生不可逆的毒性反应。

(1) 耳毒性。包括前庭神经和耳蜗神经损伤。前庭神经损伤表现为视力减退、眼球震颤、眩晕、恶心、呕吐和共济失调。不同氨基苷类药物所致前庭神经损伤的发生率依次为：新霉素>卡那霉素>链霉素>西索米星>阿米卡星≥庆大霉素≥妥布霉素>奈替米星>依替米星。耳蜗神经损伤表现为耳鸣、听力减退和永久性耳聋。不同氨基苷类药物引起耳蜗神经损伤发生率依次为：新霉素>卡那霉素>阿米卡星>西索米星>庆大霉素>妥布霉素>奈替米星>链霉素>依替米星。孕妇用药也可导致子宫内胎儿耳蜗神经损伤。药物在内耳淋巴液中的较高浓度与本类药物的耳毒性直接相关，药物可损害内耳柯蒂器内、外毛细胞的能量代谢，造成细胞膜 Na^+-K^+-ATP 酶功能障碍，最终导致毛细胞损伤。早期损伤可逆，但累积到一定程度即造成不可逆损伤。为防止和减少本类药物耳毒性的发生，用药期间应经常询问患者是否有眩晕、耳鸣等先兆症状，并定期检查患者听力。应避免与其他有耳毒性的药物合用（如万古霉素、强效利尿药、镇吐药、甘露醇等）。镇静催眠药以及其他有镇静作用的药物可掩盖患者的耳毒性症状，故应谨慎合用。

(2) 肾毒性。氨基苷类药物是诱发药源性肾衰竭的最常见原因。本类药物对肾组织有极高亲和力，可通过胞饮的方式大量积聚于肾皮质，造成肾小管尤其是近曲小管上皮细胞损伤，导致肾小管肿胀甚至组织坏死。肾毒性表现包括蛋白尿、管型尿、血尿等，严重时可出现无尿、氮质血症和肾衰竭。本类药物的肾毒性取决于各药在肾皮质中的聚积程度和对肾小管的损伤能力，根据发生率排序依次为：新霉素>卡那霉素>庆大霉素>妥布霉素>阿米卡星>奈替米星>链霉素>依替米星。为防止和减少肾毒性的发生，用药时应定期检查患者的肾功能，如出现管型尿、蛋白尿、血尿素氮和肌酐升高、尿量减少（<240 mL/8h）等现象应立即停药。有条件的地方应作血药浓度监测。肾功能减退可减慢药物排泄，使血浆药物浓度升高，从而加重肾损伤和耳毒性，因此肾功能减退患者应慎用本类药物或调整用药方案。氨基苷类药物的排泄速率随年龄增长逐渐减慢，故应根据患者具体情况调整用药剂量，也应避免合用有肾毒性的药物，如强效利尿药、顺铂、第一代头孢菌素和万古霉素等。

(3) 神经肌肉麻痹。与给药剂量和给药途径有关，最常见于大剂量腹膜内或胸膜内给药或静脉滴注速度过快时，偶见于肌肉注射后。表现为心肌抑制、血压下降、肢体无力和呼吸衰竭。原因可能是药物作用于神经肌肉接头处的突触前膜，与 Ca^{2+} 竞争受体，从而抑制突触前膜释放乙酰胆碱，阻断神经肌肉传递。不同氨基苷类药物引起神经肌肉麻痹的严重程度不同，依次为新霉素>链霉素>卡那霉素>奈替米星>阿米卡星>庆大霉素>妥布霉素>依替米星，应立即静脉注射新斯的明和钙盐抢救，也应避免合用肌肉松弛药、全麻药等。低血钙和重症肌无力患者禁用或慎用本类药物。

(4) 过敏反应。常见皮疹、发热、血管神经性水肿和口周发麻等表现。局部应用新霉素常引起接触性皮炎。链霉素可引起过敏性休克，发生率仅次于青霉素，防治措施同青霉素。

三、常用氨基苷类抗菌药的临床应用

1. 链霉素

链霉素是第一个用于临床的氨基苷类抗生素，临床常用硫酸盐。链霉素口服吸收极少，肌注吸收快。易分布至胸腔、腹腔、结核性脓腔和干酪化脓腔。本药 90%经肾小球滤过排出体外。临床主要用于：①治疗结核病（一线药）；②与四环素类联合使用治疗鼠疫和兔热病（首选）；③与青霉素联用治疗溶血性链球菌、草绿色链球菌及肠球菌等引起的心内膜炎。

2. 卡那霉素

卡那霉素是从链霉菌培养液中分离获得，有 A、B、C 三种成分，常用 A 组分。本药口服吸收极差，肌注易吸收，在胸腔液和腹腔液中分布较好，主要经肾脏排泄。对多数常见革兰氏阴性菌和结核分枝杆菌均有效，但因不良反应较重，疗效不突出，现已被同类其他药物取代。目前主要用于治疗耐药金黄色葡萄球菌及敏感革兰氏阴性杆菌感染，可与其他抗结核药联用治疗对一线药物耐药的结核，也可口服用于肝性昏迷或腹部术前准备的患者。

3. 庆大霉素

庆大霉素用于治疗各种革兰氏阴性杆菌所致的感染，对沙雷菌属的作用尤为强大，为本类药物的首选。可与青霉素或其他抗生素合用，协同治疗严重的肺炎球菌、铜绿假单胞菌、肠球菌、耐药性金黄色葡萄球菌、草绿色链球菌、大肠杆菌、变形杆菌、巴氏杆菌或沙门氏菌感染，如败血症、泌尿生殖道感染、呼吸道感染（肺炎、支气管肺炎）、胃肠道感染、乳腺炎、皮肤和软组织感染等。也可用于术前预防和术后感染，还可局部使用治疗皮肤、黏膜感染和眼、耳、鼻部感染。

4. 妥布霉素

口服难以吸收，肌注后迅速吸收。可在胸腔、腹腔和滑膜腔内达到治疗浓度。对肺炎杆菌、肠杆菌属、变形杆菌属和铜绿假单胞菌的活性强于庆大霉素。对庆大霉素耐药菌株仍有效。适用于治疗铜绿假单胞菌所致的各种感染（如败血症、脓毒血症、脑膜炎、泌尿生殖系统和肺部感染等）。常与青霉素类或头孢菌素类药物联用治疗铜绿假单胞菌感染。本药对其他革兰氏阴性杆菌的活性不如庆大霉素。在革兰氏阳性菌中，妥布霉素仅对葡萄球菌有效。

5. 阿米卡星

阿米卡星（丁胺卡那霉素）是卡那霉素的半合成衍生物。肌注后迅速吸收，主要分布于细胞外液，难以透过血脑屏障。阿米卡星抗菌谱较广，对革兰氏阴性杆菌和金黄色葡萄球菌均有较强的抗菌活性，但作用弱于庆大霉素。本药对肠道革兰氏阴性杆菌和铜绿假单胞菌所产生的多种钝化酶稳定，故能有效治疗革兰氏阴性杆菌中对卡那霉素、庆大霉素或妥布霉素耐药菌株所致的感染，常作首选。本药与 β-内酰胺类药物具有协同作用。当粒细胞缺乏或其他免疫缺陷患者发生严重革兰氏阴性杆菌感染时，联合用药比单用阿米卡星疗效更好。该药的耳毒性强于庆大霉素，但肾毒性低于庆大霉素。

案例学习

学习要点：
氨基苷类药物的抗菌谱与毒性。
关键词： 铜绿假单胞菌；耳毒性

案例

一名65岁男性糖尿病患者于五官科就诊，主诉右耳内及右耳后疼痛。体检发现外耳道水肿，有脓性渗出物，右侧面肌无力。革兰氏染色结果显示耳部渗出物包含大量革兰氏阴性杆菌和多形核细胞。渗出物样本进一步送检进行细菌培养和药敏试验。初步诊断为外耳道炎。

问答题

1. 此时如何处理最为合适？
2. 治疗约一周后，患者耳部感染症状消失，但听力减退。可能的原因是什么？应如何应对？

选择题

1. 氨基苷类药物的作用机制涉及以下哪项？（   ）
   A. 具有抑菌作用
   B. 与50S核糖体亚基结合
   C. 导致细菌mRNA模板上的密码被误读
   D. 抑制肽基转移酶
   E. 稳定多聚小体

2. 关于氨基苷类药物阿米卡星的抗菌作用，下列哪种说法正确？（   ）
   A. 细胞壁合成抑制剂会削弱其抗菌活性
   B. 抗菌作用与浓度无关
   C. 抗菌作用具有时间依赖性
   D. 药效与其血药浓度高于最小抑菌浓度的时间成正比
   E. 该药在血药浓度降低至检测限以下时仍具有抗菌作用

3. 关于氨基苷类药物的毒性，下列哪种说法正确？（   ）
   A. 庆大霉素和妥布霉素造成肾损伤的可能性最小
   B. 阿米卡星和庆大霉素引起的耳毒性包括前庭功能障碍且通常不可逆
   C. 袢利尿剂因促进氨基苷类抗生素的肾脏排泄，故可减轻后者的耳毒性
   D. 血肌酐降低是氨基苷类肾毒性的早期征兆
   E. 局部使用新霉素后出现皮肤反应罕见

4. 氨基苷类抗生素在患者体内无明显代谢，其原因是（   ）。
   A. 该类药物的化学结构使其不易被代谢
   B. 肝脏中缺乏相应的酶来降解该类药物
   C. 机体缺乏代谢氨基苷类药物所必需的辅助因子。

D. 氨基苷类药物不易进入降解酶存在的部位(如肝脏)
   E. 该类药物抑制了药物代谢酶的活性
5. 氨基苷类抗生素经常与 β-内酰胺抗生素联合使用,其依据是以下哪项?(　　)
   A. 扩大抗菌谱
   B. 两药具有协同作用
   C. 内酰胺抗生素可预防氨基苷类抗生素的毒性
   D. 可降低超级感染的发生率
   E. 减少不良反应
6. 下列药物中具有耳毒性的是(　　)。
   A. 庆大霉素　　B. 呋塞米　　C. 依他尼酸　　D. 头孢噻吩　　E. 青霉素
7. 氨基苷类主要分布于(　　)。
   A. 血浆　　B. 细胞内液　　C. 细胞外液　　D. 浆膜腔　　E. 脑脊液
8. 对氨基苷类不敏感的细菌是(　　)。
   A. 各种厌氧菌　　B. 肠杆菌　　C. 革兰氏阴性球菌
   D. 金黄色葡萄球菌　　E. 绿脓杆菌
9. 主要用于鼠疫杆菌和结核杆菌感染的抗生素为(　　)。
   A. 庆大霉素　　B. 妥布霉素　　C. 阿米卡星　　D. 卡那霉素　　E. 链霉素
10. 肾脏毒性最低的氨基苷类药物是(　　)。
    A. 卡那霉素　　B. 庆大霉素　　C. 新霉素　　D. 妥布霉素　　E. 奈替米星

Case study

Key points:

Antimicrobial spectrum and toxicity of aminoglycosides.

Key words: pseudomonas aeruginosa; ototoxicity; aminoglycosides

Case

A 65-year-old male with diabetes mellitus complained of pain within and behind the right ear. Physical examination revealed oedema of the external auditory canal with purulent exudate and weakness of the right facial muscles. Gram stain results showed that the ear exudate contained a large number of gram negative bacilli and polymorphonuclear cells. The exudate sample was further sent for bacterial culture and drug sensitivity test. A preliminary diagnosis of otitis externa was made.

◎ **Essay questions**

1. What is the most appropriate treatment at this point?
2. After treatment for about a week, the patient's ear infection disappeared, but her hearing decreased. What was the likely cause? What measure should be taken?

Multiple-choice questions

1. The mechanism of action of aminoglycosides involves which of the following? (   )
    A. Bacteriostatic
    B. Binding to the 50S ribosomal subunit
    C. Leads to misreading of the codes on the bacterial mRNA template
    D. Inhibition of peptidyl transferase
    E. Stabilize the polymeric vesicles

2. Which of the following statements is true about the antibacterial action of the aminoglycoside amikacin? (   )
    A. Inhibitors of cell wall synthesis impair their antimicrobial activity
    B. Antimicrobial effects are concentration-independent
    C. Antimicrobial action is time-dependent
    D. The efficacy of a drug is proportional to the period of time during which its blood concentration is above the minimum inhibitory concentration
    E. There is antimicrobial activity when a drug's blood concentration drops below the limit of detection

3. Which of the following statements is true about the toxicity of aminoglycosides? (   )
    A. Gentamicin and tobramycin are least likely to cause kidney damage
    B. Amikacin-induced and gentamicin-induced ototoxicity includes vestibular dysfunction and is usually irreversible
    C. Loop diuretics attenuate the ototoxicity of aminoglycoside antibiotics by facilitating their renal excretion
    D. Decreased blood creatinine is an early sign of aminoglycoside nephrotoxicity
    E. Skin reactions are very rare following topical administration of neomycin

4. Aminoglycoside antibiotics are not significantly metabolized in patients because (   ).
    A. the chemical structure of this class of drugs makes them less susceptible to metabolism
    B. lack of appropriate enzymes in the liver to degrade the drug
    C. the body lacks the cofactors necessary to metabolize aminoglycosides.
    D. aminoglycosides are not readily accessible to sites where degradative enzymes are present (e.g. the liver)
    E. aminoglycoside antibiotics inhibit drug-metabolizing enzymes

5. Aminoglycoside antibiotics are often used in combination with β-lactam antibiotics on the basis of which of the following? (   )
    A. Expanding the antimicrobial spectrum
    B. Synergistic effects of the two drugs
    C. Lactam antibiotics prevent toxicity of aminoglycoside antibiotics
    D. Reducing the incidence of superinfections

E. Reducing adverse effects
6. Which of the following drugs are ototoxic?（　　）
    A. Gentamicin
    B. Furosemide
    C. Etanercept
    D. Cefuroxime
    E. Penicillin
7. Administered aminoglycosides are mainly distributed in (　　).
    A. plasma
    B. intracellular fluid
    C. extracellular fluid
    D. plasma membrane lumen
    E. cerebrospinal fluid
8. Bacteria that are not susceptible to aminoglycosides are (　　).
    A. various anaerobic bacteria
    B. enterobacteriaceae
    C. gram-negative cocci
    D. staphylococcus aureus
    E. pseudomonas aeruginosa
9. The antibiotic primarily used for yersinia pestis and mycobacterium infections is (　　).
    A. gentamicin
    B. tobramycin
    C. amikacin
    D. kanamycin
    E. streptomycin
10. The aminoglycoside agent with the least nephrotoxicity is (　　).
    A. kanamycin
    B. gentamicin
    C. neomycin
    D. tobramycin
    E. nertilmicin

第三十七章案例学习和选择题答案

第三十八章 四环素与氯霉素类

知识要点

一、四环素类药物的主要特点

1. 抗菌作用

本类药物属快速抑菌药，具有相似的抗菌谱、抗菌作用机制和临床应用。本类药物的抗菌活性依次为：替加环素>米诺环素>多西环素>美他环素>地美环素>四环素>土霉素。四环素和土霉素的耐药菌株日益增多，加之不良反应多，两药已不再作为本类药物的首选药。但土霉素由于抑制肠道菌群代谢，使阿米巴原虫失去生长条件，从而间接发挥抗阿米巴作用，故仍可用于治疗肠内阿米巴感染（但对肠外阿米巴病无效），疗效优于其他四环素类药物。

四环素对革兰氏阳性菌的抑制作用强于阴性菌，对革兰氏阳性菌的作用不如青霉素类和头孢菌素类，对革兰氏阴性菌的作用不如氨基苷类及氯霉素。极高浓度四环素有杀菌作用。本药对伤寒杆菌、副伤寒杆菌、铜绿假单胞菌、结核分枝杆菌、真菌和病毒无效。

2. 临床应用

治疗立克次体感染（斑疹伤寒、Q热和恙虫病等）、支原体感染（支原体肺炎和泌尿生殖系统感染等）、衣原体感染（鹦鹉热、沙眼和性病性淋巴肉芽肿等）以及某些螺旋体感染（回归热等）首选四环素类药物。四环素类药物还可首选用于治疗鼠疫、布鲁菌病、霍乱、幽门螺杆菌感染引起的消化性溃疡、肉芽肿鞘杆菌感染引起的腹股沟肉芽肿以及牙龈卟啉单胞菌引起的牙周炎。使用本类药物时首选多西环素。

3. 不良反应

（1）局部刺激。口服可引起恶心、呕吐、腹泻等症状，食物可减轻这些症状，但影响药物吸收。因局部刺激，不可肌注。静脉滴注易引起静脉炎。

（2）二重感染。正常人的口、咽喉部和下消化道中存在完整的微生态系统，即正常菌群。长期口服或注射使用广谱抗菌药时，正常菌群被抑制，使得对药物不敏感的微生物得以乘机大量繁殖，由原来的劣势菌群变为优势菌群造成新的感染，称作二重感染或菌群交替症。婴儿、老年人、体弱者、使用糖皮质激素或抗肿瘤药物的患者在使用四环素时易发生二重感染。较常见的二重感染有两种：①真菌感染，多由白假丝酵母菌引起，表现为鹅口疮、肠炎，应立即停药并同时给予抗真菌治疗；②对四环素耐药的难辨杆状芽孢杆菌所致的假膜性肠炎，表现为剧烈的腹泻、发热、肠壁坏死、体液渗出甚至休克死亡，应立即停药并口服万古霉素或甲硝唑。

(3) 影响骨骼和牙齿生长。四环素类药物可与新生牙组织中的磷灰石结合形成淡黄色的四环素-磷酸钙复合物,造成恒牙出现永久性的色素沉着(俗称牙黄染)以及牙釉质发育不全。药物对新形成的骨组织也有相同的作用,可抑制胎儿、婴幼儿骨骼发育。孕妇、哺乳期妇女及8岁以下儿童禁用四环素和其他四环素类药物。

4. 其他不良反应

长期大剂量使用可造成严重肝损伤或加重原有的肾损伤,多见于孕妇特别是肾功能异常的孕妇。偶见过敏反应和交叉过敏。也可引起光敏反应和前庭反应,如头晕、恶心、呕吐等。

二、多西环素

1. 抗菌作用

多西环素属长效半合成四环素类,是目前本类药物中的首选。多西环素的抗菌谱与四环素相同,但抗菌活性更强,具有强效、速效、长效的特点。对土霉素或四环素耐药的金黄色葡萄球菌对本药仍敏感,但多西环素与其他四环素类药物存在交叉耐药。半衰期长,每日用药1次。口服吸收迅速且完全,不易受食物影响。大部分药物随胆汁排泄进入肠腔,存在肠肝循环。肠道中的药物多以无活性的结合形式或络合形式存在,故很少引起二重感染。少量药物经肾脏排泄,肾功能减退时药物经胆汁排泄增多,故肾功能衰竭时也可使用本药。

2. 临床应用

适应证与四环素相似,但特别适合肾外感染伴肾功能衰竭者以及胆道系统感染,也用于酒糟鼻、痤疮、前列腺炎和呼吸系统感染。

3. 不良反应

可引起恶心、呕吐、腹泻、舌炎、口腔炎和肛门炎。应饭后服用,并大量饮水。服药后保持直立体位30分钟以上,以避免引起食管炎。静脉注射时可能出现舌麻木及口腔异味感。有光敏反应,其他不良反应少于四环素。

三、米诺环素

1. 抗菌作用

米诺环素口服吸收率接近100%,不易受食物影响,但抗酸药或重金属离子可减少口服米诺环素的吸收。该药脂溶性高于多西环素,组织穿透力强、分布广,在脑脊液中的浓度高于其他四环素类。米诺环素可潴留于脂肪组织,其粪便及尿液中的排泄量显著低于其他四环素类。米诺环素的抗菌谱与四环素相似,抗菌活性强于其他四环素类药物。对四环素或青霉素类耐药的A群链球菌、B群链球菌、金黄色葡萄球菌和大肠埃希菌对米诺环素仍敏感。

2. 临床应用

主要用于治疗酒糟鼻、痤疮和沙眼衣原体所致的性传播疾病以及上述耐药菌引起的感染,但一般不作为首选药物使用。

3. 不良反应

除四环素类共有的不良反应外,米诺环素具有独特的前庭反应,表现为恶心、呕吐、眩晕、运动失调等。首次用药后可迅速出现，女性多于男性。很多患者因严重的前庭反应停药，停药 24~48 小时后前庭反应消失。用药期间不宜从事高空作业驾驶和机器操作。

四、氯霉素的抗菌谱、抗菌作用、临床应用和不良反应

1. 抗菌谱

氯霉素属于抑菌药，对革兰氏阴性菌的抗菌作用强于革兰氏阳性菌，对流感嗜血杆菌、脑膜炎奈瑟菌、肺炎链球菌具有杀灭作用；对革兰氏阳性菌的抗菌活性不如青霉素类和四环素类。氯霉素对结核分枝杆菌、真菌和原虫无效。

2. 抗菌作用

氯霉素与细菌核糖体 50S 亚基上的肽酰转移酶作用位点发生可逆性结合，阻止 P 位肽链的末端羧基与 A 位氨基酰 tRNA 的氨基发生反应，从而阻止肽链延伸，使蛋白质合成受阻。氯霉素的结合位点十分接近大环内酯类和克林霉素的作用位点，这些药物同时应用可能因竞争靶点而相互拮抗。

3. 临床应用

氯霉素的毒性强烈，临床已很少应用。氯霉素可能产生致命的骨髓抑制，须严格掌握适应证。当有其他抗菌药可供选择时不可使用氯霉素。用药期间应定期检查血象。适应证包括：①耐药菌诱发的严重感染；②伤寒；③立克次体感染；④联合其他药物用于腹腔或盆腔厌氧菌感染；⑤眼科局部用药，治疗眼内感染、沙眼和结膜炎等。

4. 不良反应

（1）血液系统毒性：①可逆性血细胞减少。较常见，发生率和严重程度与剂量和疗程有关，机制与大剂量氯霉素抑制骨髓造血细胞线粒体中的 70S 亚单位有关。表现为贫血、白细胞减少症或血小板减少。及时停药后造血功能可恢复，部分患者仍可能发展成致死性再生障碍性贫血或急性髓细胞性白血病。②再生障碍性贫血。发病率与用药量、疗程无关，一次用药亦可发生。发生率低，但死亡率高。发生率女性较男性高 2~3 倍，多在停药数周或数个月后发生。

（2）灰婴综合征。早产儿和新生儿肝脏缺乏葡萄糖醛酸转移酶，肾排泄功能不全，过大剂量氯霉素可致中毒，表现为循环衰竭、呼吸困难、进行性血压下降、皮肤苍白和发绀，故称灰婴综合征。一般发生于治疗的第 2~9 天，出现症状两天内的死亡率高达 40%，大龄儿童甚至成人亦可发生。

（3）肝肾功能损伤者、葡萄糖-6-磷酸脱氢酶缺陷者、新生儿、早产儿、孕妇、哺乳期妇女不宜使用氯霉素。

案例学习

学习要点：
（1）莱姆病及其病因。
（2）多西环素的抗菌谱和抗菌活性。
关键词：多西环素；莱姆病

案例

一名 30 岁的男性地质工作者，既往身体健康，没有已知的潜在疾病。他于 8 月初前往某林区考察，约 2 周后来院就诊。患者右大腿前侧可见一个红色斑丘疹，皮疹从起始部位呈圆形向外越来越红，病变中心区域有部分消退。患者的右腿和躯干也出现几个类似的皮损。患者身上没有发现节肢动物咬伤。

问答题

该患者考虑诊断何种疾病？首选哪种药物进行治疗？

选择题

1. 四环素的抗菌作用机制包括（　　）。
   A. 拮抗细菌转位酶的活性　　　　B. 与 50S 核糖体亚基结合
   C. 抑制 DNA 依赖性的 RNA 聚合酶　　D. 干扰氨基酰-tRNA 与细菌核糖体的结合
   E. 选择性抑制核糖体肽基转移酶

2. 一名 3 岁小儿误食父母用于治疗细菌性痢疾的药片后被送往医院。患儿呕吐超过 24 小时，伴腹泻且大便呈绿色。患儿精神萎靡，面色苍白，低体温、低血压和腹胀。最有可能导致这些表现的药物是（　　）。
   A. 氨苄西林　　B. 阿奇霉素　　C. 氯霉素　　D. 强力霉素　　E. 红霉素

3. 8 岁以下儿童不宜服用四环素类药物，是因为这些药物（　　）。
   A. 可导致肌腱断裂　　B. 沉积于正在钙化的组织　　C. 不能进入脑脊液
   D. 可导致再生障碍性贫血　　E. 可引起软骨损伤

4. 氯霉素可作为以下哪种疾病的首选治疗药物？（　　）
   A. 肺炎双球菌脑膜炎　　B. 病毒感染　　C. 流感嗜血杆菌引起的喉炎
   D. 痢疾　　E. 斑疹伤寒

5. 四环素类药物不良反应中没有下列哪种表现？（　　）
   A. 空腹口服易发生胃肠道反应　　B. 长期大量静脉给药可引起严重肝脏损害
   C. 长期应用后可发生二重感染　　D. 不会产生过敏反应
   E. 幼儿乳牙釉质发育不全

6. 某患者服用氯霉素一周后查血象，发现有严重贫血和白细胞、血小板减少，这种现象发生的原因是（　　）。
   A. 氯霉素破坏了红细胞　　B. 氯霉素缩短了红细胞的寿命
   C. 氯霉素抑制了线粒体铁螯合酶的活性　　D. 氯霉素抑制了高尔基体的功能
   E. 氯霉素加强了吞噬细胞的功能

7. 服用四环素引起伪膜性肠炎，应如何抢救？（　　）
   A. 服用头孢菌素　　B. 服用林可霉素　　C. 服用氯霉素
   D. 服用万古霉素　　E. 服用青霉素

8. 治疗立克次体的首选药物是（　　）。
   A. 青霉素 G　　B. 庆大霉素　　C. 链霉素　　D. 四环素　　E. 多黏菌素

9. 抗菌作用最强的四环素类药物是(　　)。
   A. 四环素　　B. 土霉素　　C. 多西环素　　D. 米诺环素　　E. 美他环素
10. 易引起灰婴综合征的药物是(　　)。
    A. 四环素　　B. 红霉素　　C. 呋喃妥因　　D. 强力霉素　　E. 氯霉素

Case study

Key points：
(1) Lyme disease and its etiology.
(2) Antimicrobial spectrum and antimicrobial activity of doxycycline.

Key words：pseudomonas aeruginosa; ototoxicity; aminoglycosides

Case

A 30-year-old male geologist was in good health and had no known underlying medical conditions. He travelled to a forested in early August and came to the hospital about 2 weeks later. A red maculopapular rash was visible on the anterior aspect of the patient's right thigh, which became increasingly reddish from the starting site in a circular pattern outwards, with partial fading in the center of the lesion. Several similar lesions were seen on the patient's right leg and torso. No arthropod bite bites were noted on the patient.

◎ **Essay question**

What disease is considered for the diagnosis of this patient? What medication is preferred for his treatment?

Multiple-choice questions

1. Mechanisms of antimicrobial action of tetracyclines include (　　).
   A. antagonism of bacterial translocase activity
   B. binding to the 50S ribosomal subunit
   C. inhibition of the DNA-dependent RNA polymerase
   D. interference with the binding of aminoacyl-tRNA to bacterial ribosomes
   E. selective inhibition of the ribosomal peptidyltransferase
2. A 3-year-old child was taken to hospital after accidentally ingesting tablets used by his parents to treat bacillary dysentery. The child had vomited for more than 24 hours and had diarrhoea with green stools. The child was depressed, pale, hypothermic, hypotensive and bloated in the abdomen. The drug most likely responsible for these signs is (　　).
   A. ampicillin　B. azithromycin　C. chloramphenicol　D. doxycycline　E. erythromycin
3. Tetracyclines should not be taken by children under 8 years of age because they (　　).
   A. can lead to tendon rupture　　　B. can deposit in calcifying tissue
   C. can't access cerebrospinal fluid　　D. can lead to aplastic anaemia

E. can cause cartilage damage

4. Chloramphenicol can be used as the treatment of choice for which of the following diseases? (   )

    A. Pneumococcal meningitis   B. Hepatitis B virus infection
    C. Laryngitis caused by Haemophilus influenzae   D. Dysentery
    E. Typhus

5. Which of the following statement is not true of tetracyclines? (   )

    A. Oral administration on an empty stomach is prone to gastrointestinal reactions
    B. Long-term intravenous administration of large amounts of drugs can cause serious liver damage
    C. Secondary infections can occur after long-term application
    D. No allergic reaction
    E. The enamel of young children's milk teeth is underdeveloped

6. A patient who had being taking chloramphenicol for a week was found to have severe anemia and decreased white blood cells and platelets. This observation was because (   ).

    A. chloramphenicol destroys red blood cells
    B. chloramphenicol shortens the life span of erythrocytes.
    C. chloramphenicol inhibits mitochondrial iron chelatase activity
    D. chloramphenicol inhibits the function of the Golgi apparatus
    E. chloramphenicol enhances the function of phagocytes

7. What is the treatment of pseudomembranous enteritis caused by use of tetracycline? (   )

    A. Cephalosporin   B. Lincomycin   C. Chloramphenicol
    D. Vancomycin   E. Penicillin

8. The drug of choice for the treatment of rickettsiae is (   ).

    A. penicillin G   B. gentamicin   C. streptomycin
    D. tetracycline   E. polymyxin

9. The tetracycline drug with the strongest antimicrobial activity is (   ).

    A. tetracycline   B. hygromycin   C. doxycycline
    D. minocycline   E. metacycline

10. The drug that can cause gray baby syndrome is (   ).

    A. tetracycline   B. erythromycin   C. furotoxin
    D. doxycycline   E. chloramphenicol

第三十八章案例学习和选择题答案

第三十九章　人工合成抗菌药

知识要点

一、喹诺酮类药物的分类

喹诺酮类药物分为4代。萘啶酸是第一代，我国已不再使用。吡哌酸是第二代药物，对大多数革兰氏阴性菌有效，口服易吸收；因其血药浓度低而尿中浓度高，仅限于治疗泌尿道和肠道感染。氟喹诺酮为第三代喹诺酮类，常用药物包括诺氟沙星、环丙沙星、氧氟沙星、左氧氟沙星、洛美沙星、氟罗沙星、司帕沙星等。新研制的氟喹诺酮类药物（如莫西沙星、加替沙星、吉米沙星和加雷沙星等）为第四代。

二、第三代喹诺酮类药物的特点

1. 抗菌作用

第三代喹诺酮（即氟喹诺酮）类药物与DNA回旋酶的亲和力和抗菌活性较前两代药物显著提高，抗菌谱显著扩大，药动学特点也显著改善。当分子结构中进一步引入环丙基后，药物对革兰氏阳性菌衣原体支原体的杀灭作用得到进一步增强，如环丙沙星、司帕沙星、莫西沙星、加替沙星和加雷沙星。特别是进一步改造的加雷沙星对革兰氏阴性菌、革兰氏阳性菌、厌氧菌、支原体、衣原体均具有与莫西沙星类似的良好活性和药动学特征，但毒性更低。

第三代喹诺酮类药物属广谱杀菌药，莫西沙星和加替沙星除保持了对革兰氏阴性菌的良好抗菌活性外，它们对革兰氏阳性菌、结核分枝杆菌、军团菌、支原体及衣原体的杀灭作用也进一步增强，特别是提高了对厌氧菌如脆弱拟杆菌、梭杆菌属、消化链球菌属和厌氧芽孢梭菌属等的抗菌活性。对于铜绿假单胞菌，环丙沙星的杀灭作用最强。

2. 作用机制

（1）DNA回旋酶是喹诺酮类抗革兰氏阴性菌的重要靶点。一般认为DNA回旋酶的A亚基是喹诺酮类的作用靶点，但二者不能直接结合。药物需嵌入断裂DNA链，形成酶-DNA-药物三元复合物从而抑制DNA回旋酶的活性，进而阻止细菌DNA的转录和复制，最终发挥杀菌作用。哺乳动物细胞内的拓扑异构酶Ⅱ在功能上类似于细菌的DNA回旋酶，但喹诺酮类需在很高浓度下才能影响该酶。

（2）拓扑异构酶Ⅳ也是喹诺酮类药物抗革兰氏阳性菌的重要靶点。喹诺酮类药物可通过抑制拓扑异构酶Ⅳ来干扰细菌DNA复制。

(3)喹诺酮类还可诱导细菌 DNA 的 SOS 修复,引起 DNA 错误复制而致细菌死亡。高浓度药物尚可抑制细菌 RNA 及蛋白质的合成。

(4)喹诺酮类药物也具有显著的抗生素后效应,即某些细菌与喹诺酮类药物接触后即使未被立即杀灭,但在 2~6 小时内会失去增殖能力;此持续时间的长短与喹诺酮类药物的浓度成正比。

3. 临床应用

氟喹诺酮类抗菌谱广、抗菌活性强、口服吸收良好、较少出现与其他种类抗菌药的交叉耐药。

(1)尿生殖系统感染。首选环丙沙星、氧氟沙星或 β-内酰胺类用于治疗单纯性淋病奈瑟菌性尿道炎或宫颈炎,但对非特异性尿道炎或宫颈炎疗效差。治疗铜绿假单胞菌性尿道炎首选环丙沙星。氟喹诺酮类对敏感菌所致的急、慢性前列腺炎以及复杂性前列腺炎,均有较好疗效。

(2)呼吸系统感染。对青霉素高度耐药的肺炎链球菌所致感染,首选左氧氟沙星或莫西沙星与万古霉素联用。对于支原体肺炎、衣原体肺炎或嗜肺军团菌引起的军团病,氟喹诺酮类(诺氟沙星除外)可替代大环内酯类。

(3)肠道感染与伤寒。志贺菌引起的急慢性和中毒性痢疾,以及鼠伤寒沙门菌、猪霍乱沙门菌、肠炎沙门菌引起的胃肠炎(食物中毒),首选喹诺酮。对沙门菌引起的伤寒或副伤寒,应首选氟喹诺酮类或头孢曲松。也可用于旅行腹泻。

(4)氟喹诺酮类对脑膜炎奈瑟菌具有强大的杀菌作用。因其在鼻咽分泌物中浓度高,可用于流行性脑脊髓膜炎鼻咽部带菌者的根除治疗。对其他抗菌药物无效的儿童重症感染可选用氟喹诺酮类;囊性纤维化患儿感染铜绿假单胞菌时应选用环丙沙星。

(5)骨、关节和软组织感染。对于敏感菌株引起的慢性骨髓炎,可用氟喹诺酮类药物进行长期治疗(数周至数月)。由革兰氏阴性杆菌、厌氧菌、链球菌和葡萄球菌等多种细菌感染引起的糖尿病足部感染,需将喹诺酮类药物与其他药物联合应用。

4. 不良反应

(1)胃肠道反应。可见胃部不适、恶心、呕吐、腹痛、腹泻等,一般不严重。

(2)中枢神经系统毒性。常见失眠、头晕、头痛,重者可出现精神异常、抽搐、惊厥等。发生率依次为:氟罗沙星>诺氟沙星>司帕沙星>环丙沙星>依诺沙星>氧氟沙星>培氟沙星>左氧氟沙星。依诺沙星、环丙沙星、诺氟沙星、培氟沙星与茶碱合用时,可使茶碱血药浓度升高。有精神病或癫痫病史者、合用茶碱或非甾体抗炎药者易产生中枢毒性。

(3)光敏反应(光毒性)。喹诺酮类药物在紫外线照射下可生成活性氧,激活皮肤成纤维细胞中的蛋白激酶 C 和酪氨酸激酶,引起皮肤炎症。表现为光照部位的皮肤出现瘙痒性红斑甚至皮肤糜烂、脱落。光敏反应最常见于司帕沙星、洛美沙星、氟罗沙星等。其他药物光敏反应的发生率依次为:依诺沙星>氧氟沙星>环丙沙星>莫西沙星=加替沙星。

(4)心脏毒性。表现为 Q-T 间期延长、尖端扭转型室性心动过速(TdP)、室颤等,罕见但后果严重。TdP 的发生率依次为:司帕沙星>加替沙星>左氧氟沙星>氧氟沙星>环沙星。

(5)软骨损害。药物可与软骨组织中的镁离子形成络合物并沉积于关节软骨,造成局部镁离子缺乏而致软骨损伤。儿童用药后可出现关节痛和关节水肿。

(6)其他不良反应。包括横纹肌溶解、跟腱炎、肝毒性、替马沙星综合征、过敏反应、血糖异常等。

三、磺胺类药物的特点

1. 抗菌作用

磺胺类对大多数革兰氏阳性菌和阴性菌有良好的抗菌活性,尤其是 A 群链球菌肺炎链球菌、脑膜炎奈瑟菌、淋病奈瑟球菌、鼠疫耶尔森菌和诺卡菌属,也可抑制沙眼衣原体、原虫、卡氏肺孢子虫和弓形虫滋养体,但对支原体、立克次体和螺旋体无效,甚至可促进立克次体生长。磺胺嘧啶银对铜绿假单胞菌有效。

2. 抗菌机制

对磺胺类敏感的细菌在增殖过程中不能利用现成的叶酸,必须以蝶啶和对氨基苯甲酸为原料在二氢蝶酸合酶的作用下生成二氢蝶酸,二氢蝶酸与谷氨酸反应生成二氢叶酸,后者经二氢叶酸还原酶催化生成四氢叶酸。活化的四氢叶酸作为一碳基团载体的辅酶参与合成嘧啶核苷酸和嘌呤。磺胺类药物与对氨基苯甲酸的结构相似,可与其竞争二氢蝶酸合酶,抑制二氢叶酸的合成,从而发挥抑菌作用。哺乳动物类细胞能直接利用食物来源的叶酸,因此磺胺类药物不影响人体细胞的核酸代谢。

四、磺胺嘧啶和磺胺甲噁唑的临床应用

磺胺嘧啶属中效磺胺,口服易吸收,易透过血-脑脊液屏障,在脑脊液中的浓度最高可达血药浓度的 80%。磺胺嘧啶或磺胺甲噁唑是预防流行性脑脊髓膜炎的首选药。对于普通型流行性脑脊髓膜炎以及诺卡菌属引起的肺部感染、脑膜炎和脑脓肿,亦可首选磺胺嘧啶。磺胺嘧啶也可用于敏感菌引起的泌尿道感染和上呼吸道感染。磺胺嘧啶与乙胺嘧啶合用可治疗弓形虫病。使用磺胺嘧啶时应多饮水,必要时同服等量碳酸氢钠以碱化尿液。

磺胺甲噁唑(新诺明)属中效类磺胺,其脑脊液浓度低于磺胺嘧啶,但仍可用于预防流行性脑脊髓膜炎。磺胺甲噁唑在尿液中的浓度与磺胺嘧啶相似,也适用于大肠埃希菌等敏感菌诱发的泌尿系统感染(如肾盂肾炎、膀胱炎、单纯性尿道炎等),主要与甲氧苄啶合用,产生协同抗菌作用,同时扩大适应证。

五、甲氧苄啶的抗菌作用与作用机制

甲氧苄啶是细菌二叶酸还原酶的抑制剂,其抗菌谱与磺胺甲噁唑相似。甲氧苄啶是抑菌药,抗菌活性强于磺胺甲噁唑,与其他磺胺类药物(如磺胺嘧啶、磺胺甲噁唑)或某些抗生素联用有增效作用,故称为抗菌增效剂,但单用甲氧苄啶易产生耐药。甲氧苄啶口服吸收迅速、完全,体内分布广,脑脊液中浓度较高(脑炎时接近血药浓度)。甲氧苄啶对细菌二氢叶酸还原酶的亲和力比哺乳动物二氢叶酸还原酶高 5 万~10 万倍,故本药对人体毒性微弱。但在敏感患者仍可引起叶酸缺乏,导致巨幼细胞贫血、白细胞减少及血小板减少等。反应一般较轻,停药即可恢复。

六、复方新诺明的抗菌作用与临床应用

复方磺胺甲噁唑(复方新诺明)是磺胺甲噁唑和甲氧苄啶按 5∶1 比例制成的合剂。磺胺甲噁唑抑制二氢蝶酸合酶,甲氧苄啶抑制二氢叶酸还原酶,两者协同阻断四氢叶酸的合成。相较两药单用,两药联用的抗菌活性可增强数倍至数十倍,甚至呈现杀菌作用。两药合用也扩大了抗菌谱,并可减少细菌耐药的发生。对磺胺耐药的细菌如大肠埃希菌、伤寒沙门菌和志贺菌属仍对复方新诺明敏感。目前复方新诺明仍广泛用于大肠埃希菌、变形杆菌和克雷伯菌引起的泌尿道感染,肺炎链球菌、流感嗜血杆菌及大肠埃希菌引起的上呼吸道感染或支气管炎,肉芽肿荚膜杆菌引起的腹股沟肉芽肿,霍乱弧菌引起的霍乱,伤寒沙门菌引起的伤寒,志贺菌属引起的肠道感染,卡氏肺孢子虫引起的肺炎,诺卡菌属引起的诺卡菌病等。

七、甲硝唑的抗菌作用、作用机制与临床应用

甲硝唑(灭滴灵)属于硝基咪唑类药物,同类药物还有替硝唑和奥硝唑。其分子中的硝基在无氧环境中可被还原成氨基抑制 DNA 的合成,从而发挥抗厌氧菌作用。甲硝唑对脆弱拟杆菌的活性尤为强大,对滴虫、阿米巴滋养体以及破伤风梭杆菌也有很强的杀灭作用,但对需氧菌或兼性需氧菌无效。口服吸收良好,体内分布广,可进入感染病灶和脑脊液。主要用于治疗厌氧菌引起的口腔、腹腔、女性生殖系统、下呼吸道、骨和关节等部位的感染。对幽门螺杆菌感染引起的消化性溃疡以及对四环素耐药的难辨梭状芽孢杆菌感染所致的假膜性肠炎有特殊疗效。甲硝唑也是治疗阿米巴病、滴虫病和破伤风的首选药物。

案例学习

学习要点:
(1)喹诺酮类药物的抗菌谱与抗菌活性。
(2)复方新诺明的组成和用途。
关键词: 肺孢子虫;复方新诺明;衣原体;喹诺酮

案例一

一名 26 岁男子因腹部穿刺伤被送至急诊室。病人入院时意识清醒,体检发现肠内容物溢出。随后发现该男子人体免疫缺陷病毒(HIV)检测结果呈阳性。其 $CD4^+$ 细胞计数为 $200/mm^3$,病毒载量为 15000 拷贝/mL。该男子同时还有淋病症状,该病常与沙眼衣原体感染有关。

◎ 问答题

1. 现有克林霉素、氨曲南、庆大霉素、青霉素、阿奇霉素和四环素,宜选择哪种抗生素来治疗脆弱杆菌感染?

2. 现有环丙沙星、克林霉素、甲氧苄啶加磺胺甲噁唑和复方新诺明,可使用哪种药物预防肺孢子虫感染?

3. 哪一代喹诺酮类抗生素是治疗沙眼衣原体感染的最佳药物？

案例二

一名 58 岁的女性在过去两天里突发急性前额头痛，且早晨加重。患者鼻腔有浓稠淡黄色分泌物流出，伴有鼻塞和发热。前额尤其是中部有按压痛，头面 X 光片显示双侧额窦炎。患者此前一周内有感冒和咳嗽。患者 3 个月前罹患抑郁症，故每日睡前服用阿米替林片，目前精神状态稳定。医生决定连续 10 天给予莫西沙星治疗感染，同时每 8 小时给予 1 次扑热息痛以及每天两次氧甲唑啉液滴鼻以缓解鼻塞。

◎ 问答题

医生所选用的抗生素是否合适？如果是，选择莫西沙星的考虑因素是什么？如果不适合，请说明原因，并建议使用哪种抗生素？

选择题

1. 关于磺胺类药物的临床应用，下列哪种说法是错误的？（   ）
   A. 对沙眼衣原体有效，可局部用于治疗眼部衣原体感染
   B. 对前列腺炎单用无效
   C. 可用于治疗斑疹伤寒
   D. 细菌可通过增加合成 PABA 来产生耐药性
   E. 细菌可通过减少药物摄取来产生耐药性

2. 以下关于氟喹诺酮类药物的说法，正确的是（   ）。
   A. 抗酸剂可增加其口服生物利用度
   B. 肝功能不全患者禁用
   C. 治疗 6 岁泌尿道感染患儿首选氟喹诺酮类药物
   D. 淋球菌对氟喹诺酮类药物的耐药性可能涉及 DNA 螺旋酶的改变
   E. 当肌酐清除率低于 50 mL/min 时，患者需要调整莫西沙星的剂量

3. 一名患者发生对环丙沙星耐药的绿脓杆菌的下呼吸道感染。细菌通过以下哪种机制获得对喹诺酮类药物的耐药性？（   ）
   A. 过量产生对氨基苯甲酸(PABA)   B. DNA 螺旋酶的合成发生改变
   C. 质粒介导的外排转运系统的改变   D. 抑制细菌细胞壁中肽聚糖亚基的合成
   E. 阻断叶酸合成过程中的不同环节

4. 外耳道炎患者使用甲氧苄啶-磺胺甲噁唑(TMP-SMX)治疗。以下哪一项是磺胺类药物的基本作用机制？（   ）
   A. 选择性抑制对氨基苯甲酸(PABA)进入人细胞参与叶酸合成
   B. 竞争性抑制 PABA 参与微生物叶酸的合成
   C. 抑制细菌细胞壁合成中的转肽反应
   D. 改变 DNA 螺旋酶和主动外排转运系统，导致药物的渗透性降低
   E. 改变二氢叶酸合酶的结构及过量合成 PABA

5. 一名 28 岁男性因咳嗽、脓痰和气短 5 天来院就诊。诊断为社区获得性肺炎。该者对

氨苄西林严重过敏,可考虑采用以下哪种药物治疗?( )
   A. 左氧氟沙星   B. 环丙沙星   C. 青霉素   D. 硝基呋喃妥因   E. 红霉素
6. 体外抗菌活性最强的氟喹诺酮类药物是( )。
   A. 诺氟沙星   B. 环丙沙星   C. 依诺沙星   D. 左氧氟沙星   E. 氟罗沙星
7. 痰中分布浓度高,对结核杆菌有效的喹诺酮类药物是( )。
   A. 氟哌酸   B. 氟啶酸   C. 环丙氟哌酸   D. 甲氟哌酸   E. 左氧氟沙星
8. 治疗流行性脑脊髓膜炎的首选药物是( )。
   A. 磺胺甲噁唑   B. 磺胺嘧啶   C. 磺胺异噁唑   D. 依诺沙星   E. 磺胺米隆
9. 适用于烧伤和大面积创伤后感染的磺胺类药物是( )。
   A. 磺胺甲噁唑   B. 磺胺嘧啶   C. 磺胺异噁唑   D. 依诺沙星   E. 磺胺嘧啶银
10. 既能抗阿米巴原虫,又有抗厌氧菌作用的药物是( )。
    A. 甲硝唑   B. 环丙沙星   C. 呋喃妥因   D. 氨苄西林   E. 头孢拉定

Case study

Key points:
(1) Antimicrobial spectrum and antimicrobial activity of quinolones.
(2) Composition and use of TMP-SMX (Bactrim).

Key words: pneumocystis; TMP-SMX (Bactrim); chlamydia; quinolone

Case 1

A 26-year-old man was admitted to the emergency department with an abdominal puncture. The patient was conscious on admission and physical examination revealed spilled bowel contents. The man was subsequently found to be positive for human immunodeficiency virus (HIV). His CD4+ cell count was 200/mm^3 and his viral load was 15,000 copies/mL. The man also had symptoms of gonorrhoea, which is often associated with Chlamydia Trachomatis infection.

◎ **Essay questions**

1. Which antibiotic would be appropriate for the treatment of mycobacterium fragilis infections?
2. In addition to anti-HIV treatment, what other drugs could be used to prevent pneumocystis carinii infection?
3. Which quinolone antibiotic would be the best treatment for Chlamydia Trachomatis infection?

Case 2

A 58-year-old woman presented with a sudden onset of acute frontal headache over the past two days that worsened in the morning. The patient had thick yellowish nasal discharge with nasal congestion and fever. There was tenderness upon pressing on the forehead, especially in the center, and cephalometric radiographs showed bilateral frontal sinusitis. The patient had had a cold and cough in the previous week. The patient had suffered from depression 3 months ago and was taking amitriptyline tablets daily at bedtime and was now mentally stable. The doctor decided to give moxifloxacin for 10 consecutive days to treat the infection, along with paracetamol every 8 hours and oxymetazoline nasal drops twice daily to relieve nasal congestion.

◎ **Essay questions**

Was the antibiotic chosen by the physician appropriate? If yes, what were the considerations for choosing moxifloxacin? If not appropriate, please explain why and which antibiotic should be recommended?

Multiple-choice questions

1. Which of the following statements is false regarding the clinical use of sulfonamides? ( )
   A. Effective against Chlamydia Trachomatis and can be used topically to treat ocular chlamydial infections
   B. Single use is ineffective for prostatitis
   C. Can be used to treat typhus
   D. Bacteria can develop resistance by increasing their synthesis of para-aminobenzoic acid (PABA)
   E. Bacteria can develop resistance by reducing drug uptake

2. Which of the following statements about fluoroquinolones are correct? ( )
   A. Antacids increase their oral bioavailability
   B. Prohibited in patients with hepatic insufficiency
   C. Fluoroquinolones are preferred for the treatment of urinary tract infections in a 6-year old child
   D. Gonococcal resistance to fluoroquinolones may involve DNA helicase gaibian
   E. When creatinine clearance is less than 50 mL/min, the patient needs a dose adjustment of moxifloxacin

3. A patient develops a lower respiratory tract infection by ciprofloxacin-resistant Pseudomonas Aeruginosa. By which of the following mechanisms does the bacteria develop resistance to quinolones? ( )
   A. Overproduction of para-aminobenzoic acid (PABA)
   B. Altered synthesis of DNA helicase
   C. Alterations in the plasmid-mediated efflux transport system
   D. Inhibition of peptidoglycan subunit synthesis in bacterial cell walls
   E. Blocking different parts of the folate synthesis process

4. A boy diagnosed with otitis externa is given methotrexate/sulfamethoxazole (TMP-SMX). Which of the following is the basic mechanism of action of sulfonamides? ( )
   A. Selective inhibition of p-aminobenzoic acid (PABA) entry into human cells for folate synthesis
   B. Competitive inhibition of PABA involvement in microbial folate synthesis

C. Inhibition of transpeptidation in bacterial cell wall synthesis

D. Alteration of DNA helicase, and active efflux transporter systems leading to reduced drug permeability

E. Alteration of the structure of dihydrofolate synthase and over-synthesis of PABA

5. A 28-year-old male presented to the hospital with a 5-day history of cough, purulent sputum and shortness of breath. The diagnosis was community-acquired pneumonia. The patient was severely allergic to ampicillin. Which of the following medications might be considered for treating the patient? (   )

   A. Levofloxacin   B. Ciprofloxacin   C. Penicillin VK
   D. Nitrofurantoin   E. Erythromycin

6. The fluoroquinolone with the highest in vitro antimicrobial activity is (   ).

   A. norfloxacin   B. ciprofloxacin   C. enoxacin
   D. ofloxacin   E. fleroxacin

7. A quinolone that has a high concentration in sputum and is effective against Mycobacterium Tuberculosis is (   ).

   A. haloperidol   B. fludioxonil   C. ciprofluoperazine
   D. mefluoperazine   E. ofloxacin

8. The drug of choice for the treatment of epidemic cerebrospinal meningitis is (   ).

   A. sulfamethoxazole   B. sulfadiazine   C. sulfisozole
   D. enoxacin   E. sulfamylon

9. The sulfonamide that is indicated for burns and large post-traumatic infections is (   ).

   A. sulfamethoxazole   B. sulfadiazine   C. sulfisozole
   D. enoxacin   E. silver sulfadiazine

10. The drug that has both anti-amoeba and anti-anaerobic activities is (   ).

    A. metronidazole   B. ciprofloxacin   C. furotoxin
    D. ampicillin   E. cefradine

第三十九章案例学习和选择题答案

第四十章 抗真菌药和抗病毒药

知识要点

一、抗真菌药的分类

(1) 抗生素类,包括两性霉素 B、制霉菌素、非多烯类如灰黄霉素。两性霉素 B 活性最强,是唯一可用于治疗深部和皮下真菌感染的多烯类药物,其他多烯类只限于局部应用治疗浅表真菌感染。

(2) 唑类,包括咪唑类和三唑类。药理作用是抑制真菌细胞色素 P450,干扰真菌细胞中麦角固醇的生物合成,使真菌细胞膜缺损,增加膜通透性,进而抑制真菌生长或使真菌死亡。与咪唑类相比,三唑类对人体细胞色素 P450 的亲和力较低,因此毒性较小,且抗菌活性更高。咪唑类药物包括酮康唑、咪康唑、益康唑、克霉唑和联苯苄唑等。酮康唑可作为浅表真菌感染治疗的首选药物。三唑类包括伊曲康唑、氟康唑和伏立康唑等,可作为治疗深部真菌感染的首选药物。

(3) 丙烯胺类,包括萘替芬和特比奈芬。药物作用是非竞争性可逆地抑制鲨烯环氧化酶将鲨烯转化为羊毛固醇,进而阻断麦角固醇的生成,导致真菌细胞膜的结构和功能破坏。

(4) 嘧啶类,如氟胞嘧啶。

二、不同抗真菌药的药理作用与临床应用

1. 两性霉素 B

两性霉素 B(庐山霉素)是治疗各种严重真菌感染的首选药之一,但毒性较大。新剂型如脂质体剂型、脂质体复合物、胶样分散剂型等可提高其疗效,并降低其毒性。两性素 B 为广谱抗真菌药,几乎对所有真菌均有活性。对新型隐球菌、白念珠菌、芽生菌、荚膜组织胞浆菌、粗球孢子菌、孢子丝菌等有较强的抑菌作用,高浓度时有杀菌作用。两性霉素 B 选择性地与真菌细胞膜中的麦角固醇结合改变细胞膜通透性,细胞内小分子物质(如氨基酸、甘氨酸等)和电解质(特别是离子)因此外泄,导致真菌停止增殖或死亡。细菌细胞膜不含固醇,故两性霉素 B 无抗细菌作用。两性霉素 B 对真菌细胞膜上麦角固醇的亲和力大于哺乳动物细胞膜固醇,故对哺乳动物细胞的毒性相对较低。哺乳动物的红细胞、肾小管上皮细胞的胞浆膜含有较多固醇,故两性霉素 B 可致溶血、肾损害等毒性反应。真菌很少对两性霉素 B 产生耐药性。本药静脉滴注用于治疗深部真菌感染。真菌性脑膜

炎时，除静脉滴注外还需鞘内注射。口服仅用于肠道真菌感染。局部应用治疗皮肤、指甲及黏膜等表浅部真菌感染。

2. 制霉菌素

制霉菌素抗真菌作用和机制与两性素 B 相似，对念珠菌属活性较强，不易产生耐药性，主要局部外用治疗皮肤、黏膜浅表真菌感染。口服吸收很少，仅适于肠道白念珠菌感染。毒性大，不宜注射给药。

3. 灰黄霉素

灰黄霉素口服吸收较少，高脂饮食可增加其吸收。广泛分布于深部各组织，皮肤、毛发、指甲、脂肪及肝脏等组织含量较高，可诱导细胞色素 P450 酶。灰黄霉素杀灭生长旺盛的真菌，但抑制静止状态的真菌。活性主要针对各种皮肤癣菌如表皮癣菌属、小芽孢菌属和毛菌属，对念珠菌属以及其他引起深部感染的真菌无效。灰黄霉素可沉积在皮肤、毛发及指（趾）甲的角蛋白前体细胞中，阻断敏感真菌中的微管蛋白聚合成微管，从而抑制其有丝分裂。此外，灰黄霉素是鸟嘌呤的类似物，可竞争性抑制真菌细胞 DNA 的合成。本药主要用于各种皮肤癣菌的治疗。对头癣疗效较好，指（趾）甲癣疗效较差。因静止状态的真菌仅被抑制，病变的清除依赖于角质的新生和受感染角质的脱落，故疗程需数周至数个月。该药毒性较大，临床已少用。

4. 酮康唑

酮康唑是第一个广谱口服抗真菌药，可有效地治疗深部、皮下及浅表真菌感染。亦可局部用药治疗表浅部真菌感染。酮康唑口服生物利用度个体差异较大，而且溶解和吸收都需要胃酸，故食物、抗酸药或抑制胃酸分泌的药物可降低酮康唑的生物利用度。在少数男性患者，酮康唑可引起内分泌异常，表现为乳房发育。

5. 特比奈芬

特比奈芬比奈替芬活性更高、毒性更低。对曲霉菌、镰孢和其他丝状真菌有良好活性。口服吸收快速良好，可在毛囊、毛发、皮肤和甲板等处长时间维持较高浓度。外用或口服治疗甲癣和其他一些浅表部真菌感染。与唑类药物或两性霉素 B 合用，对深部曲霉菌、侧孢、假丝酵母菌和肺隐球酵母菌所致感染可获良好效果。

6. 氟胞嘧啶

氟胞嘧啶是人工合成的广谱抗真菌药，进入菌体后经过一系列反应生成 5-氟尿嘧啶脱氧核苷，后者抑制胸腺嘧啶核苷合成酶，阻断尿嘧啶脱氧核苷转变为胸腺嘧啶核苷，从而抑制 DNA 的合成。中间代谢产物 5-氟尿嘧啶还能掺入真菌的 RNA，影响蛋白质合成。哺乳动物细胞缺乏胞嘧啶脱氨酶，不能将 5-氟胞嘧啶转变为 5-尿嘧啶，因此人体组织细胞代谢不受影响。本药主要用于隐球菌、念珠菌和着色霉菌所致感染，疗效不如两性霉素 B。易透过血脑屏障，对隐球菌性脑膜炎疗效较好，但应与两性霉素 B 合用。

三、主要抗病毒药物的作用机制、临床用途及评价

1. 利巴韦林

利巴韦林是人工合成的鸟苷类广谱抗病毒药，对多种 RNA 和 DNA 病毒有效，包括甲型肝炎病毒和丙型肝炎病毒，对腺病毒、疱疹病毒和呼吸道合胞病毒的也有效。本品并不

影响病毒吸附、侵入和脱壳，也不诱导干扰素的产生。药物进入被病毒感染的细胞后迅速磷酸化，其产物抑制肌苷单磷酸脱氢酶、流感病毒 RNA 多聚酶和 mRNA 鸟苷转移酶，减少细胞内鸟苷三磷酸的生成，从而干扰病毒 RNA 和蛋白的合成，最终抑制病毒的复制与传播。利巴韦林对呼吸道合胞病毒肺炎和支气管炎疗效最佳，通常气雾剂给药，流感也适用气雾剂给药。治疗其他大多数病毒感染时通常采用静脉注射。本药对急性甲型和丙型肝炎也有一定疗效。

2. 干扰素

干扰素为广谱抗病毒药，对病毒的穿膜、脱壳、mRNA 合成、蛋白翻译后修饰、病毒颗粒组装和释放等步骤均有抑制作用。但在不同病毒，干扰素的主要作用环节有所不同，不同病毒对干扰素的敏感性也有较大差异。干扰素影响相关基因的表达使细胞表达抗病毒蛋白。已知干扰素可诱导 3 种酶来抑制病毒蛋白的合成、翻译和装配：①蛋白激酶：抑制病毒肽链启动；②寡腺苷酸合成酶：激活 RNA 酶，降解病毒 mRNA；③磷酸二酯酶：降解 RNA 末端核苷，抑制病毒肽链延长。干扰素还可通过免疫效应发挥抗病毒作用。干扰素具有广谱抗病毒活性，临床主要用于治疗急性病毒感染性疾病（如流感及其他上呼吸道感染性疾病、病毒性心肌炎、流行性腮腺炎、乙型脑炎等）和慢性病毒性感染（如慢性活动性肝炎、巨细胞病毒感染等）。也广泛用于肿瘤治疗。

3. 阿昔洛韦

阿昔洛韦为广谱高效抗病毒药，是目前最有效的抗Ⅰ型和Ⅱ型单纯疱疹病毒药物之一，对水痘带状疱疹病毒和 EB 病毒等其他疱疹病毒也有效。阿昔洛韦对正常细胞几乎无影响，但在被感染的细胞内，阿昔洛韦在病毒胸苷激酶和细胞激酶的催化下转变为三磷酸无环鸟苷，对病毒 DNA 多聚酶具有强大的抑制作用，从而抑制病毒 DNA 的合成。病毒可通过改变病毒胸苷激酶或 DNA 多聚酶而对阿昔洛韦产生耐药。阿昔洛韦为单纯疱疹病毒感染的首选药。可局部应用治疗疱疹性角膜炎、单纯疱疹和带状疱疹。口服或静注可有效治疗单纯疱疹脑炎、生殖器疱疹、免疫缺陷病人单纯疱疹感染等。

案例学习

学习要点：
（1）机会致病菌感染及其处理。
（2）抗真菌药物的不良反应。
关键词：机会致病菌；白色念珠菌；两性霉素；不良反应

案例一

一名 35 岁女性白血病患者，在接受静脉化疗期间发生全身性机会致病菌感染。患者插管部位未见红斑或水肿，但阴道有白色分泌物。对血、尿和阴道分泌物等取样行体外培养，随即经验性地静脉给予庆大霉素、萘夫西林和替卡西林进行治疗。治疗持续 3 天后患者的感染病情未见明显好转。患者出现喉咙疼痛，咽部出现白色斑块。第 4 天返回的阴道分泌物培养结果显示无细菌生长，但患者的血液和尿中均检出白色念珠菌。

◎ 问答题

1. 此时是否应继续使用当前的抗生素？此时应考虑使用何种抗真菌药物？
2. 如果用两性霉素 B 进行治疗，可采用哪些药物预处理病人以控制不良反应？
3. 念珠菌是引起院内血流感染的主要原因，是否可使用药物预防机会性念珠菌感染？

案例二

一名艾滋病患者此前接受茚地那韦、地达诺辛和齐多夫定的三药联合治疗，同时还在使用西多福韦、氟康唑、利福布汀和甲氧苄啶-磺胺甲噁唑以预防机会性致病原感染。患者后来发生疱疹感染和口腔念珠菌病，遂服用阿昔洛韦和酮康唑治疗。患者现主诉厌食、恶心、呕吐和腹痛，上腹部有压痛。实验室结果显示淀粉酶活性为 220 U/L，初步诊断为急性胰腺炎。

◎ 问答题

1. 哪种药物可有效抑制疱疹病毒感染并预防巨细胞病毒视网膜炎？
2. 该患者使用的茚地那韦剂量高于常规剂量，原因是什么？
3. 该患者的急性胰腺炎可能是上述哪一种药物引起的？立即停用该药后，可以用哪种药物代替？

◎ 选择题

1. 下列哪种药物可与细胞膜成分相互作用，形成由药物分子中亲水基团构成的孔隙？
   (   )
   A. 卡泊芬净   B. 氟尿嘧啶   C. 格列齐特   D. 制霉菌素   E. 特比萘芬
2. 关于氟康唑下列说法中正确的是(   )。
   A. 不能透过血脑屏障　　　　　　　B. 是治疗曲霉菌病的首选药物
   C. 能诱导肝脏药物代谢酶　　　　　D. 在所有唑类药物中对药物代谢的影响最小
   E. 口服生物利用度低于酮康唑
3. 使用抗组胺药阿司咪唑或特非那定的患者同时服用哪种药物会出现严重的心脏反应？
   (   )
   A. 两性霉素 B   B. 灰黄霉素   C. 酮康唑   D. 特比萘芬   E. 伏立康唑
4. 关于抗病毒药物的作用机制，下列说法中准确的是(   )。
   A. 阿昔洛韦不需要磷酸化激活
   B. 更昔洛韦抑制病毒 DNA 聚合酶，但不会终止 DNA 链延长
   C. α 干扰素可增加宿主细胞核糖核酸酶的活性，从而降解病毒 mRNA
   D. 膦甲酸在单纯疱疹病毒感染的细胞中活化的第一步是被胸苷激酶磷酸化
   E. 艾滋病毒逆转录酶对福沙那韦抑制作用的敏感性是宿主细胞 DNA 聚合酶的 30～50 倍
5. 关于 α 干扰素，以下说法中错误的是(   )。
   A. 用药初始大多数病人会出现流感症状   B. 适应证包括治疗生殖器疣
   C. 可用于治疗乙型和丙型肝炎   D. 拉米夫定会干扰其抗乙型肝炎的活性

E. 毒性包括骨髓抑制
6. 艾滋病病毒感染者需要服用一种抑制病毒成熟的药物。这类药物通常会有下列哪种不良反应？（   ）
   A. 贫血   B. 胰腺炎   C. 神经精神反应   D. 周围神经病变   E. 脂肪营养不良
7. 下列哪种药物主要用于口腔、皮肤、阴道念珠菌感染？（   ）
   A. 红霉素   B. 灰黄霉素   C. 制霉菌素   D. 两性霉素   E. 多黏菌素
8. 静脉滴注时常见寒颤、高热、呕吐的药物是（   ）。
   A. 灰黄霉素   B. 克霉唑   C. 志军霉素   D. 两性霉素   E. 氟胞嘧啶
9. 无抗真菌作用的咪唑类药物是（   ）。
   A. 克霉唑   B. 甲硝唑   C. 氟康唑   D. 酮康唑   E. 咪康唑
10. 兼有抗震颤麻痹作用的抗病毒药是（   ）。
    A. 利巴韦林   B. 阿糖腺苷   C. 阿昔洛韦   D. 金刚烷胺   E. 碘苷

Case study

Key points：
（1）Opportunistic pathogenic infections and their management.
（2）Adverse effects of antifungal drugs.

Key words：opportunistic pathogens；Candida albicans；amphotericin；adverse reactions

Case 1

A 35-year-old female leukaemia patient developed a systemic opportunistic pathogenic bacterial infection while receiving intravenous chemotherapy. There was no erythema or oedema at the cannula site, but there was a white vaginal discharge. Blood, urine, and vaginal secretions were sampled for in vitro culture, followed by empirical intravenous treatment with gentamicin, nafcillin, and ticarcillin. The patient's infection did not improve significantly after 3 days of treatment. The patient developed a sore throat and began to have white patches in the pharynx. Culture result of vaginal secretions returned on day 4 showing no bacterial growth, but Candida Albicans was detected in the patient's blood and urine.

◎ **Essay questions**

1. Should the current antibiotic be continued or stopped now? What antifungal medications should be considered now?
2. If treated with amphotericin B, the patient should be pretreated with what drugs to ward off adverse effects?
3. Candida is the leading cause of nosocomial bloodstream infection. What drugs can be used to prevent opportunistic Candida infections?

Case 2

A patient with AIDS had previously been receiving a three-drug combination of indinavir, didanosine and zidovudine, and also using cidofovir, fluconazole, rifabutin and trimethoprim-sulphamethoxazole for the prevention of opportunistic pathogenic infections. The patient subsequently developed herpes infection and oral candidiasis, which was treated with acyclovir and ketoconazole. The patient now complained of anorexia, nausea, vomiting and abdominal pain with tenderness in the upper abdomen. Laboratory results showed an amylase activity of 220 U/L and a preliminary diagnosis of acute pancreatitis was made.

◎ **Essay questions**

1. Which is the drug that inhibits herpesvirus infection and prevents cytomegalovirus retinitis?
2. Why is this patient's indinavir dose higher than the usual doses?
3. Which drug might have caused this patient's acute pancreatitis? The drug should be stopped immediately and could be replaced with what drug?

Multiple-choice questions

1. Which of the following drugs can interact with cell membrane components to form pores made up of hydrophilic groups in the drug molecule? (   )
    A. Caspofungin   B. Fluorouracil   C. Gliclazide
    D. Mycotoxins   E. Terbinafine
2. Which of the following statements about fluconazole is correct? (   )
    A. Inability to cross the blood-brain barrier
    B. Drug of choice for the treatment of aspergillosis
    C. Induction of hepatic drug-metabolising enzymes
    D. Minimal effect on drug metabolism among all azoles
    E. Lower oral bioavailability than ketoconazole
3. Patients using the antihistamines astemizole or terfenadine, who are taking which of the following drug at the same time will experience a serious cardiac reaction? (   )
    A. Amphotericin B   B. Colistin   C. Ketoconazole
    D. Terbinafine   E. Voriconazole
4. Regarding the mechanisms of action of antiviral drugs, which of the following statements is accurate? (   )
    A. Acyclovir does not require phosphorylation for activation
    B. Ganciclovir inhibits viral DNA polymerase but does not terminate DNA chain elongation
    C. Interferon-α increases the activity of host cell ribonuclease which degrades viral mRNAs
    D. The first step in the activation of Foscarnet in herpes simplex virus-infected cells is phosphorylation by the thymidine kinase
    E. HIV reverse transcriptase is 30~50 times more sensitive to fosamprenavir inhibition than

host cell DNA polymerase

5. With respect to interferon-α, which of the following statements is incorrect (　　).
   A. the majority of patients will experience influenza symptoms at the start of the drug administration
   B. indications include treatment of genital warts
   C. can be used to treat hepatitis B and C
   D. lamivudine interferes with its anti-hepatitis B activity
   E. toxicity includes myelosuppression

6. A person infected with HIV needs to take a drug that inhibits the maturation of the virus. Which of the following adverse effects is usually associated with this type of drugs? (　　)
   A. Anaemia　　　　　　B. Pancreatitis　　　　　　C. Neuropsychiatric responses
   D. Peripheral neuropathy　　E. Adipose malnutrition

7. Which of the following drugs is used primarily for oral, skin, and vaginal Candida infections? (　　)
   A. Erythromycin　　　　B. Gray yellows　　　　C. Mycotoxin
   D. Amphotericin　　　　E. Polymyxin

8. Chills, high fever, and vomiting are common occurrences during intravenous infusion of (　　).
   A. gray penicillin　　　　B. clotrimazole　　　　C. amphotericin
   D. amphotericin　　　　E. flucytosine

9. The imidazole that do not have antifungal effects is (　　).
   A. clotrimazole　　　　B. metronidazole　　　　C. fluconazole
   D. ketoconazole　　　　E. miconazole

10. The antiviral drug that also acts as an antitremor paralytic is (　　).
    A. ribavirin　　　　　B. vidarabine　　　　　C. acyclovir
    D. amantadine　　　　E. idoxuridine

第四十章案例学习和选择题答案

第四十一章　抗结核药及抗麻风病药

知识要点

一、抗结核病一线、二线药物的分类和主要作用机制

1. 分类

(1) 一线药物：疗效好、不良反应较少、患者易耐受，包括异烟肼、利福平、乙胺丁醇、链霉素、吡嗪酰胺等。

(2) 二线药物：毒性较大、疗效较差，主要用于对一线药物耐药的病患或用于与其他抗结核药配伍使用，包括对氨基水杨酸钠、氨硫脲、卡那霉素、阿米卡星、乙硫异烟胺、卷曲霉素、环丝氨酸等。

(3) 新一代药物：疗效较好、毒副作用相对较小的新一代抗结核药，如利福喷丁、利福定、左氧氟沙星、莫西沙星、加替沙星、新大环内酯类等，在耐多药结核病的治疗中起重要作用。利奈唑胺和氯法齐明（氯苯吩嗪）对耐多药结核病甚至是广泛耐药结核病具有良好的治疗效果，已被 WHO 列入治疗结核的核心药物。

2. 作用机制

(1) 阻碍细菌细胞壁合成，如环丝氨酸、乙硫异烟胺。

(2) 干扰结核杆菌代谢，如对氨基水杨酸钠。

(3) 抑制 RNA 合成，如利福平。

(4) 抑制结核杆菌蛋白合成，如链霉素、卷曲霉素和紫霉素。

(5) 多种作用机制共存或机制未明，如异烟肼、乙胺丁醇。

二、抗结核病药物的应用原则

合理用药的目的是提高药物疗效，降低不良反应，原则为早期、联合、适量、规律及全程用药。

(1) 早期用药是指结核病一旦确诊应立即用药治疗。早期活动性病灶处于渗出阶段，病灶内结核杆菌生长旺盛，对药物作用敏感，易被抑制或杀灭。患病初期机体抵抗力也较强，局部病灶血运丰富，药物浓度高，能促进炎症吸收从而获得较好疗效。晚期则由于病灶纤维化、干酪化或空洞形成，病灶内血液循环不良，导致药物分布差，疗效不佳。

(2) 联合用药是指根据病情和药物特点联合使用两种或两种以上药物，以增强疗效并可避免严重不良反应和延缓耐药性的产生。常根据病情采取二联、三联甚至四联的

用药方案。轻症肺结核通常选用异烟肼和利福平联合应用,重症者则采取四联或更多药物联用。

(3)适量用药是指用药剂量要适当。剂量不足时,药物难以在病灶组织内达到有效浓度,且易诱发细菌耐药,使治疗失败。药物剂量过大则易产生严重不良反应而使治疗难以继续。

(4)坚持全程规律用药。结核病的治疗必须做到有规律长期用药,不可随意改变药物剂量或药物种类,否则难以获得疗效。过早停药会使已被抑制的细菌再度繁殖或迁延,导致治疗失败病情复发。因此,规律全程用药,不过早停药是治疗成功的关键。轻症肺结核应持续治疗9~12个月,中度及重度肺结核应持续治疗18~24个月或根据患者的病情调整用药方案。

三、主要抗结核药物的特点

1. 异烟肼

1)临床应用

异烟肼对各种类型的结核病均为首选药物。早期轻症肺结核或预防用药时可单独使用,规范化治疗时必须联合其他抗结核药物使用,以防止或延缓耐药性的产生。对粟粒性结核和结核性脑膜炎应加大剂量并延长疗程,必要时应注射给药。

2)不良反应

异烟肼不良反应的产生与用药剂量及疗程有关,应谨慎使用和及时调整用药剂量,以避免发生严重不良反应。

(1)神经毒性。常见反应为周围神经炎,表现为手脚麻木、肌肉震颤和步态不稳等。大剂量时可出现头痛、头晕、兴奋和视神经炎,严重时可导致中毒性脑病和精神病。此作用是由于异烟肼促进维生素 B_6 排泄而使机体缺乏 B_6 所致。另外,维生素 B_6 缺乏也会使中枢 γ-氨基丁酸减少,导致中枢兴奋。因此使用异烟肼时应注意补充维生素 B_6。癫痫患者同时使用苯妥英钠和异烟肼和可引起过度镇静或运动失调。

(2)肝脏毒性。异烟肼可损伤肝细胞,引起转氨酶升高,少数患者可出现黄疸,严重者可出现肝小叶坏死,故用药期间应定期检查肝功能。乙酰化快代谢型患者对异烟肼敏感,慎用异烟肼。

(3)其他不良反应。可引起皮疹、发热、胃肠道反应、粒细胞减少、血小板减少和溶血性贫血。亦可出现脉管炎及关节炎综合征。

2. 利福平

1)临床应用

(1)利福平与其他抗结核药联合使用可用于治疗各种类型的结核病,包括初治和复发患者。与异烟肼合用治疗初发患者可降低结核性脑膜炎的病死率并减少后遗症。与乙胺丁醇及吡嗪酰胺联用对复发患者疗效较好。

(2)可用于治疗麻风病和耐药金黄色葡萄球菌及其他敏感细菌所致的感染。

(3)利福平在胆汁中浓度较高,故也可用于治疗重症胆道感染。

(4)局部用药可用于治疗沙眼、急性结膜炎及病毒性角膜炎。

2) 不良反应

(1) 胃肠道反应。常见恶心、呕吐、腹痛、腹泻，多不严重。

(2) 肝脏毒性。长期大量使用利福平可出现黄疸、肝肿大、肝功能减退等，严重时可致死。肝毒性多见于慢性肝病者、酒精中毒者、老年或者使用异烟肼者。用药期间应定期检查肝功能。严重肝病、胆道阻塞患者禁用利福平。

(3) "流感综合征"。大剂量间隔使用利福平时可出现发热、寒战、头痛、肌肉酸痛等类似感冒的症状，其发生频率与用药剂量和间隔时间有明显关联，因此间隔给药方案现已不采用。

(4) 其他不良反应。个别患者可出现皮疹、药热等重症反应。偶见疲乏、嗜睡、头晕和运动失调等。动物实验显示该药有致畸作用，妊娠早期妇女禁用利福平。

3) 药物相互作用

利福平是肝药酶诱导剂，可加速自身及许多药物的代谢，如洋地黄毒苷、奎尼丁、普萘洛尔、维拉帕米、巴比妥类、口服抗凝血药、氯贝丁酯、美沙酮、磺酰脲类口服降血糖药、口服避孕药、糖皮质激素和茶碱等。利福平与这些药物同时使用时应调整剂量。

3. 乙胺丁醇

1) 药理作用

乙胺丁醇对繁殖期结核分枝杆菌有较强的抑制作用，对其他细菌无效。其作用机制为与镁离子络合，阻止菌体内亚精胺与镁离子结合，从而干扰分枝杆菌 RNA 的合成。单独使用易产生耐药，因此常与其他抗结核药联合使用，目前无交叉耐药现象。

2) 临床应用

用于治疗各型肺结核和肺外结核。与异烟肼和利福平合用治疗初治患者，与利福平和卷曲霉素合用治疗复发患者。特别适用于链霉素和异烟肼无效的患者和不能耐受对氨基水杨酸钠的患者。因其疗效明确、不良反应少、耐药发生慢，目前已取代对氨基水杨酸钠成为一线抗结核药。

4. 吡嗪酰胺的药理作用和临床应用

吡嗪酰胺在酸性环境中对结核分枝杆菌有较强的抑制和杀灭作用。单独使用易出现耐药，与异烟和利福平合用有协同作用，与其他抗结核药无交叉耐药。长期、大量使用吡嗪酰胺可引发严重肝损害，出现转氨酶升高、黄疸甚至肝坏死。用药期间应定期检查肝功能，肝功能不良者慎用。吡嗪酰胺还能抑制尿酸盐排泄，诱发或加重痛风。

四、抗麻风病药

砜类化合物是目前临床最重要的抗麻风病药，常用药有氨苯砜、苯丙砜和醋氨苯砜。氨苯砜是治疗麻风的首选药物。该药在小肠吸收后通过肠肝循环重吸收，故循环时间较长，可达 10~50 小时，宜采用周期性间隔给药方案，以免发生蓄积中毒。本药抗菌谱与磺胺类药相似，其抗菌机制也可能与磺胺类相同。氨苯砜单用易产生耐药性，与利福平联合使用可延缓耐药性的产生。以小剂量开始治疗，直至最适剂量。一般用药 3~6 个月，症状开始改善，细菌完全消失至少需 1~3 年。因此在治疗过程中不应随意减少剂量或过早停药。氨苯砜较常见的不良反应是溶血性贫血和发绀，葡萄糖-6-磷酸脱氢酶（G-6-PD）

缺乏者较易发生。其次为高铁血红蛋白血症。本药对肝脏亦有一定毒性，应定期检查血象及肝功能。治疗早期或药物剂量增加过快可引起"砜综合征"，表现为发热、不适、剥脱性皮炎、黄疸伴肝坏死、淋巴结肿大、贫血等。

案例学习

学习要点：
(1) 结核病的一线用药和联合用药。
(2) 异烟肼的不良反应和代谢(能力)多态性。
(3) 抗结核药与其他药物和食物的相互作用。
关键词： 一线抗结核药物；结核药物原则；异烟肼；代谢多态性；不良反应

案例

某少数民族30岁女性入院就诊，主诉最近一个月持续感觉疲倦，食欲不振，体重下降。近几日有咳嗽且咳出绿色的痰，痰中不时带有血丝。除了左上肺叶闻及啰音，体检未见其他异常。查血显示白细胞计数为12000/μL，血细胞比容为33%。胸部X光片显示肺左上叶有浸润性改变，有空腔。痰液革兰氏染色涂片显示多菌群混合，无优势菌种，抗酸染色显示很多粉红色细棒状杆菌。医生初步诊断为肺结核，痰液采样送实验室进行培养，并将病人收入院治疗。

问答题

1. 请提出一种药物方案开始对患者进行治疗。
2. 该患者使用异烟肼治疗，但使用了高于常规的维持剂量，依据可能是什么？用药期间，患者每日服用吡哆醇，其目的是什么？患者某日在进食含酪胺的食物后，出现呼吸困难、潮红、心悸和出汗等症状，可能的原因是什么？患者是否有发生肝毒性的风险？
3. 患者出院后仍需继续维持治疗。医生告诉患者需要避孕，但不能仅依靠口服避孕药，因为她使用的抗结核药物可能会干扰口服避孕药的作用。哪种一线抗结核药最可能有此作用？

选择题

1. 药物联用治疗结核病最主要目的是(　　)。
   A. 延缓或防止出现耐药性　B. 确保病人遵守用药方案　C. 协同提高抗菌活性
   D. 预防其他细菌感染　　　E. 降低不良反应的发生率
2. 一名28岁男性结核病患者在接受药物治疗1个月后复诊，诉视力下降影响阅读书报。此状况最可能由以下哪种药物所致？(　　)
   A. 异烟肼　　　B. 利福平　　　C. 吡嗪酰胺　　　D. 乙胺丁醇　　　E. 链霉素
3. 正在接受肺结核治疗的男子突发低烧、右脚大脚趾疼痛和肿胀。患者体检符合痛风性关节炎的特征，且有高尿酸血症。这种情况可能是哪种药物引起的？(　　)
   A. 环丝氨酸　　B. 氨硫脲　　　C. 吡嗪酰胺　　　D. 利福平　　　E. 对氨基水杨酸钠

4. 用于治疗麻风病的一种药物会使尿液变成橙红色。该药抑制细菌中哪种成分的合成？（   ）
   A. 霉菌酸   B. 糖蛋白   C. 膜脂质   D. 核糖核酸   E. 叶酸
5. 关于氯苯吩嗪治疗麻风病，以下说法中正确的是（   ）。
   A. 缺乏葡萄糖-6-磷酸脱氢酶（G-6-PD）的患者不应使用氯苯吩嗪（氯法齐明）
   B. 该药最常见的不良反应是周围神经病变
   C. 长期服用可能导致皮肤变色。
   D. 用药会增加出现麻风结节红斑的风险
   E. 该药具有较强的肾毒性
6. 对细菌及结核分枝杆菌感染有效的药物是（   ）。
   A. 异烟肼   B. 利福平   C. 乙胺丁醇
   D. 对氨基水杨酸   E. 氨苄西林
7. 应用异烟肼治疗结核病时，常合用维生素 B_6，其目的是（   ）。
   A. 增强疗效   B. 防治周围神经炎   C. 延缓抗药性
   D. 减轻肝损伤   E. 延长作用时间
8. 一线抗结核药不包括（   ）。
   A. 异烟肼   B. 利福平   C. 利福定   D. 乙胺丁醇   E. 链霉素
9. 抗结核病短期疗法的疗程为（   ）。
   A. 1到3个月   B. 1个月   C. 6到9个月   D. 3到6个月   E. 12个月
10. 某60岁男性患者，因患骨结核就医，医生推荐三联药物疗法。最有可能是下列哪种方案？（   ）
    A. 异烟肼、利福平、环丝氨酸   B. 利福平、链霉素、卷曲霉素
    C. 利福定、乙胺丁醇、对氨水杨酸   D. 异烟肼、乙胺丁醇、链霉素
    E. 利福平、利福定、乙硫异烟胺

Case study

Key points：

(1) First-line drugs and combinations in the treatment of tuberculosis.

(2) Adverse effects and metabolic (capacity) polymorphisms of isoniazid.

(3) Interactions of anti-tuberculosis drugs with other drugs and food.

Key words：first-line anti-tuberculosis drugs；tuberculosis drug principles；isoniazid；metabolic polymorphisms；adverse reactions

Case

A 30-year-old woman from an ethnic minority group in a southwestern province was admitted to the hospital complaining of persistent fatigue, loss of appetite and weight loss in the past month. She had a cough in the last several days and coughed up green sputum occasionally with blood in the sputum. Physical examination revealed no abnormalities except for rales in the left upper lobe of the lungs. A blood test showed a white blood cell count of 12,000/μL and a hematocrit of 33%. Chest X-ray film showed infiltrative changes in the left upper lobe of the lungs with cavities. Gram stain of sputum smear showed a mixture of multiple bacterial colonies without dominant microorganisms, and antacid staining showed many pink fine rod-shaped bacilli. The physician made a preliminary diagnosis of tuberculosis and sputum samples were sent to the laboratory for culture and the patient was admitted to the hospital for treatment.

◎ **Essay questions**

1. Please propose a drug regimen to for treatment of the patient.
2. This patient is treated with isoniazid but is on a higher than usual maintenance dose, on what possible basis? What is the purpose of the patient's daily dose of pyridoxine during the medication period? The patient develops dyspnea, flushing, palpitations, and sweating one day after eating a tyramine-containing food. What are the possible causes? Is the patient at risk of hepatotoxicity?
3. The patients is discharged from the hospital with maintenance therapy. Her doctor tells the patient that she needs to avoid pregnancy but cannot solely rely on oral contraceptives because the anti-tuberculosis drugs she is using may interfere with the action of oral contraceptives. Which first-line antituberculosis drug is most likely to have this effect?

Multiple-choice questions

1. The most important objective of drug combination therapy for tuberculosis is (　　).
    A. delaying or preventing the emergence of drug resistance
    B. ensuring patient compliance with medication regimens
    C. achieving synergistic enhancement of antimicrobial activity
    D. preventing other bacterial infections
    E. reducing the incidence of adverse reactions
2. A 28-year-old male patient with tuberculosis returns to the clinic one month after receiving medication and complains of vision loss that interferes with reading books and newspapers. Which of the following drugs is most likely to be responsible for this condition? (　　)
    A. Isoniazid 　　　B. Rifampicin 　　　C. Pyrazinamide
    D. Ethambutol 　　E. Streptomycin
3. A man on tuberculosis therapy presented with sudden onset of low fever, pain and swelling of the big toe of the right foot. The patient's physical examination is consistent with gouty arthritis and he has hyperuricaemia. Which medication could have caused this condition? (　　)
    A. Cycloserine 　　B. Ammonia thiourea 　　C. Pyrazinamide
    D. Rifampicin 　　E. Aminosalicylic acid
4. A drug used to treat leprosy causes urine to turn orange-red. The drug inhibits the synthesis of which component in the bacteria? (　　)

A. Mycolic acid B. Glycoproteins C. Membrane lipids
D. Ribonucleic acid E. Folic acid

5. Which of the following statements regarding the treatment of leprosy with clofazimine is correct? ( )

   A. Clofazimine should not be used in patients with glucose-6-phosphate dehydrogenase (G-6-PD) deficiency
   B. The most common adverse effect of the drug is peripheral neuropathy
   C. Prolonged use may cause skin discolouration
   D. Drug use increases the risk of developing erythema nodosum leprosum
   E. The drug is highly nephrotoxic

6. A drug that is both effective against bacterial and Mycobacterium tuberculosis infections ( ).

   A. isoniazid B. rifampin C. ethambutol
   D. para-aminosalicylic acid E. ampicillin

7. Isoniazid is often combined with vitamin B_6 in the treatment of tuberculosis to ( ).

   A. enhance the efficacy of treatment B. prevent peripheral neuritis
   C. delay drug resistance D. reduce liver damage
   E. prolong the duration of action

8. The first-line antituberculosis drugs do not include ( ).

   A. isoniazid B. rifampicin C. rifampicin
   D. ethambutol E. streptomycin

9. The course of short-term antituberculosis therapy lasts ( ).

   A. 1 to 3 months B. 1 month C. 6 to 9 months
   D. 3 to 6 months E. 12 months

10. A 60-year-old male patient is in the clinic for bone tuberculosis, and the physician recommends a triple drug regimen. Which of the following regimens are most likely the physician's recommendation? ( )

    A. Isoniazid, rifampin, cycloserine
    B. Rifampin, streptomycin, and colistin
    C. Rifampicin, ethambutol, p-aminolevulinic acid
    D. Isoniazid, ethambutol, streptomycin
    E. Rifampicin, rifampicin, ethylthioisonicotinamide

第四十一章案例学习和选择题答案

第四十二章 抗寄生虫药

知识要点

一、抗疟药的分类

(1)主要用于控制症状的药物,如氯喹、奎宁、甲氟喹、青蒿素等。该类药均能杀灭红细胞内期裂殖体,控制症状发作和预防性抑制疟疾症状发作。

(2)主要用于控制远期复发和传播的药物,如伯氨喹。该类药能杀灭肝脏中的休眠子,控制疟疾的复发,并能杀灭各种疟原虫的配子体,控制疟疾传播。

(3)主要用于病因预防的药物,如乙胺嘧啶。该类药能杀灭红细胞外期的子孢子,发挥病因性预防。

二、主要抗疟药的特点

1. 主要用于控制症状的抗疟药

1)氯喹

(1)抗疟作用:氯喹可富集于红细胞内尤其是被疟原虫入侵的红细胞,对各种疟原虫的红细胞内期裂殖体均有较强的杀灭作用,可迅速有效地控制疟疾的临床发作。但氯喹对子孢子、休眠子和配子体无效,不能用于病因预防以及控制远期复发和传播。氯喹起效快、疗效强,通常用药后24~48小时内临床症状消退,48~72小时血中疟原虫消失。氯喹大量分布于肝、肺等内脏,缓慢释放入血,其代谢与排泄都较为缓慢,故药效持久。氯喹的抗疟机制涉及抑制疟原虫对血红蛋白的消化,干扰其对血红素的代谢,减少疟原虫必需氨基酸的来源。氯喹也能抑制血红素聚合酶,阻止血红素转化为疟色素,从而减少对人体的毒性。

(2)预防性用药:在进入疫区前1周和离开疫区后4周内,每周服药一次可预防疟疾症状。

(3)治疗肠道外阿米巴病:氯喹可富集于肝脏并杀死其中的阿米巴滋养体,可用于甲硝唑无效的阿米巴肝脓肿患者。

(4)免疫抑制:大剂量氯喹能抑制免疫反应,可用于治疗类风湿关节炎、系统性红狼疮等自身免疫疾病。

2)青蒿素

青蒿素可快速杀灭各种疟原虫的红细胞内期裂殖体,用药后48小时内疟原虫从血中消失，但对红细胞外期疟原虫无效。主要用于治疗耐氯喹或多药耐药的恶性疟。因可透过血脑屏障，对脑性疟的抢救有较好的效果。

2. 主要用于控制远期复发和传播的抗疟药：伯氨喹

伯氨喹对间日疟和卵形疟在肝脏中的休眠子有较强杀灭作用，是防治疟疾远期复发的主要药物。伯氨喹与红细胞内期抗疟药合用能根治良性疟并减少耐药的发生。伯氨喹也能杀灭各种疟原虫的配子体，阻止疟疾传播，但对红细胞内期的疟原虫无效。一次给予标准剂量的伯氨喹多无法完全清除肝内耐药虫株，需加倍剂量并延长疗程至两周。治疗剂量的伯氨喹不良反应较少。可引起剂量依赖性的胃肠道反应，停药后消失。大剂量（60~240 mg/d）时可引起高铁血红蛋白血症，伴有紫绀。葡萄糖-6-磷酸脱氢酶（G-6-PD）缺乏者使用伯氨喹后可发生急性溶血。

3. 主要用于病因性的抗疟药：乙胺嘧啶

乙胺嘧啶抑制二氢叶酸还原酶，使二氢叶酸不能转变为四氢叶酸，核酸合成障碍，从而抑制疟原虫的增殖。乙胺嘧啶对已发育成熟的裂殖体无效，通常在用药后疟原虫的第 2 个无性增殖期才能显效，故本药控制疟疾症状起效缓慢。一般用于病因性预防，作用持久，一周服药一次。乙胺嘧啶常与磺胺类或砜类药物合用，在叶酸代谢的两个环节上发挥双重阻抑作用。乙胺嘧啶不能直接杀灭配子体，但含药血液随配子体被按蚊吸食后，能阻止疟原虫在蚊体内发育产生配子体，故能起到阻断疟原虫传播的作用。

三、主要抗阿米巴病药和抗滴虫病药的特点

1. 甲硝唑

（1）抗阿米巴。对肠内、肠外阿米巴滋养体有强大杀灭作用，治疗急性阿米巴痢疾和肠道外阿米巴感染效果显著。此药对肠腔内阿米巴原虫和包囊则无明显作用，主要用于组织感染，不能根治肠腔病原体，也不用于治疗无症状的包囊携带者。

（2）抗滴虫。甲硝唑是治疗阴道毛滴虫感染的首选药物，口服后可分布于阴道分泌物、精液和尿液中，对阴道毛滴虫有直接杀灭作用，对阴道内正常菌群无影响，对男女感染者均有良好疗效。

（3）抗厌氧菌。甲硝唑对革兰氏阳性或革兰氏阴性厌氧杆菌和球菌都有较强的抗菌作用，脆弱拟杆菌感染尤为敏感。常用于厌氧菌引起的产后盆腔炎、败血症和骨髓炎等的治疗，也可与抗菌药合用防止妇科手术、胃肠外科手术时的厌氧菌感染。

（4）抗贾第鞭毛虫。甲硝唑可有效治疗贾第鞭毛虫病感染，治愈率达 90%。

2. 二氯尼特

二氯尼特为目前最有效的杀阿米巴包囊药，单用对无症状的阿米巴包囊携带者有良好效果。对于急性阿米巴痢疾，用甲硝唑控制症状后再用本品可肃清肠腔内包囊，可有效防止复发。对肠外阿米巴病无效。

3. 巴龙霉素

氨基苷类抗生素，通过抑制蛋白质合成直接杀灭阿米巴滋养体。也可通过抑制共生菌群的代谢间接抑制肠道阿米巴原虫的生存与繁殖。临床用于治疗急性阿米巴痢疾。口服吸收少，肠道浓度高。

4. 氯喹

氯喹为抗疟药，也可杀灭肠外肝和肺阿米巴滋养体。仅用于甲硝唑无效或禁忌的阿米巴肝炎或肝脓肿。对肠内阿米巴病无效，应与肠内抗阿米巴病药合用以防止复发。口服吸收迅速，肝中浓度高。

四、主要抗血吸虫病药和抗丝虫病药的特点

1. 吡喹酮

对日本血吸虫、埃及血吸虫、曼氏血吸虫单一感染或混合感染均有良好疗效，迅速强效杀灭血吸虫成虫，对幼虫也有较弱作用。对其他吸虫如华支睾吸虫、姜片吸虫、肺吸虫也有显著杀灭作用。对各种绦虫感染和其幼虫引起的囊虫病、包虫病也有不同程度的疗效。有效浓度可引起虫体痉挛麻痹失去吸附能力，导致虫体脱离宿主组织，使血吸虫从肠系膜静脉迅速移至肝脏。较高治疗浓度时可引起虫体表膜损伤，抗原暴露，在宿主免疫机制的共同作用下导致虫体破坏、死亡。吡喹酮对哺乳动物细胞膜无上述作用。本药可用于治疗各型血吸虫病。适用于急性、慢性、晚期及有并发症的血吸虫病患者。也可用于肝脏华支睾吸虫病、肠吸虫病（如姜片虫病、异形吸虫病、横川后殖吸虫病等）、肺吸虫病及绦虫病等。

2. 乙胺嗪

乙胺嗪可杀灭班氏丝虫和马来丝虫，对马来丝虫的作用优于班氏丝虫，对微丝蚴的作用强于成虫。体外乙胺嗪对两种丝虫的微丝蚴和成虫并无直接杀灭作用，其杀虫作用依赖于宿主免疫机制的参与。乙胺嗪分子中的哌嗪基团可使微丝蚴的肌组织超极化，发生弛缓性麻痹，从而从寄生部位脱离，迅速发生"肝移"，并易被网状内皮系统捕获。乙胺嗪也可破坏微丝蚴表膜的完整性，使抗原暴露，从而受到宿主免疫机制的攻击。

五、主要抗蠕虫病药的特点

1. 甲苯达唑

甲苯达唑（甲苯咪唑）为广谱驱肠虫药，对蛔虫、钩虫、蛲虫、鞭虫、绦虫和粪类圆线虫等肠道蠕虫均有效。本药影响虫体多种代谢，尤其是能量代谢，从而抑制虫体生存和繁殖。药效缓慢，需数日才能将虫体排出。甲苯达唑对蛔虫卵、钩虫卵、鞭虫卵及幼虫有杀灭和抑制发育作用，可用于治疗上述肠蠕虫单独或混合感染。

2. 阿苯达唑

阿苯达唑是高效、低毒的广谱驱肠虫药，能杀灭多种肠道线虫、绦虫和吸虫的成虫及虫卵，用于多种线虫混合感染，疗效优于甲苯咪唑，也可用于治疗棘球蚴病（包虫病）与囊虫病，对肝片吸虫病及肺吸虫病也有良好疗效。

3. 哌嗪

哌嗪是常用驱蛔虫药，对蛔虫、蛲虫具有较强的驱虫作用，主要通过改变虫体肌细胞膜对离子的通透性引起膜超极化，阻断神经-肌肉接头，导致虫体弛缓麻痹，使虫体随粪便排出体外。哌嗪也能抑制琥珀酸合成，干扰虫体糖代谢，阻断能量合成。哌嗪可减少虫体游走移行，主要用于驱除肠道蛔虫、治疗蛔虫所致的不完全性肠梗阻和早期胆道蛔虫。

4. 左旋咪唑

左旋咪唑可选择性抑制虫体肌肉中的琥珀酸脱氢酶，抑制虫体肌肉的无氧代谢，减少能量产生。

5. 氯硝柳胺

氯硝柳胺可杀灭多种绦虫成虫，包括牛肉绦虫、猪肉绦虫、鱼绦虫、阔节裂头绦虫、短膜壳绦虫等。药物与虫体接触后杀死虫体头节和近端节片，虫体随后脱离肠壁，随肠蠕动排出体外。抗虫机制为抑制虫体细胞线粒体的氧化磷酸化，抑制 ATP 生成。对虫卵无效，死亡节片易被肠腔内蛋白酶消化分解释放出虫卵，有致囊虫病的危险。本药可杀灭钉螺和日本血吸虫尾蚴，可防止血吸虫传播。

6. 吡喹酮

吡喹酮为广谱抗吸虫药和驱绦虫药，不仅对多种吸虫有强大杀灭作用，对绦虫感染和囊虫病也有良好疗效。本药是治疗各种绦虫病的首选。治疗脑型囊虫病时，可因虫体死亡后的炎症反应引起脑水肿、颅内压升高，宜同时使用脱水药和糖皮质激素以预防。

案例学习

学习要点：
(1) 神经囊肿病的治疗。
(2) 阿米巴病的药物治疗。

关键词： 神经囊虫病；阿苯达唑；阿米巴病；甲硝唑；二氯尼特

案例一

一名 40 岁男子，3 天内出现 2 次癫痫样发作。既往无癫痫或神经系统病史，也没有癫痫或精神病家族史。患者此前一个多月一直诉头痛，服用扑热息痛后有缓解。根据患者妻子的描述，患者的发作表现符合强直阵挛发作的特征。她还提到患者近两个月也有一些行为改变，比如发作后会出现行为混乱和嗜睡，持续 2~3 个小时。核磁共振扫描显示患者脑部皮质有 4 个活动性实质囊尾蚴，诊断为神经囊虫病。

◎ **问答题**

该患者应如何进行药物治疗？

案例二

一名男子因下腹不适、胀气和偶发性腹泻就诊。诊断为肠道阿米巴病，并在其腹泻粪便中发现溶组织埃希氏菌。医生给该患者开处了一种口服药，减轻其肠道症状。患者后来又出现严重痢疾、右上腹痛、体重减轻、发烧和肝脏肿大。患者被确诊为阿米巴肝脓肿，随即被收入院治疗。患者最近服用过抗心律失常药物。

◎ **问答题**

1. 对于患者的初始病情（为轻至中度），考虑患者接受的首选治疗药物是什么？
2. 对于该患者严重的肠外疾病，最有效的药物治疗方案是什么？

选择题

1. 以下哪种药物的作用是抑制线粒体中二磷酸腺苷的磷酸化？（　　）
   A. 阿苯达唑　　B. 甲苯咪唑　　C. 氯硝柳胺　　D. 吡喹酮　　E. 二氯尼特
2. 哪种蠕虫感染对吡喹酮无效？（　　）
   A. 包虫病　　B. 蛔虫病　　C. 副线虫病　　D. 猪肉绦虫感染　　E. 血吸虫病
3. 哪种药物能增强 γ-氨基丁酸在线虫体内的作用使其肌肉麻痹？（　　）
   A. 阿苯达唑　　B. 二乙基卡马嗪　　C. 伊维菌素　　D. 奥沙尼喹　　E. 双羟萘酸噻嘧啶
4. 哪种寄生虫对氯硝柳胺敏感？（　　）
   A. 蛔虫　　B. 疏螺旋体　　C. 肝吸虫　　D. 美洲钩虫　　E. 猪肉绦虫
5. 关于抗原虫药物，哪种说法是准确的？（　　）
   A. 氯喹是疟原虫二氢叶酸还原酶的抑制剂
   B. 甲氟喹可杀死继发性红细胞外裂殖体
   C. 伯氨喹可杀死血液裂殖体但不影响继发性组织裂殖体
   D. 氯胍与双链 DNA 形成复合物阻止 DNA 复制
   E. 甲氧苄啶-磺胺甲噁唑是治疗肺孢子菌肺炎的首选药物
6. 疟原虫对氯喹产生耐药性的原因是（　　）。
   A. 受体结构改变
   B. 药物在食物泡中富集减少
   C. DNA 修复机制增强
   D. 二氢叶酸还原酶合成增加
   E. 诱导药物失活酶
7. 甲硝唑对以下哪种疾病无效？（　　）
   A. 阿米巴病　　B. 脆弱拟杆菌感染　　C. 肺囊虫感染
   D. 假膜性结肠炎　　E. 滴虫病
8. 主要用于根治疟疾，控制复发的药物是（　　）。
   A. 氯喹　　B. 乙胺嘧啶　　C. 青蒿素　　D. 伯氨喹　　E. 奎宁
9. 治疗蛲虫病的首选药物是（　　）。
   A. 甲苯咪唑　　B. 槟榔　　C. 槟榔+南瓜子　　D. 噻嘧啶　　E. 恩波维铵
10. 长期大量应用可干扰人体叶酸代谢的药物是（　　）。
    A. 氯喹　　B. 乙胺嘧啶　　C. 青蒿素　　D. 伯氨喹　　E. 奎宁

Case study

Key points：
(1) Treatment of neurocysticercosis.
(2) Pharmacologic treatment of amebiasis.

Key words：neurocysticercosis; albendazole; amoebiasis; metronidazole; diclonide

Case 1

A 40-year-old man presents with 2 epilepsy-like seizures in the past 3 days. The patient has no past history of epilepsy or neurological conditions, and no family history of epilepsy or psychosis. The patient have been complaining of headaches for more than a month, which could be relieved by paracetamol. the patient's seizure presentation was consistent with tonic clonic seizures judged from the patient's companion's description. She also mentioned that the patient had some behavioural changes in the last two months, such as confusion and drowsiness after the seizures, which lasted for 2-3 hours. An MRI scan shows 4 active parenchymal cysticerci in the cortex of the patient's brain, and a diagnosis of neurocysticercosis is made.

◎ **Essay questions**

What medications should be given to this patient?

Case 2

A man presented with lower abdominal discomfort, flatulence and occasional diarrhoea. A diagnosis of intestinal amebiasis was made and Escherichia histolytica was found in his diarrhoeal stools. The doctor prescribed an oral medication that alleviated the patient's intestinal symptoms. The patient later developed severe dysentery, right upper abdominal pain, weight loss, fever and hepatomegaly. The patient was diagnosed with an amoebic liver abscess and was then admitted into the hospital. The patient had recently taken antiarrhythmic medications.

◎ **Essay questions**

1. Please propose an appropriate treatment for the patient's initial condition (mild to moderate).
2. What would be the most effective pharmacological treatment option for this patient's severe parenteral disease?

Multiple-choice questions

1. Which of the following drugs acts by inhibiting the phosphorylation of adenosine diphosphate in mitochondria? ( )
   A. Albendazole　　　　B. Mebendazole　　　　C. Clonidine
   D. Praziquantel　　　　E. Diloxanide
2. Which helminth infection does not respond to praziquantel? ( )
   A. Borrelia　　　　B. Ascariasis　　　　C. Paragonimiasis
   D. Pork tapeworm infection　　E. Schistosomiasis
3. Which drug enhances the action of γ-aminobutyric acid in nematodes to paralyse their muscles? ( )
   A. Albendazole　　　　B. Diethylcarbamazine　　　　C. Ivermectin
   D. Oxamniquine　　　　E. Thiamphenicol bis(hydroxynaphthenate)
4. Which parasite is sensitive to niclosamide? ( )

A. Roundworms B. Borrelia C. Liver fluke
   D. Hookworm of America E. Pork tapeworm
5. Which statement about the antiprotozoal drugs is accurate? (   )
   A. Chloroquine as an inhibitor of dihydrofolate reductase in Plasmodium vivax
   B. Mefloquine kills secondary extra-erythrocytic schizonts
   C. Primaquine kills blood clefts but does not affect secondary tissue clefts
   D. Clonidine forms a complex with double-stranded DNA to prevent DNA replication.
   E. Methotrexate-sulfamethoxazole is the drug of choice for the treatment of Pneumocystis carinii pneumonia
6. Resistance to chloroquine in plasmodium falciparum is due to (   ).
   A. structural changes in receptors   B. decreased enrichment of drugs in food vesicles
   C. enhanced DNA repair mechanisms   D. increased synthesis of dihydrofolate reductase
   E. induction of drug-inactivating enzymes
7. Metronidazole is not effective against which of the following infection? (   )
   A. Amebiasis   B. Mycobacterium avium infection
   C. Pneumocystis infection D. Pseudomembranous colitis
   E. Trichomoniasis
8. The drug primarily used to eradicate malaria and to control relapses is (   ).
   A. chloroquine   B. pyrimethamine   C. artemisinin
   D. primaquine   E. quinine
9. The drug of choice for the treatment of pinworms is (   ).
   A. mebendazole   B. betel nut   C. betel nut + pumpkin seeds
   D. thiamphenicol   E. enbuvium
10. The drug that can interfere with folate metabolism when used in large quantities over a long period of time is (   ).
    A. chloroquine   B. ethylaminopyrimidine   C. artemisinin
    D. primaquine   E. quinine

第四十二章案例学习和选择题答案

第四十三章 抗恶性肿瘤药物

知识要点

一、抗恶性肿瘤药的分类

抗肿瘤药可分为细胞毒类和非细胞毒类抗肿瘤药两大类。细胞毒类抗肿瘤药主要干扰肿瘤细胞的核酸和蛋白质的结构与功能，直接抑制肿瘤细胞增殖和(或)诱导肿瘤细胞死亡，如抗代谢药和抗微管蛋白药等。非细胞毒类抗肿瘤药作用于肿瘤分子病理过程的关键调控分子，如调节体内激素平衡药物、分子靶向药物和肿瘤免疫治疗药物等。

二、细胞毒类抗肿瘤药的作用机制

1. 分子水平(生化机制)

(1)干扰核酸生物合成。药物抑制DNA生物合成的不同环节，这类药物又称为抗代谢药物，主要包括：①二氢叶酸还原酶抑制剂，如甲氨蝶呤等；②胸苷酸合成酶抑制剂，如氟尿嘧啶等；③嘌呤核苷酸互变抑制剂，如巯嘌呤等；④核苷酸还原酶抑制剂，如羟基脲等；⑤DNA多聚酶抑制剂，如阿糖胞苷等。

(2)破坏DNA的结构与功能。药物破坏DNA的结构或抑制拓扑异构酶，影响DNA的复制和修复。主要药物有：①DNA交联剂如氮芥、环磷酰胺和塞替派等烷化剂；②破坏DNA的铂类配合物，如顺铂；③破坏DNA的抗生素，如丝裂霉素和博来霉素；④拓扑异构酶抑制剂，如喜树碱类和鬼臼毒素衍生物。

(3)干扰RNA转录和抑制RNA合成。药物嵌入DNA碱基对干扰转录、阻止mRNA的形成。主要药物包括多柔比星、柔红霉素等蒽环类抗生素和放线菌素D等。

(4)抑制蛋白质的合成与功能。药物抑制微管蛋白的聚合、抑制核糖体或影响氨基酸的供应。主要药物有：①微管蛋白抑制剂，如长春碱类和紫杉醇类等；②核糖体抑制剂，如三尖杉生物碱；③影响氨基酸供应的药物，如L-门冬酰胺酶。

2. 细胞水平

肿瘤细胞群包括增殖细胞和静止细胞(G_0期)。增殖的肿瘤细胞的一次分裂周期(即一个细胞周期)包含4个时相，即DNA合成前期(G_1期)、DNA合成期(S期)、DNA合成后期(G_2期)和有丝分裂期(M期)。根据药物作用的细胞周期或时相特异性，可将药物分为：

(1)细胞周期非特异性药物，如烷化剂、抗肿瘤抗生素及铂类配合物等。这类药物作用较强，能杀死处于增殖周期各时相甚至G_0期的肿瘤细胞。

（2）细胞周期（时相）特异性药物仅作用于处于增殖周期的某些时相的肿瘤细胞，如抗代谢药物作用于 S 期细胞，长春碱类作用于 M 期细胞。处于其他时相和 G_0 期的肿瘤细胞则对药物作用不敏感。此类药物的作用多数较弱，需要一段时间显效。

三、非细胞毒类抗肿瘤药的作用机制

以肿瘤分子病理过程的关键调控分子等为靶点的药物，如改变激素平衡失调状态的某些激素或其拮抗药、以细胞信号转导分子为靶点的蛋白酪氨酸激酶抑制药、丝裂原活化蛋白激酶信号转导通路抑制药和细胞周期调控剂、针对某些与增殖相关细胞信号转导受体的单克隆抗体可破坏或抑制新生血管生成，有效地阻止肿瘤生长和转移的新生血管生成抑制药、减少癌细胞脱落黏附和基底膜降解的抗转移药、以端粒酶为靶点的抑制药、促进恶性肿瘤细胞向成熟分化的分化诱导剂、通过重新启动并维持肿瘤-免疫循环，恢复机体正常的抗肿瘤免疫反应，从而控制与杀伤肿瘤的免疫治疗药物等。

四、肿瘤产生耐药性的机制

肿瘤细胞对抗肿瘤药物产生耐药是化疗失败的重要原因。有些肿瘤细胞对某些抗肿瘤药物具有天然耐药性（即不敏感），如处于非增殖的 G_0 期肿瘤细胞一般对多数抗肿瘤药不敏感。有的肿瘤细胞在经过治疗一段时间后对原来敏感的药物变得不敏感，这称之为获得性耐药性。耐药性产生的原因十分复杂，同一种药物可有多种耐药机制，肿瘤细胞也可经过同一种机制对不同药物产生耐药。多药耐药性是指肿瘤细胞在接触一种抗肿瘤药后，对多种结构不同、作用机制各异的其他抗肿瘤药的产生耐药。多药耐药性的形成机制比较复杂：①药物的转运或摄取障碍；②药物的活化障碍；③靶点的改变；④药物入胞后产生新的代谢途径；⑤分解酶的增加；⑥损伤修复机制增强；⑦膜外排转运蛋白表达增加，细胞排出药物增多；⑧DNA 链间或链内的交联减少。另外，肿瘤细胞中众多信号转导通路存在复杂的交互和代偿机制，这也使得肿瘤细胞对分子靶向药物产生耐药。

五、常用的抗恶性肿瘤药物

1. 甲氨蝶呤

甲氨蝶呤的化学结构与叶酸相似，它与二氢叶酸还原酶的亲和力比叶酸大 10^6 倍，对该酶产生强大而持久的竞争性抑制，使二氢叶酸不能变成四氢叶酸。该药主要用于治疗儿童急性白血病和绒毛膜上皮癌。鞘内注射可用于中枢神经系统白血病的预防和缓解症状。不良反应包括消化道反应如口腔炎、胃炎、腹泻、便血；骨髓抑制最为突出，可出现白细胞、血小板减少，严重者可有全血细胞减少；长期大量用药可导致肝损害；妊娠早期使用可致畸胎、死胎。为减轻甲氨蝶呤的骨髓毒性，可在应用大剂量甲氨蝶呤一定时间后肌注亚叶酸钙以保护正常骨髓细胞。

2. 巯嘌呤

巯嘌呤在体内经过酶催化变成硫代肌苷酸，后者阻止肌苷酸转变为腺苷酸及鸟苷酸，从而干扰嘌呤代谢，阻碍核酸合成。本药对 S 期肿瘤细胞作用最显著，对 G_1 期有延缓作用。肿瘤细胞对巯嘌呤可产生耐药，机制可能是耐药肿瘤细胞中酶的改变导致巯嘌呤不易

转变成硫代肌苷酸，或产生的硫代肌苷酸被迅速降解。巯嘌呤起效慢，主要用于急性淋巴细胞白血病的维持治疗。大剂量巯嘌呤对绒毛膜上皮癌亦有较好疗效。不良反应常见骨髓抑制和消化道黏膜损害，少数患者可出现黄疸和肝功能损害。

3. 羟基脲

羟基脲抑制核酸还原酶，阻止胞苷酸转变为脱氧胞苷酸，从而抑制 DNA 的合成，对 S 期肿瘤细胞有选择性毒性。对成人急性粒细胞白血病有显著疗效，可暂时缓解黑色素瘤。可使肿瘤细胞集中于 G_1 期，可用作同步化药物以增加肿瘤对化疗或放疗的敏感性。该药的主要毒性为骨髓抑制，有轻度消化道反应。肾功能不良者慎用。可致畸胎，孕妇忌用。

4. 环磷酰胺

环磷酰胺体外无活性，进入体内后经肝微粒体细胞色素 P450 酶氧化生成中间产物磷胺，后者在肿瘤细胞内分解出磷酰胺氮芥发挥作用。环磷酰胺为烷化剂类广谱抗肿瘤药，对恶性淋巴瘤疗效显著，对多发性骨髓瘤、急性淋巴细胞白血病、肺癌、乳腺癌、卵巢癌、神经母细胞瘤和睾丸肿瘤等均有一定疗效。该药的常见不良反应有骨髓抑制、恶心、呕吐、脱发等。大剂量环磷胺可引起出血性膀胱炎，可能与大量代谢物丙烯醛经泌尿道排泄有关，同时应用美司钠可预防发生。

5. 氟尿嘧啶

氟尿嘧啶在细胞内转变为 5-氟尿脱氧核苷酸，后者阻断脱氧胸苷酸合成酶，抑制脱氧鸟苷酸甲基化转变为脱氧胸苷酸，最终干扰 DNA 的合成。此外氟尿嘧啶可转化为 5-氟尿嘧啶核苷掺入 RNA 中干扰蛋白质的合成，故本药对其他各期肿瘤细胞也有作用。氟尿嘧啶需静脉给药，全身分布，在肝和肿瘤组织中浓度较高。消化系统（食管癌癌、肠癌、胰腺癌、肝癌）和乳腺癌疗效较好，对宫颈癌、卵巢癌、绒毛膜上皮癌、膀胱癌、头颈部肿瘤也有效。骨髓和消化道毒性较大，如出现血性腹泻应立即停药。该药可引起脱发、皮肤色素沉着等，肝、肾损害偶见。

6. 多柔比星（阿霉素）

多柔比星（阿霉素）能嵌入 DNA 碱基对之间并紧密结合到 DNA 上，阻止 RNA 转录，抑制 RNA 合成，也能阻止 DNA 复制。多柔比星属于细胞周期非特异性药物，S 期细胞对该药更为敏感。多柔比星抗肿瘤谱广、作用强，主要用于对其他药物耐药的急性淋巴细胞白血病或粒细胞白血病、恶性淋巴肉瘤、乳腺癌、卵巢癌、小细胞肺癌、胃癌、肝癌及膀胱癌等。多柔比星最严重的毒性反应为心肌退行性病变和心肌间质水肿，毒性机制可能与自由基生成有关。右丙亚胺可预防多柔比星引起的心脏毒性。多柔比星还可引起骨髓抑制、消化道反应、皮肤色素沉着及脱发等不良反应。

案例学习

学习要点：

（1）细胞毒性药物的抗癌机制和不良反应。

（2）细胞周期特异性和细胞周期非特异性药物。

关键词：细胞毒性药物；细胞周期特异性

案例一

一名女性乳腺癌患者在乳房切除术和邻近淋巴结清扫后接受化疗，使用的药物有多柔比星、环磷酰胺、甲氨蝶呤、氟尿嘧啶。由于患者的肿瘤细胞为激素受体阳性，因此还使用辅助药物他莫昔芬。

◎ 问答题

1. 氟尿嘧啶的抗癌作用机制是什么？
2. 该患者接受化疗后发生急性出血性膀胱炎，该毒性最可能是由哪种药物所致？
3. 患者经过几个周期的化疗后出现静息脉搏加快。无创放射性核素扫描提示心肌病。最有可能引起心脏毒性的药物是哪一种？

案例二

一名霍奇金淋巴瘤患者曾接受甲氯雷他敏、长春新碱、泼尼松和丙卡巴嗪（方案 A）治疗后疗效不佳。患者改用多柔比星、博来霉素、长春新碱和达卡巴嗪（方案 B）治疗获得成功。

◎ 问答题

1. 该患者使用的哪一类抗癌药物具有细胞周期特异性，并同时用于方案 A 和方案 B？
2. 患者在接受方案 B 治疗期间出现呼吸困难、无痰咳嗽和间歇性发热。胸部 X 光片显示肺部浸润性改变。哪种药物最有可能引起这些肺部症状？

选择题

1. 在同类抗肿瘤药物中，抗癌谱最广的氮芥类药物是（　　）。
   A. 异环磷酰胺　B. 环磷酰胺　C. 盐酸氮芥　D. 苯丁酸氮芥　E. 左旋苯丙氨酸氮芥
2. 哪种药物在女性滋养细胞绒毛膜癌的治疗中首次显示了化疗能治愈人类癌症？（　　）
   A. 苯丁酸氮芥　B. 塞替哌　C. 甲氨蝶呤　D. 左旋苯丙氨酸氮芥　E. 卡氮芥
3. 以下哪一类药物能结合微管蛋白并使细胞停滞于分裂期？（　　）
   A. 长春生物碱　B. 氮芥　C. 烷化剂　D. 抗雌激素药物　E. 抗代谢药物
4. 以下哪种化疗药物对女性乳腺癌具有特异性？（　　）
   A. 环磷酰胺　B. 多柔比星　C. 氟甲睾酮　D. 甲氨蝶呤　E. 曲妥珠单抗
5. 癌细胞可通过以下哪种机制对长春新碱和甲氨蝶呤均产生耐药性？（　　）
   A. 目标酶的特性发生改变　　　B. 激活酶的活性降低
   C. 增加 P-糖蛋白转运体的表达　　D. 增加产生药物捕获分子
   E. 参与 DNA 修复的蛋白质增加
6. 甲氨蝶呤是常用的抗恶性肿瘤药，为减轻其骨髓抑制毒性反应，保护正常骨髓，常与下列那种药合用？（　　）
   A. 叶酸　B. 维生素 B_{12}　C. 碳酸氢钠　D. 巯乙磺酸钠　E. 甲酰四氢叶酸钙
7. 下列药物中可预防环磷酰胺引起出血性膀胱炎的是（　　）。

A. 叶酸　　　B. 维生素 B_{12}　　C. 碳酸氢钠　　D. 巯乙磺酸钠　　E. 甲酰四氢叶酸钙

8. 恶性肿瘤化疗后易于复发，其原因是(　　)。
   A. M 期细胞对抗肿瘤药物不敏感　　　　B. S 期细胞对抗肿瘤药物不敏感
   C. G1 期细胞对抗肿瘤药物不敏感　　　　D. G0 期细胞对抗肿瘤药物不敏感
   E. G2 期细胞对抗肿瘤药物不敏感

9. 环磷酰胺在体内转化成为烷化作用强的代谢物而起到抗恶性肿瘤的作用，该代谢物是(　　)。
   A. 4-酮基环磷酰胺　　　　B. 4-羟基环磷酰胺　　　　C. 磷酰胺氮芥
   D. 羧磷酰胺　　　　　　　E. 丙烯醛

10. 下列抗恶性肿瘤药物中，对骨髓造血功能没有抑制作用的是(　　)。
    A. 植物碱类　　B. 激素类　　C. 抗生素类　　D. 烷化剂　　E. 抗代谢类

Case study

Key points：
（1）Anti-cancer mechanisms and adverse effects of cytotoxic drugs.
（2）Cell cycle specific and cell cycle non-specific drugs.

Key words：cytotoxic drugs；cell cycle specificity

Case 1

A female breast cancer patient is on adjuvant chemotherapy comprising doxorubicin and cyclophosphamide/methotrexate/fluorouracil after mastectomy and dissection of adjacent lymph nodes. The patient is also given the adjuvant medication tamoxifen because her tumour cells are positive of hormone receptors.

◎ **Essay questions**

1. What is the mechanism of anticancer action of fluorouracil?
2. This patient developed acute haemorrhagic cystitis after receiving chemotherapy. Which drug was the most likely cause of this toxicity?
3. The patient presents with an accelerated resting pulse after several cycles of chemotherapy. A noninvasive radionuclide scan suggests cardiomyopathy. Which drug most likely caused this cardiotoxicity?

Case 2

A patient with Hodgkin's lymphoma was treated with metoclopramide, vincristine, prednisone and procarbazine (regimen A) without success. Then, the patient was successfully treated with doxorubicin, bleomycin, vincristine and dacarbazine (regimen B).

◎ **Essay questions**

1. Which class of anticancer drug with cell cycle specificity is used in this patient and in both

regimens A and B?
2. The patient developed dyspnoea, a sputumless cough and intermittent fever during treatment of regimen B. The patient's chest X-ray film showed pulmonary infiltrates. Which drug was most likely to cause these pulmonary symptoms?

Multiple-choice questions

1. Among antineoplastic drugs of the same class, the nitrogen mustard with the broadest anticancer spectrum is (　　).
   A. isocyclophosphamide
   B. cyclophosphamide
   C. nitrogen mustard hydrochloride
   D. nitrogen mustard phenylbutyrate
   E. levophenylalanine nitrogen mustard

2. Which drug, when used in the treatment of female trophoblastic choriocarcinoma, showed for the first time the potential of chemotherapy to cure human cancer? (　　)
   A. Nitrogen mustard phenylbutyrate
   B. Thiotepa
   C. Methotrexate
   D. Levophenylalanine nitrogen mustard
   E. Carmustine

3. Which of the following classes of drugs binds to microtubule proteins and arrests cells in division? (　　)
   A. Vincristine
   B. Nitrogen mustard
   C. Alkylating agents
   D. Anti-estrogen drugs
   E. Antimetabolites

4. Which of the following chemotherapeutic agents is specific for female breast cancer? (　　)
   A. Cyclophosphamide
   B. Doxorubicin
   C. Fluoromethyltestosterone
   D. Methotrexate
   E. Trastuzumab

5. By which of the following mechanisms can cancer cells become resistant to both vincristine and methotrexate? (　　)
   A. Changes in the properties of the target enzyme
   B. Reduced activity of activated enzymes
   C. Increased expression of P-glycoprotein transporters
   D. Increased production of drug-trapping molecules
   E. Increase in proteins involved in DNA repair

6. Methotrexate is a commonly used anti-malignant drug. In order to reduce its myelosuppressive toxicity and protect bone marrow, it is often used in combination with which one of the following drugs? (　　)
   A. Folic acid
   B. Vitamin B_{12}
   C. Bicarbonate or soda
   D. Sodium mercaptoethanesulfonate
   E. Calcium formyltetrahydrofolate

7. Which of the following drugs may prevent hemorrhagic cystitis caused by cyclophosphamide? (　　)
   A. Folic acid
   B. Vitamin B_{12}
   C. Sodium bicarbonate

D. Sodium mercaptoethanesulfonate E. Calcium formyltetrahydrofolate

8. Malignant tumors are prone to relapse after chemotherapy because which of the following reasons? (   )

    A. M-phase cells are not sensitive to antitumor drugs

    B. S-phase cells are not sensitive to antitumor drugs

    C. G1 phase cells are not sensitive to antitumor drugs

    D. G0-phase cells are not sensitive to anti-tumor drugs

    E. G2 phase cells are insensitive to anti-tumor drugs

9. Cyclophosphamide is converted in vivo to an alkylating metabolite that acts against malignant tumors. This metabolite is (   ).

    A. 4-ketocyclophosphamide B. 4-hydroxycyclophosphamide

    C. phosphoramidonium nitrogen mustard D. carboxyphosphoramide

    E. acrolein

10. Which of the following antimalignant drugs does not inhibit bone marrow hematopoiesis? (   )

    A. Plant bases B. Hormones C. Antibiotics

    D. Alkylating agents E. Antimetabolites

第四十三章案例学习和选择题答案

第四十四章　影响免疫功能的药物

知识要点

一、主要的免疫病理反应类型

当机体免疫功能异常时可出现免疫病理反应，包括变态反应（过敏反应）、自身免疫性疾病、免疫缺陷病和免疫增殖病等，表现为机体免疫功能低下或免疫功能过度增强，严重时可导致机体死亡。影响免疫功能的药物通过影响上述一个或多个环节而发挥免疫抑制或免疫增强作用，从而防治免疫功能异常所导致的疾病。

（1）过敏反应：异常的、过高的免疫应答。机体与抗原性物质在一定条件下相互作用，产生致敏淋巴细胞或特异性抗体，如与再次进入的抗原结合，可导致机体生理功能紊乱和组织损害的免疫病理反应。又称为变态反应。

（2）自身免疫病：机体对自身抗原产生免疫反应而导致组织损害所引起的疾病。具有以下特点：①病因多不明，女性多于男性；②血液中存在高滴度自身抗体和（或）自身抗体组织成分起反应的致敏淋巴细胞；③病情反复发作或慢性迁延；④有明显的家族倾向性，多与 HLA 抗原相关。

（3）免疫缺陷病：一组由于免疫系统发育不全或受损，导致免疫功能缺陷引起的疾病。有两类：①原发性免疫缺陷病，又称先天性免疫缺陷病，与遗传有关，多发生于婴幼儿时期；②继发性免疫缺陷病，又称获得性免疫缺陷病，可发生在任何年龄，多因严重感染，尤其是直接侵犯免疫系统的感染、恶性肿瘤、应用免疫抑制剂、放射治疗和化疗等原因引起。

（4）免疫增殖病：免疫器官、免疫组织或免疫细胞（包括淋巴细胞和单核-巨噬细胞）异常增生（包括良性或恶性）所致的一组疾病，表现包括免疫功能异常及免疫球蛋白质和量的变化。

二、免疫抑制药的种类

免疫抑制药是一类具有免疫抑制作用的药物，临床主要用于器官移植的排斥反应和自身免疫反应性疾病。大多数免疫抑制药主要作用于免疫反应的感应期，抑制淋巴细胞增殖，也有一些作用于免疫反应的效应期。其作用可分为以下几类：①抑制 IL-2 生成及其活性，如环孢素、他克莫司等；②抑制细胞因子表达，如糖皮质激素；③抑制嘌呤或嘧啶合成，如硫唑嘌呤等；④阻断 T 淋巴细胞表面信号分子，如单克隆抗体等。近年来出现了针对鞘氨醇-1-磷酸、淋巴细胞特异性酪氨酸蛋白激酶、Janus 激酶 3、哺乳类动物雷帕霉素靶蛋白等特异靶点新型免疫抑制剂。

三、免疫增强药的种类

免疫增强药是指单独或与抗原同时使用时能增强机体免疫应答的药物，主要用于免疫缺陷病、慢性感染性疾病，也常作为肿瘤的辅助治疗药物。免疫增强药种类繁多，包括提高巨细胞吞噬功能的药物(如卡介苗等)，提高细胞免疫功能的药物(如左旋咪唑、转移因子及其他免疫核糖核酸、胸腺素等)，提高体液免疫功能的药物(如丙种球蛋白等)。

案例学习

学习要点：
(1) 移植排斥反应的类型和治疗药物。
(2) 药物引起的病理免疫反应。

关键词： 移植物抗宿主免疫反应；过敏反应；自身免疫反应

案例一

某患者在接受骨髓移植四周后出现黄疸，四肢和面部皮疹，时有呕吐和腹泻。生化检查显示患者的血清肝酶(LDH、ALT)和胆红素水平升高。

◎ 问答题

这些症状最可能的原因是什么？应如何治疗？

案例二

一名患者因细菌感染接受青霉素治疗。在青霉素注射几分钟后，患者出现严重的支气管收缩、喉头水肿和低血压。立即注射肾上腺素抢救后患者幸存。一年后患者在接受抗精神病药物治疗时又出现粒细胞减少。

◎ 问答题

青霉素注射引发了哪种免疫反应？而抗精神病药物又可能引发了哪种类型的免疫反应？

选择题

1. 以下哪种用于预防异体移植排斥反应的药物会引起高脂血症？(　　)
   A. 硫唑嘌呤　　B. 巴利昔单抗　　C. 贝拉西普　　D. 霉酚酸酯　　E. 西罗莫司
2. 以下哪种药物可特异性抑制活化的 T 淋巴细胞中的钙调磷酸酶？(　　)
   A. 巴利昔单抗　　B. 他克莫司　　C. 泼尼松　　D. 西罗莫司　　E. 霉酚酸酯
3. 以下哪项最准确地描述了环孢素的免疫抑制作用？(　　)
   A. 激活 NK 细胞　　　　　　　　　B. 阻断组织对炎症介质的反应
   C. 促进 IgG 抗体的降解　　　　　　D. 抑制白细胞介素的基因转录

E. 干扰T细胞的MHC II肽激活

4. 关于环孢素的副作用，以下哪项描述准确？（ ）
   A. 白细胞减少、低血压、溶血性贫血
   B. 肾毒性、神经毒性、多毛症
   C. 血小板减少、低钾血症
   D. 出血性膀胱炎、低血糖症
   E. 循环免疫复合物增加、心律失常

5. 硫唑嘌呤等细胞毒性药物具有免疫抑制活性，这是因为这些药物（ ）。
   A. 与循环免疫复合物结合并使其失活
   B. 特异性抑制IL-2基因转录
   C. 通过抑制嘌呤合成阻止T细胞和B细胞的克隆扩增
   D. 诱导抗独特型抗体的合成
   E. 烷化和交联DNA，抑制细胞芽生

6. 以下哪一项免疫抑制剂的联合应用不合理？（ ）
   A. 巴利昔单抗、贝拉西普、霉酚酸酯和泼尼松
   B. 胸腺球蛋白、环孢素、硫唑嘌呤和强的松
   C. 他克莫司、霉酚酸酯和泼尼松
   D. 他克莫司、环孢素和强的松
   E. 他克莫司、西罗莫司和泼尼松

7. 以下哪种药物能抑制细胞免疫、抑制前列腺素和白三烯的合成，并增加IgG抗体的降解？（ ）
   A. 环磷酰胺   B. 环孢素   C. 英夫利西单抗   D. 霉酚酸酯   E. 泼尼松

8. 以下哪种免疫调节剂能增加慢性肉芽肿病患者巨噬细胞的吞噬能力？（ ）
   A. 醛白细胞介素   B. γ干扰素   C. 淋巴细胞免疫球蛋白
   D. 泼尼松   E. 曲妥珠单抗

9. 西罗莫司和环孢素具有相似的免疫抑制作用，但两种药物的毒性不同。与环孢素相比，西罗莫司更容易引起以下哪种毒性反应？（ ）
   A. 过敏性反应   B. 高血压   C. 骨质疏松症   D. 肾功能不全   E. 血小板减少

10. 一名男性患者在接受肾移植手术后开始服用环孢素。但48小时后该患者出现严重的恶心和腹泻，转氨酶也突然升高。换用他克莫司后，患者仍然有恶心症状，并出现头晕和呼吸困难。此时可换用哪种免疫抑制剂？（ ）
    A. 霉酚酸酯   B. 依那西普   C. 托西珠单抗   D. 秋水仙碱   E. 巴利昔单抗

Case study

Key points：
(1) Types of transplant rejection responses and therapeutic agents.
(2) Drug-induced pathologic immune responses.

Key words： graft-versus-host immune reaction; allergic reaction; autoimmune response

Case 1

A patient developed jaundice, skin rash on the extremities and face, occasional vomiting and diarrhoea four weeks after receiving a bone marrow transplant. Biochemical tests showed elevated serum liver enzymes (LDH, ALT) and bilirubin levels in the patient.

◎ **Essay question**

What is the most likely cause of these symptoms? What treatment should be adopted for the patient?

Case 2

A patient was treated with penicillin for a bacterial infection. A few minutes after the penicillin injection, the patient developed severe bronchoconstriction, laryngeal oedema and hypotension. The patient survived after immediate resuscitation with epinephrine. One year later the patient developed agranulocytopenia while receiving antipsychotic medications.

◎ **Essay question**

What immune response was triggered by the penicillin injection? What type of immune response may have been triggered by the antipsychotic drugs?

Multiple-choice questions

1. Which of the following drugs used to prevent allograft rejection causes hyperlipidaemia? ( )
   A. Azathioprine   B. Baliximab   C. Beelzebub   D. Mycophenolate mofetil   E. Sirolimus
2. Which of the following drugs specifically inhibits the calcineurin in activated T lymphocytes? ( )
   A. Baliximab   B. Tacrolimus   C. Prednisone   D. Sirolimus   E. Mycophenolate mofetil
3. Which of the following most accurately describes the immunosuppressive effects of cyclosporine? ( )
   A. Activation of NK cells
   B. Blocking tissue response to inflammatory mediators
   C. Increased catabolism of IgG antibodies
   D. Inhibition of interleukin gene transcription
   E. Interference with MHC II peptide activation in T cells
4. Which of the following is an accurate description of the side effects of cyclosporine? ( )
   A. Leukopenia, hypotension, haemolytic anaemia
   B. Nephrotoxicity, neurotoxicity, hirsutism
   C. Thrombocytopenia, hypokalaemia
   D. Haemorrhagic cystitis, hypoglycaemia
   E. Increased circulating immune complexes, cardiac arrhythmias

5. Cytotoxic drugs such as azathioprine have immunosuppressive activity because they (   ).
   A. bind and inactivate circulating immune complexes
   B. specifically inhibit IL-2 gene transcription
   C. block clonal expansion of T and B cells by inhibiting purine synthesis
   D. inducw the synthesis of anti-unique antibodies
   E. alkylate and cross-link DNA to inhibit cell budding
6. Which of the following combinations of immunosuppressive agents is not reasonable? (   )
   A. Baliximab, berazep, mycophenolate mofetil and prednisone
   B. Thymoglobulin, cyclosporine, azathioprine and prednisone
   C. Tacrolimus, mycophenolate mofetil and prednisone
   D. Tacrolimus, cyclosporine and prednisone
   E. Tacrolimus, sirolimus and prednisone
7. Which of the following drugs suppresses cellular immunity, inhibits prostaglandin and leukotriene synthesis, and increases the breakdown of IgG antibodies? (   )
   A. Cyclophosphamide   B. Cyclosporine   C. Infliximab
   D. Mycophenolate mofetil   E. Prednisone
8. Which of the following is an immune modulator that increases phagocytosis by acrophages in patients with chronic granulomatous disease? (   )
   A. Aldesleukin   B. Interferon-γ   C. Lymphocyte immune globulin
   D. Prednisone   E. Trastuzumab
9. Although sirolimus and cyclosporine have similar immunosuppressant effects, their toxicity profiles differ. Which of the following toxicities is more likely to be associated with sirolimus than with cyclosporine? (   )
   A. An anaphylactic reaction   B. Hypertension   C. Osteoporosis
   D. Renal insufficiency   E. Thrombocytopenia
10. Following a kidney transplant, a male patient is placed on cyclosporine but after 48 hours complains of serious nausea and diarrhea and has a sudden increase in transaminases. You switch him to tacrolimus but the nausea persists and he complains of getting dizzy and has dyspnea. Which of the following immunosuppressive agents would be an alternate drug in this scenario? (   )
    A. Mycophenolate mofetil   B. Etanercept   C. Tocilizumab
    D. Colchicine   E. Basiliximab

第四十四章案例学习和选择题答案

参 考 文 献

[1] YEN C Y, CHEN C C, TSENG P C. Role of pilocarpine use following laser peripheral iridotomy in eyes with refractory acute angle closure glaucoma: a case report and literature review[J]. Medicine (Baltimore), 2022, 101(27): e29245.

[2] CAO Y, SUN J, WANG X, et al. The double-edged nature of nicotine: toxicities and therapeutic potentials[J]. Frontiers in Pharmacology, 2024, 15:1427314.

[3] ELDUFANI J, BLAISE G. The role of acetylcholinesterase inhibitors such as neostigmine and rivastigmine on chronic pain and cognitive function in aging: a review of recent clinical applications[J]. Alzheimer's & Dementia, 2019, 5:175-183.

[4] PATEL A, CHAVAN G, NAGPAL A K. Navigating the Neurological Abyss: A Comprehensive Review of Organophosphate Poisoning Complications[J]. Cureus Journal of Medical Science, 2024, 16 (2): e54422.

[5] CHEN P J, HSIA Y, TSAI T H, et al. Impact of atropine use for myopia control on intraocular pressure in children: a comprehensive review including postpupil dilation intraocular pressure changes[J]. Taiwan Journal of Ophthalmology, 2024, 14 (2): 179-189.

[6] ZHANG Y X, NIU X Y, XIAO Z Y, et al. Scopolamine for patients with motion sickness: a systematic review and meta-analysis with trial sequential analysis[J]. Acta oto-laryngologica, 2024, 144 (7-8):429-438.

[7] BARRONS R W, NGUYEN L T. Succinylcholine-Induced Rhabdomyolysis in Adults: Case Report and Review of the Literature[J]. Journal of Pharmacy practice, 2020, 33 (1): 102-107.

[8] SHOENBERGER J M, MALLON W K. Rocuronium Versus Succinylcholine Revisited: Succinylcholine Remains the Best Choice[J]. Annals of Emergency Medicine, 2018, 71 (3): 398-399.

[9] GHASEMI M, MEHRANFARD N. Neuroprotective actions of norepinephrine in neurological diseases[J]. Pflugers Archiv: European Journal of Physiology, 2024, 476(11):1703-1725.

[10] CALOGIURI G, SAVAGE M P, CONGEDO M, et al. Is Adrenaline Always the First Choice Therapy of Anaphylaxis? An Allergist-cardiologist Interdisciplinary Point of View [J]. Current Pharmaceutical Design, 2023, 29 (32): 2545-2551.

[11] SARDANA D, LEE J, YIU C K, et al. Effectiveness of phentolamine mesylate in reversal of local anesthesia: systematic review and meta-analysis[J]. Journal of Evidence-Based Dental Practice, 2023, 23 (3): 10186.

[12] CUESTA A M, GALLARDO-VARA E, CASADO-VELAJ, et al. The Role of Propranolol as a Repurposed Drug in Rare Vascular Diseases[J]. International Journal OF Molecular, 2022, 23(8): 4217.

[13] HOPKINS P M, GIRARD T, DALAYS, et al. Malignant hyperthermia 2020: Guideline from the Association of Anaesthetists[J]. Anaesthesia, 2021, 76(5): 655-664.

[14] BRUNTON L, KNOLLMANN B. Goodman & Gilman's The Pharmacological Basis of Therapeutics[M]. 14th ed. New York: McGraw Hill, 2023.

[15] KINSELLA S M, CARVALHO B, DYER R A, et al. Consensus Statement Collaborators: international consensus statement on the management of hypotension with vasopressors during caesarean section under spinal anaesthesia[J]. Anaesthesia, 2018, 73(1): 71-92.

[16] MOHTA M, R L, CHILKOTI G T, AGARWAL R, et al. A randomised double-blind comparison of phenylephrine and norepinephrine for the management of postspinal hypotension in pre-eclamptic patients undergoing caesarean section[J]. European Journal of Anaesthesiology, 2021, 38(10): 1077-1084.

[17] BAO Y, PHAN M, ZHU J, et al. Alterations of Cytochrome P450-Mediated Drug Metabolism during Liver Repair and Regeneration after Acetaminophen-Induced Liver Injury in Mice[J]. Drug Metabolism and Disposition, 2022, 50(5): 694-703.

[18] FUKASAWA T, SUZUKI A, OTANI K. Effects of genetic polymorphism of cytochrome P450 enzymes on the pharmacokinetics of benzodiazepines[J]. Journal of Clinical Pharmacy and Therapeutics, 2007, 32(4): 333-341.

[19] THIJS R D, SURGES R, O'BRIEN T J, et al. Epilepsy in adults[J]. Lancet, 2019, 393(10172): 689-701.

[20] COCK H R. Drug-induced status epilepticus[J]. Epilepsy & Behavior, 2015, 49: 76-82.

[21] MICHAEL T H. Parkinson's Disease and Parkinsonism[J]. American Journal of Medicine, 2019, 132(7): 802-807.

[22] KALIA V L, Lang A E. Parkinson's disease[J]. Lancet, 2015, 386(9996): 896-912.

[23] LEUCHT S, LEUCHT C, HUHN M, et al. Sixty Years of Placebo-Controlled Antipsychotic Drug Trials in Acute Schizophrenia: Systematic Review, Bayesian Meta-Analysis and Meta-Regression of Efficacy Predictors[J]. American Journal of Psychiatry, 2017, 174(10): 927-942.

[24] ZHANG Y, BECKER T, M A Y, et al. A systematic review of Chinese randomized clinical trials of SSRI treatment of depression[J]. BMC Psychiatry, 2014, 14: 245.

[25] VOWLES K E, MCENTEE M L, JULNES P S, et al. Rates of opioid misuse, abuse, and addiction in chronic pain: a systematic review and data synthesis[J]. Pain, 2015, 156(4): 569-576.

[26] ALI S, TAHIR B, JABEEN S, et al. Methadone Treatment of Opiate Addiction: A Systematic Review of Comparative Studies[J]. Innovations in Clinical Neuroscience, 2017, 14(7-8): 8-19.

[27] US PREVENTIVE SERVICES TASK FORCE, DAVIDSON K W, BARRY M J, et al. Aspirin Use to Prevent Cardiovascular Disease: US Preventive Services Task Force Recommendation Statement[J]. JAMA, 2022, 327(16): 1577-1584.

[28] COSTA B R, PEREIRA T V, SAADAT P, et al. Effectiveness and safety of non-steroidal anti-inflammatory drugs and opioid treatment for knee and hip osteoarthritis: network meta-analysis[J]. BMJ: British medical journal / British Medical Association, 2021, 375: n2321.

[29] STEVENS C. Brenner and Stevens' Pharmacology[M]. 6th ed. Philadelphia, Elsevier, 2022.

[30] KATZUNG B G, VANDERAH T W. Katzungs Basic and Clinical Pharmacology[M]. 16th ed. Arizona, McGraw Hill, 2023.

[31] LAURENT S. Antihypertensive drugs[J]. Pharmacological Research, 2017, 124: 116-125.

[32] ANGELICO-GONCALVES A, LEITE A R, NEVES J S, et al. Changes in health-related quality of life and treatment effects in chronic heart failure: a meta-analysis[J]. International Journal of Cardiology, 2023, 386: 65-73.

[33] ROGER V L. Epidemiology of Heart Failure: A Contemporary Perspective[J]. Circulation Research, 2021, 128(10): 1421-1434.

[34] TSU L V, CARROLL K, KATEE K, et al. Pharmacological Management of Hyperlipidemia in Older individuals[J]. Senior Care Pharmacist, 2021, 36(6): 284-303.

[35] NG J Y, DSOUZA M, HUTANIF, et al. Management of Heparin-Induced Thrombocytopenia: A Contemporary Review[J]. Journal of Clinical Medicine, 2024, 13(16): 4686.

[36] NELSON M R, BLACK J A. Aspirin: latest evidence and developments[J]. Heart, 2024, 110(17): 1069-1073.

[37] CIPRANDIG. The updated role of budesonide in managing children and adolescents with allergic rhinitis[J]. Minerva Pediatrics, 2024, 76(4): 526-536.

[38] MARQUES L, VALE N. Salbutamol in the Management of Asthma: A Review[J]. International Journal of Molecular Sciences, 2022, 23(22): 14207.

[39] KAMBOJ A K, PATEL D A, YADLAPATI R. Long-Term Proton Pump Inhibitor Use: Review of Indications and Special Considerations[J]. Clinical Gastroenterology and Hepatology, 2024, 22(7): 1373-1376.

[40] TANAKA M, BANBA M, JOKOA, et al. Pharmacological and therapeutic properties of lafutidine (stogar and protecadin), a novel histamine H_2 receptor antagonist with gastroprotective activity[J]. Nihon Yakurigaku Zasshi, 2001, 117(6): 377-386.

[41] 中国防治恶性高热专家共识工作组. 中国防治恶性高热专家共识(2020版)[J]. 中华麻醉学杂志, 2021, 41(1): 20-25.